Mission Statement of IASP Press®

The International Association for the Study of Pain (IASP) is a nonprofit, interdisciplinary organization devoted to understanding the mechanisms of pain and improving the care of patients with pain through research, education, and communication. The organization includes scientists and health care professionals dedicated to these goals. The IASP sponsors scientific meetings and publishes newsletters, technical bulletins, the journal *Pain,* and books.

The goal of IASP Press is to provide the IASP membership with timely, high-quality, attractive, low-cost publications relevant to the problem of pain. These publications are also intended to appeal to a wider audience of scientists and clinicians interested in the problem of pain.

Progress in Pain Research and Management
Volume 35

Pain in Older Persons

Editors

Stephen J. Gibson, PhD

National Ageing Research Institute, Parkville, Victoria;
Department of Medicine, University of Melbourne,
Melbourne, Victoria; Caulfield Pain Management
and Research Center, Caulfield, Victoria, Australia

Debra K. Weiner, MD

Division of Geriatric Medicine, Department of Medicine,
University of Pittsburgh; Pain Evaluation and Treatment
Institute, University of Pittsburgh Medical Center,
Pittsburgh, Pennsylvania, USA

IASP PRESS® • SEATTLE

Library of Congress Cataloging-in-Publication Data

Pain in older persons / editors, Stephen J. Gibson, Debra K. Weiner.
    p. ; cm. -- (Progress in pain research and management ; v. 35)
  Includes bibliographical references and index.
  ISBN 0-931092-59-0 (alk. paper)
  1. Pain in old age.
  [DNLM: 1. Pain--diagnosis--Aged. 2. Pain--therapy--Aged. WL 704 P14578 2005]
  I. Gibson, Stephen J., 1959- II. Weiner, Debra K. III. Series.
  RB127.P322265 2005

                    2005052016

Published by:

IASP Press
International Association for the Study of Pain
909 NE 43rd Street, Suite 306
Seattle, WA 98105-6020 USA
Fax: 206-547-1703
www.iasp-pain.org
www.painbooks.org

Printed in the United States of America

Contents

Contributing Authors

Robert Arnold, MD *Institute for Doctor-Patient Communication, Section of Palliative Care and Medical Ethics, Division of General Internal Medicine, University of Pittsburgh, Pittsburgh, Pennsylvania, USA*

Cheryl Bernstein, MD *Department of Anesthesiology, University of Pittsburgh School of Medicine, Pittsburgh, Pennsylvania, USA*

Danelle Cayea, MD *Division of Geriatric Medicine, Department of Medicine, University of Pittsburgh Medical Center, Pittsburgh, Pennsylvania, USA; currently Division of Geriatric Medicine, Johns Hopkins University School of Medicine, Baltimore, Maryland, USA*

Robert H. Dworkin, PhD *Department of Anesthesiology, University of Rochester School of Medicine and Dentistry, Rochester, New York, USA*

Robert R. Edwards, PhD *Department of Psychiatry and Behavioral Sciences, Johns Hopkins University School of Medicine, Baltimore, Maryland, USA*

Michael J. Farrell, PhD *Howard Florey Institute and Centre for Neuroscience, University of Melbourne, Melbourne, Victoria; National Ageing Research Institute, Parkville, Victoria, Australia*

Perry Fine, MD *University of Utah Pain Management Center, Salt Lake City, Utah, USA*

Lucia Gagliese, PhD *School of Kinesiology and Health Science, York University, Toronto, Ontario; Department of Anaesthesia and Pain Management, University Health Network, Toronto General Hospital, Toronto, Ontario; Departments of Anaesthesia and Psychiatry, University of Toronto, Toronto, Ontario, Canada*

Stephen J. Gibson, PhD *National Ageing Research Institute, Parkville, Victoria; Department of Medicine, University of Melbourne, Melbourne, Victoria; Caulfield Pain Management and Research Centre, Caulfield, Victoria, Australia*

David R.P. Guay, PharmD *Institute for the Study of Geriatric Pharmacotherapy, Department of Experimental and Clinical Pharmacology, College of Pharmacy, University of Minnesota, Minneapolis, Minnesota; Partnering Care Senior Services, Health Partners Inc., Minneapolis, Minnesota, USA*

Thomas Hadjistavropoulos, PhD *Department of Psychology, University of Regina, Regina, Saskatchewan, Canada*

Joseph T. Hanlon, PharmD, MS *Division of Geriatric Medicine, Department of Medicine, School of Medicine, and Department of Pharmacy and Therapeutics, School of Pharmacy, University of Pittsburgh, Pittsburgh, Pennsylvania; and Center for Health Equity Research and Promotion, Veterans Administration Pittsburgh Health Care System, Pittsburgh, Pennsylvania, USA*

Keela A. Herr, PhD, RN, FAAN *Adult and Gerontological Nursing, College of Nursing, The University of Iowa, Iowa City, Iowa, USA*

Timothy J. Ives, PharmD, MPH *Division of Pharmacotherapy, School of Pharmacy, University of North Carolina, Chapel Hill, North Carolina, USA*

Gareth T. Jones, PhD *The Unit of Chronic Disease Epidemiology, and the Arthritis Research Campaign (ARC) Epidemiology Unit, Division of Epidemiology and Health Sciences, The University of Manchester, Manchester, United Kingdom; currently Epidemiology Group, Department of Public Health, University of Aberdeen, Aberdeen, United Kingdom*

Benny Katz, MBBS, FRACP, FFPMANZCA *Consultant Geriatrician, Austin Health, Heidelberg, Victoria, Australia*

Francis J. Keefe, PhD *Department of Psychiatry and Behavioral Medicine, Duke University Medical Center, Durham, North Carolina, USA*

Linda A. King, MD *Section of Palliative Care and Medical Ethics, Division of General Internal Medicine, University of Pittsburgh, Pittsburgh, Pennsylvania, USA*

Bud Lateef, MD *Department of Pain Medicine, University of Pittsburgh School of Medicine, Pittsburgh, Pennsylvania, USA*

Susan J. Lieber, MS, OTR/L *Department of Anesthesiology and Pain Evaluation and Treatment Institute, University of Pittsburgh, Pittsburgh, Pennsylvania, USA*

Gary J. Macfarlane, PhD *The Unit of Chronic Disease Epidemiology, and the Arthritis Research Campaign (ARC) Epidemiology Unit, Division of Epidemiology and Health Sciences, The University of Manchester, Manchester, United Kingdom; currently Epidemiology Group, Department of Public Health, University of Aberdeen, Aberdeen, United Kingdom*

Margo McCaffery, MS, RN, FAAN *Clinical consultant, Los Angeles, California, USA*

Patricia A. Parmelee, PhD *Emory Center for Health in Aging, Emory University School of Medicine, and Birmingham/Atlanta Geriatric Research, Education and Clinical Center, Atlanta Veterans Affairs Medical Center, Atlanta, Georgia, USA*

Chris Pasero, MS, RN, FAAN *Clinical consultant, El Dorado Hills, California, USA, John A. Hartford Foundation Building Academic Geriatric Nursing Capacity Scholar, Iowa City, Iowa, USA; Clinical Consultant, Los Angeles, California, USA*

Gisèle Pickering, MD, PhD, DPharm *Clinical Pharmacology Center, University Hospital, Medical Faculty, Clermont-Ferrand, France*

Karen Prestwood, MD *Center on Aging, University of Connecticut Health Center, Farmington, Connecticut, USA*

Barbara Rakel, RN, PhD *John A. Hartford Foundation Building Academic Geriatric Nursing Capacity Scholar, Department of Nursing Services and Patient Care, University of Iowa Hospitals and Clinics, Iowa City, Iowa, USA*

Thomas E. Rudy, PhD *Departments of Anesthesiology, Psychiatry, and Biostatistics and Pain Evaluation and Treatment Institute, University of Pittsburgh, Pittsburgh, Pennsylvania, USA*

Rhonda J. Scudds, PhD, PT *Department of Rehabilitation Sciences, Faculty of Health and Social Sciences, Hong Kong Polytechnic University, Kowloon, Hong Kong; currently Health and Rehabilitation Sciences Research Institute, Faculty of Life and Health Sciences, University of Ulster, Newtonabbey, County Antrim, Northern Ireland, United Kingdom*

Roger A. Scudds, PhD, PT *Department of Rehabilitation Sciences, Faculty of Health and Social Sciences, Hong Kong Polytechnic University, Kowloon, Hong Kong; currently Health and Rehabilitation Sciences Research Institute, Faculty of Life and Health Sciences, University of Ulster, Newtonabbey, County Antrim, Northern Ireland, United Kingdom*

Sam Scherer, MBBS, DGM *Pain Management Clinic for the Elderly, Melbourne Health, Parkville, Victoria, Australia*

Kenneth E. Schmader, MD *Division of Geriatrics, Department of Medicine and the Center for the Study of Aging and Human Development, Duke University Medical Center, Durham, North Carolina; Geriatric Research, Education and Clinical Center, Durham VA Medical Center, Durham, North Carolina, USA*

Sandra J. Waters, PhD *Department of Psychiatry and Behavioral Medicine, Duke University Medical Center, Durham, North Carolina, USA*

Debra K. Weiner, MD *Division of Geriatric Medicine, Department of Medicine, University of Pittsburgh; Pain Evaluation and Treatment Institute, University of Pittsburgh Medical Center, Pittsburgh, Pennsylvania, USA*

Julia T. Woodward, PhD *Department of Psychiatry and Behavioral Medicine, Duke University Medical Center, Durham, North Carolina, USA*

Foreword

But no matter how they make you feel, you should always watch elders carefully. They were you and you will be them. You carry the seeds of your old age in you at this very moment, and they hear the echoes of their youth each time they see you.

Kent Nerburn, U.S. theologian, artist, and author.
Letters to My Son (1993).

The world's population is aging, and most of the current generation can expect to survive to the eight or ninth decade or beyond. Future generations can expect an even longer life, as with each passing year human life expectancy increases by another couple of weeks or so. For most of us, longevity is a cherished ambition, but just how old age will be for us personally depends on many factors—our genetics, lifestyle, socioeconomic status, personal attributes, environment, and the presence (or absence) of disease or accidents. Indeed, we carry the seeds of our old age within us, but how they will eventually translate may or may not be how we would anticipate or wish.

Old age can be a mixed blessing. On one hand, it can provide a reflective time, an integration of life experiences, a time of accepting things as they are instead of how they could have been—the development of wisdom. On the other, a longer lifespan increases susceptibility to chronic, disabling diseases, many of which are painful. If only we could have the benefits of wisdom and cultural knowledge that aging is known to foster, without the troublesome effects of physical decline! In late life, "survivorship" can take on new meaning, including coping with the challenges of disability and the trials of chronic pain. In reality, it is very hard to be reflective, perceptive, and wise when organ systems don't work as they should, everything hurts, and breakdown in one area seems to lead to problems in another! Multiple studies have shown that those older people who have poorer psychological adaptation to aging problems have less life satisfaction and poorer quality of life and are likely to have a greater burden of disease and disability (Smith and Baltes 1999). Not all diseases in late life are painful, but many are very painful indeed, and pain is a major contributor to disability and depression (Parmelee 1997). While some studies have shown that older people can live well and have a reasonable sense of well-being despite illness or disability, virtually none show a similar resilience in older persons with persistent pain.

Pain in old age presents many challenges, not only to those in pain, but also to their family, social network, and health care providers. Pain has profound psychosocial effects that influence the person far beyond any immediate physiological impact. Disregarding, denying, or neglecting pain has adverse consequences, not just physically, but also on psychological adjustment, mood state, and quality of life. What should be quality time with families at the end of a long life can become distressing and intolerable.

Pain has different meanings for different people. While some stoics view aches and pains as an expected consequence of aging, others may suffer in silence, mistaken in a belief that pain signals a dread disease or that they might be admitted to hospital, or worse, an institution. Nor does persistent pain in older people just belong to those directly afflicted; it often affects family caregivers who provide instrumental and emotional support, sometimes harming their own mental health. A pain problem can become emotionally overwhelming, overshadowing everything else in life, becoming a stage for interpersonal and intrapersonal dynamics to be acted out to the detriment of all involved.

An older person with persistent pain needs to be understood in his or her own biopsychosocial context. It is disease, not aging, that initiates persistent pain. While this may seem self-evident, it is surprising how often pain is thought to be a "normal" part of the aging process by elders themselves, by their caregivers, and unfortunately also by their clinicians. Pathology becomes entwined with physiology as late life progresses, modified in turn by psychosocial factors, each component influencing the others. A good understanding of contextual factors increases the individual's appreciation of the complexity of pain and helps the clinician to be more empathic to patients' problems.

Aging and *pain* are not synonymous. While aging is inevitable, pain in old age is not. Given appropriate knowledge and skills, much is available to alleviate pain and suffering, improving the quality of life for many older people. In recent years, the gerontological literature has been interested in "successful ageing," defined simply as "doing the best one can with what one has" (Baltes and Carstensen 1996). Older people have their own ideas as to what they consider "successful ageing," such as retaining their ability to adapt, focusing on gains rather than losses, and having a sense of psychological well-being and social engagement (Phelan et al. 2004). Older people value these characteristics far more than maintaining physical or cognitive functioning. It is much more likely that older persons will achieve the attributes they desire if they are without pain, or if any pain that they have is well controlled. Thus, the rewards for good management of pain in persons of advanced age are potentially great. The relief of discomfort allows older persons to engage more with their families and communities, to have a better chance of developing a sense of personal well-being, and to be more likely to gain that much-cherished quality time at the end of their days.

So far, despite acknowledging that increased longevity will be accompanied by a concomitant increase in the prevalence of painful diseases, we seem to be focusing little effort on controlling pain in older people. About 60–71% of community-dwelling older people report feeling pain somewhere, with over 33% reporting daily persistent pain (Brochet 1998). The extent to which pain interferes with daily activities increases incrementally with age. Yet while the prevalence of pain may be high in elders, the prevalence of pain actually treated is shockingly low. This discrepancy is seen in community-dwelling elders without dementia who are more functional and better able to articulate their pain (Pitkala et al. 2002), in community-dwelling individuals with dementia (Mäntyselkä et al. 2004), and especially in institutionalized elders (Ferrell 2004).

One fundamental reason for the relative neglect of pain in older people is lack of education in the assessment and management of pain in geriatric curriculae, thus turning out health professionals lacking the knowledge and skills to treat pain in their older patients. Another cause is the unfortunate nihilistic attitudes of some health professionals to pain associated with aging, leading them to undertreat because they believe there is little point. Yet another involves the numerous myths that abound about pain in older people, such as the notion of presbyalgia or that prescription of regular analgesics leads to addiction and a lack of long-term efficacy, or the belief that failure to express pain complaints means they do not exist. Pain is complex, but so is aging. That is why the current volume on *Pain in Older Persons* is so necessary and timely. We need to educate, to dispel the myths, to highlight the important issues, to explore the intricacy of the relationship between pain and aging, and to provide information on the practicalities of pain management.

A mere intellectual acknowledgement of the issues related to pain and aging, including epidemiology, notable age differences, and methods of assessment and treatment, may still be viewed as a limited response to the massive problem of pain and suffering in old age. Knowledge and empathy are not enough without a commitment for action, but they are an important start. As Nerburn reminds us so significantly: "You should always watch elders carefully. They were you and you will be them. You carry the seeds of your old age in you at this very moment."

Not only does each one of us carry the seeds of our own old age, but collectively, health professionals interested in the management of persistent pain carry the kernels of knowledge about optimal pain management for the aged. *Pain in Older Persons* has been written to help us cultivate that knowledge so that we can develop a suitable climate of professional consideration, compassion, and commitment to allow those seeds to germinate and grow.

REFERENCES

Baltes M, Carstensen L. The process of successful aging. *Ageing Soc* 1996; 16:397–422.

Brochet B, Michel P, Barberger-Gateau P, Dartigues J. Population-based study of pain in elderly people: a descriptive survey. *Age Ageing* 1998; 27:279–284.

Ferrell BA. The management of pain in long-term care. *Clin J Pain* 2004; 20(4):240–243.

Mäntyselkä P, Hartikainen S, Louhivuori-Laako K, Sulkava R. Effects of dementia on perceived daily pain in home-dwelling elderly people: a population-based study. *Age Ageing* 2004; 33:496–499.

Parmelee P. Pain and psychological function in late life. In: Mostofsky D, Lomrantz J (Eds). *Handbook of Pain and Aging*. New York: Plenum Press, 1997, pp 207–226.

Nerburn K. *Letters to My Son: Reflections on Becoming a Man*. San Rafael, CA: New World Library, 1993.

Phelan E, Anderson L, Lacroix A, Larson E. Older adults' views of "successful aging." How do they compare with researchers' definitions? *J Am Geriatr Soc* 2004; 52:211–216.

Pitkala KH, Strandberg TE, Tilvis RS. Management of nonmalignant pain in home-dwelling older people: a population-based survey. *J Am Geriatr Soc* 2002: 50(11):1861–1865.

Smith J, Baltes P. Profiles of psychological functioning in the old and oldest old. *Psychol Aging* 1997; 12:458–472.

PAMELA S. MELDING, MB, CHB, FFARCS, FRANZCP, DIPHSM
Senior Lecturer in Psychiatry of Old Age
Department of Psychological Medicine
Faculty of Medical and Health Sciences
University of Auckland
Consultant in Psychiatry of Old Age
Waitemata District Health Board
North Shore Hospital
Takapuna, Auckland
New Zealand

Preface

The average human life expectancy continues to rise with falling mortality in infancy and childhood as well as advances in social policy, public health measures, and improved medical care across the adult lifespan. For the first time in history the number of older persons now exceeds the number of children in many developed countries. A prolonged lifespan has much merit and provides many new opportunities, but longevity is only a blessing if one can maintain reasonable health. Bothersome or chronic pain is a major problem in older segments of the population because it can have a profound negative impact on physical functioning, psychosocial health, and quality of life, and it is one of the most prevalent health problems affecting older persons. The IASP recognized the importance of this topic with the timely release of a volume entitled *Pain in the Elderly* in 1996. This publication, edited by Bruce and Betty Ferrell, had an international team of contributors and comprised 11 chapters. In the 10 years since the IASP's first volume on the problem of pain and aging, the field has flourished with an accumulation of new knowledge regarding the neurophysiology and neurobiology of pain in older adults, further testing of age differences in pain perception and report, the development of age-appropriate pain assessment tools, new ways of treating pain disorders common in advanced age, and the identification of areas that require more study in order to further improve the care of older pain patients.

Pain in Older Persons attempts to update our understanding of these areas and highlight the major accomplishments that have occurred since the first IASP publication on this topic. The book comprises 19 chapters, divided into five main sections. Part I provides an introduction to the field through discussion of the epidemiology of common painful disorders from which older adults suffer. The four chapters in Part II focus on age differences in pain, including differences in the neurobiology of pain processing and behavior in animals and humans, the unique aspects of clinical pain states as manifested in older adults, studies on pain threshold and age differences in the sensitivity to experimental pain stimuli, and age-related psychological and cognitive differences in pain and its impact. This section provides important background material to aid in understanding pain as it affects older persons.

Part III includes four chapters that critically review the literature on psychometric and behavioral pain assessment as it specifically relates to older adults. Many assessment tools are developed in young adult populations and are then applied to older segments without formal validation or consideration of age-specific needs. The authors review the age-appropriate evidence base regarding valid approaches to the assessment of pain severity in cognitively intact and cognitively impaired older persons, the assessment of pain-related physical functioning, and the monitoring of psychosocial aspects of chronic pain. Part IV presents pain-related treatment modalities that apply to a wide range of pain conditions, including oral analgesics, physical therapy techniques and exercise, cognitive-behavioral therapy, interventional pain management procedures, complementary and alternative medicine applications, and multidisciplinary pain management clinics. Once again, the emphasis is on a critical evaluation of age-appropriate treatment modalities with due consideration to the specific needs of older persons with bothersome pain. Part V includes four chapters that discuss evaluation and treatment approaches to various pain conditions common in advanced age, including low back pain and its contributors (osteoarthritis, fibromyalgia, myofascial pain, osteoporosis, and sacroiliac joint syndrome), neuropathic pain, postoperative pain, and cancer pain. Bothersome pain in older persons represents a major public health problem for our society, and this problem will become even more pressing with the demographic shift in the age composition of the world's population. It is our hope that this volume not only will help to update the field as a whole, but will stimulate new thinking and contribute to new developments in this critical area of investigation.

STEPHEN J. GIBSON, PhD
DEBRA K. WEINER, MD

Part I

Overview

Pain in Older Persons, Progress in Pain Research and Management, Vol. 35, edited by Stephen J. Gibson and Debra K. Weiner, IASP Press, Seattle, © 2005.

1

Epidemiology of Pain in Older Persons

Gareth T. Jones and Gary J. Macfarlane

The Unit of Chronic Disease Epidemiology, and the Arthritis Research Campaign (ARC) Epidemiology Unit, Division of Epidemiology and Health Sciences, The University of Manchester, Manchester, United Kingdom

Epidemiology—the study of disease occurrence and distribution—has two main elements: (1) Descriptive epidemiology—the study of the distribution of disease in the population: How does the occurrence of disease vary between groups: by age and sex, and across time, by geography and socioeconomic strata? (2) Analytical epidemiology—the study of disease etiology: What are the risk factors (or risk markers) for disease? What factors are protective against disease?

It is beyond the scope of this chapter to provide a comprehensive review of *all* epidemiological literature relating to the occurrence of pain in older persons. Rather, we will present information from the key papers in this area, covering first the descriptive and then the analytical literature. However, it is evident that the etiological information available specifically on pain in older persons is relatively limited, particularly in the very oldest age groups. Where is it lacking, we will draw on the epidemiology of pain at all ages. First, however, we provide some brief discussion of the pertinent methodological issues to consider in reviewing epidemiological literature.

This chapter focuses primarily on the epidemiology of pain associated with musculoskeletal disorders. The reader is referred to other chapters in this volume for a discussion of the epidemiology of neuropathic pain states (Chapter 17), cancer pain (Chapter 19) and osteoporosis (Chapter 16).

METHODOLOGICAL ISSUES

PAIN

Several problems make it difficult to define pain for epidemiological research. Being a subjective phenomenon, pain sensation is extremely difficult to measure. The researcher has to rely on self-report, and there are no gold standard clinical tools by which the subjective pain experience can be verified. Relying on clinical diagnoses, as an alternative, also has a number of inherent difficulties. First, for many pain syndromes, only a small proportion of sufferers consult health service providers about their pain. For example, in a large prospective cohort study in the United Kingdom, Papageorgiou et al. (1998) found that more than one-third of 2715 study participants initially free of low back pain (LBP) reported a new episode of LBP over a 12-month period, although only approximately 4% consulted their family practitioner with these symptoms. Second, there is often only a weak association between clinical measurements and the subjective pain experience. For example, a recent study demonstrated that 10% of LBP patients presenting in primary care were completely free of limitation in all planes of measurement (Thomas et al. 1998), and other researchers have shown that only 15% of persons who report knee pain have any radiological evidence of disease (Hannan et al. 2000).

Added to the subjectivity of pain perception, the reporting of pain is subject to an individual's norms and values and dependent on a number of societal and cultural influences. Therefore, a major problem of studying pain in the clinic is that the epidemiology of the symptoms and the epidemiology of consultation behavior cannot be distinguished. Even in population-based studies, it is not the epidemiology of pain per se that is being studied, but rather the study of pain reporting.

MEASURING PAIN OCCURRENCE

There are two main measures of disease occurrence that can be used in epidemiological study: prevalence and incidence. Knowledge of prevalence can provide information about the population disease burden and, therefore, can aid in planning the allocation of health care and other resources. The prevalence of a disease is the proportion of persons with disease within the population of interest at a given point or period in time. Rather than relating to disease presence or absence, incidence is a measure of the disease onset, i.e., the number of new cases of disease within the population of interest within a specified period of time.

One problem in pain epidemiology is that small differences in definitions can result in large changes in the estimates of pain occurrence. In a comprehensive review of the epidemiological literature on shoulder pain, van der Windt and Croft (1999) reported that prevalence estimates range from approximately 7% to 61%. They noted that "the results of the studies are difficult to compare because of the wide variation in study setting, target population, case definition, and response rate." Similarly, Scher et al. (1999) pointed out that as much as 36% of all variation in migraine prevalence estimates across 24 studies was due to difference in case definition alone (with a further 34% being accounted for by demographic differences between study populations). Studies that examine, for example, the 1-year prevalence of pain will, by definition, yield higher estimates of occurrence than those that examine 1-month prevalence. Studies also vary with respect to precise anatomical definitions: in one U.K. population-based sample aged 18–75 years, Pope et al. (1997) demonstrated that the prevalence of shoulder pain varied between 31% and 48% depending on which of four different definitions were employed.

Some authors have proposed standardized definitions for what constitutes an "episode" of pain: for example, for LBP: "a period of pain in the lower back lasting for more than 24 hours, preceded and followed by a period of at least one month without LBP" (de Vet et al. 2002). However, the strength of such definitions lies more in the aiding of comparability between studies than in any a priori rationale.

In this chapter we will discuss data available on the occurrence and etiology of regional pain conditions and widespread body pain. Pain is a remarkably prevalent condition. Hunt et al. (1999), in a large community-based survey in northwest England, reported that the prevalence of bodily pain "lasting for at least 24 hours on any day in the past month" varied from 8% in the forearm and abdomen to around 28% in the low back, thigh, and hip. Further, these authors also demonstrated that approximately 13% of persons reported chronic widespread pain. Like many biological phenomena, pain occurrence varies with age. Urwin et al. (1998), in a similar study also in northwest England, examined the occurrence of pain lasting "more than one week in the past month." These authors reported that pain prevalence varied from 6% in the elbow to 23% in the back, for persons of all ages. The age-related changes in the prevalence of pain at different sites, reported by these authors, can be seen in Table I. In older persons (those aged 75 years and older), prevalence ranged from 7% in the elbow to 31% in the knee, and pain prevalence was higher in these individuals than in younger persons at the majority of sites. Further, older persons were more likely to

Table I

Crude prevalence of regional pain ("any pain . . . for more than one week in the past month") in persons in the United Kingdom

	Prevalence of Pain (%)							
	Back	Neck	Shoulder	Elbow	Hip	Knee	Hand	Pain in ≥ 3 Areas
Women								
16–44 years	20	12	12	5	4	10	7	9
45–64 years	27	19	19	8	15	23	19	23
65–74 years	32	23	26	6	20	32	21	31
≥ 75 years	30	21	24	9	20	35	20	31
Men								
16–44 years	20	7	9	3	3	15	7	8
45–64 years	24	15	19	13	11	21	12	18
65–74 years	20	17	16	6	13	27	14	20
≥ 75 years	17	18	20	6	11	27	12	19

Source: Data from Urwin et al. (1998).

report pain at multiple sites: nearly one-third of men and one-half of women aged 75 years and older reported pain at two or more sites of the body.

MUSCULOSKELETAL PAIN

LOW BACK PAIN

Low back pain is the most common regional musculoskeletal pain syndrome. The 1-month period prevalence of the condition has been estimated to be around 20% (Croft and Rigby 1994), although other estimates are nearer 40% (Papageorgiou et al. 1995). Further, some authors have estimated that as many as 80% of the population will experience symptoms at some point in life (Dionne 1999). Prevalence is higher in women than men, and increases with age to around the seventh decade, beyond which it decreases in later life (Papageorgiou et al. 1995).

There is little literature examining the prevalence of LBP specifically in older persons. To examine pain in these age groups one has to study the older age groups of larger population surveys. Hillman et al. (1996) reported the 1-year prevalence of LBP in persons aged 55–64 years to be 39%. Croft and Rigby (1994) reported the 1-month prevalence in the same age group to be 21%, increasing slightly in older age groups to 26% in those aged 75 years and older. In contrast, Thomas et al. (2004), in a large population-based study of pain in persons aged 50 years and older, found that the prevalence of LBP "in the past four weeks ... for one day or longer" decreased in older age groups from 36% in persons aged 50–59 years to 27% in those aged 80 years and older. Using a narrower definition, Urwin et al. (1998) reported a similar occurrence. These authors demonstrated that, in persons aged 75 years and older, 23% report back pain lasting for "more than one week in the past month." These studies also showed that, in older age groups, as in all age groups, prevalence is higher in women than men. Weiner et al. (2003), in a large community-based study of Americans aged 70–79 years, reported the 1-year prevalence of back pain to be 36%. Further, these authors provided some information on back pain severity: approximately two-thirds of these individuals reported back pain of (at least) moderate intensity, and one-fifth experienced back pain occurring "very often," commonly with pain at other sites.

Much of the etiological literature pertaining to LBP has concentrated on occupational risk factors. Prospective studies have shown that, in the absence of pain, factors such as lifting heavy weights, standing or walking for more than 2 hours per day, and flexion or rotation of the trunk significantly increase the risk of future symptoms (Macfarlane et al. 1997; Hoogendoorn et al. 2000; Harkness et al. 2003b). Also, several studies have shown that individuals who are dissatisfied with their working environment are more likely to develop LBP than other individuals (Papageorgiou et al. 1997; Power et al. 2001), and others have reported associations between LBP and several other negative work-related psychosocial characteristics: low levels of support, perceived high demands, and low decision-making latitude (Josephson et al. 1996; Latza et al. 2000; Hoogendoorn et al. 2001).

Although data are scarce on the etiology of LBP in older persons, it is possible that lifetime cumulative exposure to detrimental mechanical factors may result in an increase in the risk of symptoms in older age groups. Alternatively, it may be that the psychosocial elements that play a role in the onset of LBP also contribute to the persistence of symptoms.

UPPER LIMB PAIN

Most studies of shoulder pain have been conducted in specific populations—workers, patient populations, or athletes—whereas comparatively few have been conducted in the general population. These studies have examined a broad age range, and few have studied pain in older persons in any detail. Urwin et al. (1998) studied a large population sample including more than 1000 persons aged 75 years or older. These authors measured self-reported pain that occurred for "more than one week in the past month" and demonstrated an increase in the prevalence of shoulder pain with age to 20%

in men and 24% in women (Table I). Other authors, however, have noted a decrease in the prevalence of shoulder/upper arm pain at older ages. Thomas et al. (2004) reported a decrease in the 1-month prevalence of pain from 31% in individuals aged 50–59 years to 25% in those aged 80 years and older, and van Schaardenburg et al. (1994) reported that shoulder pain occurred on "most days in the preceding month" in 29% of women and 19% of men aged 85 years and older. Similarly, Vogt et al. (2003) also reported a high prevalence in individuals aged 70–79 years: the 1-month prevalence of shoulder pain was 19%, and 67% of those reporting shoulder pain rated their pain as moderate or extreme.

Other than in the shoulder, there are few studies of pain in the upper limb. Thomas et al. (2004) reported a steady decrease in the prevalence of forearm pain from 23% in individuals aged 50–59 years to 12% in those aged 80 years and older. Macfarlane et al. (2000) showed that in a U.K. population sample, 8.3% of subjects reported pain in their forearms, all of whom had been free of pain at this location 2 years previously. These authors also demonstrated an increase in the prevalence of new onset of forearm pain with age, ranging from 5.2% in 18–39-year-old men to 13% in men over 60 years old, although no such relationship was observed in women, with an increase of only 6% to 7% in the respective age groups. Regarding pain in the hand, Thomas et al. (2004) demonstrated that the 1-month period prevalence decreases from 24% in persons aged 50–59 years to 17% in individuals aged 80 years and older. Urwin et al. (1998) reported that the 1-month prevalence of hand pain in individuals over 75 years was 20% in women but only 12% in men and that it is relatively stable, in both groups, from around the fifth decade of life (Table I).

A number of studies have examined the etiology of shoulder pain across the adult age-range, frequently in the occupational environment. Studies have highlighted the importance of a number of mechanical factors (Miranda et al. 2001; Harkness et al. 2003a) and adverse psychological and psychosocial factors (Fredriksson et al. 1999; Harkness et al. 2003a). There are few etiological studies of shoulder pain among older persons. Vogt et al. (2003) reported that in individuals aged 70–79 years, shoulder pain was associated with lower educational level, poor self-rated health, and a history of both cardiovascular and depressive symptoms. However, this study was cross-sectional therefore unable to identify whether these factors preceded or followed the shoulder symptoms.

Pain felt in the shoulder may arise from other nearby structures including the spine or viscera. In older persons particularly, the involvement of degenerative disease may play a role, and several authors have demonstrated shoulder involvement in patients with rheumatic diseases (Coari et al. 1999;

Olofsson et al. 2003). Further, van Schaardenburg et al. (1994) reported that in a study of individuals aged 85 years and older, 27% of women and 25% of men had a shoulder disorder (frozen shoulder being the most common diagnosis).

In older persons, pain in the hand is often associated with arthritis and has been shown to follow a diurnal pattern in patients with both rheumatoid and osteoarthritis (Bellamy et al. 1991, 2002). Regarding environmental influences, the literature is sparse. In a population sample of individuals aged 18–65 years, Macfarlane et al. (2000) found that, in addition to repetitive movements of the arm or wrist, high levels of psychological distress, the occurrence of two or more somatic symptoms, and a perceived lack of support from work colleagues were risk factors for the future development of forearm pain. Further, Fredriksson et al. (1999) demonstrated that unsatisfactory leisure time 24 years previously was a strong predictor of consultation and treatment for disorders of the hands or wrists at age 42–59 years. However, the specific role of these factors in an older population has not been evaluated.

HIP PAIN

Several studies have examined the occurrence of hip pain in the general population. In a U.K. study, 14% of participants reported hip pain on most days for at least 1 month in the preceding year (Frankel et al. 1999) and other authors, in the United Kingdom and The Netherlands, have reported the 1-month period prevalence of the condition to be between 8.3% and 13% (Odding et al. 1996; Urwin et al. 1998; Pope et al. 2003). Hip pain is more common in women than men, and several studies have shown an increase in hip pain with age (Urwin et al. 1998; Frankel et al. 1999; Pope et al. 2003), although others have demonstrated a plateau in older age groups (Unwin et al. 1998; Thomas et al. 2004).

Few authors have studied hip pain specifically in an older population. Christmas et al. (2002) surveyed 6596 individuals in the United States aged 60 years and older as part of the third National Health and Nutrition Examination Survey. These authors reported that the 6-week period prevalence of hip pain was 12% in men and 16% in women. In the United Kingdom, in individuals of the same age, Pope et al. (2003) reported a combined 1-month period prevalence of 16%, and Urwin et al. (1998) demonstrated that, in those at least 75 years old, hip pain for more than one week in the past month was reported by 11% of men and 20% of women. Meanwhile, Frankel et al. (1999), examining pain in the past year in either hip "on most days for one month or longer," reported a prevalence of 13% in men aged 65–74 years and 14% in those aged 75 years and older. In women, prevalence was higher in both groups, at over 21%.

A recent population-based study of individuals aged 18–85 years demonstrated that a number of lifestyle and occupational activities significantly and independently predicted the onset of hip pain: sitting for prolonged periods at work, lifting weights of >50 pounds (22.68 kg), and walking as a leisure activity (Pope et al. 2003). In older age groups, hip pain is commonly associated with a number of inflammatory and degenerative diseases, such as osteoarthritis (OA). Birrell et al. (2000b) reported that nearly half of all patients in primary care with a new onset episode of hip pain had OA, noting that 17% had advanced disease. These authors demonstrated no significant difference between women and men, but showed that OA was more common in older individuals (50% and 36% in persons aged >63 years and <63 years, respectively) and in those reporting a longer duration of hip pain at presentation. Some studies have found evidence of structural damage of the hip joint in patients with hip pain: Birrell et al. (2000b) found that 44% of persons consulting in primary care with a new episode of hip pain had OA of the hip. Further, although structural damage of the hip joint was poorly correlated with quality of life (Birrell et al. 2000a), nearly one-quarter of patients required surgery 4 years later. Birrell et al. (2003) also showed that, in a population with a mean age of 63 years, the greatest predictors of hip replacement (or rather, being on a waiting list for hip replacement) 2 years after first consultation were restriction of internal rotation, pain duration, and the use of a walking stick.

KNEE PAIN

Knee pain in the general population is relatively common. The 1-month period prevalence of the condition was found to be 18% in individuals aged over 55 years in The Netherlands (Odding et al. 1996). In the United Kingdom, Jinks et al. (2002) demonstrated the 1-year prevalence to be 47% in those aged >50 years, nearly one-third of whom reported severe pain, and two-fifths (20% of the total sample) had "severe difficulty" with at least one component of physical functioning. Knee pain is more common in females than males, and prevalence increases with age (McAlindon et al. 1992; Odding et al. 1996; Urwin et al. 1998; Jinks et al. 2002). In a study of persons aged 55 years or older, Odding et al. (1996) reported that 13% of subjects years had had knee pain at some point in the previous month, and Urwin et al. (1998) demonstrated that 27% of men and 35% of women aged 75 years or older experienced knee pain "for more than one week in the past month." Further, McAlindon et al. (1992) demonstrated that the prevalence of "any knee pain during the last year" increased in older women from 23% in those aged 55–59 years to 39% in those aged 85 years or older. In men, however, these authors demonstrated a nonlinear relationship, with knee pain prevalence peaking at 30% at age 70–74 years, then decreasing to 19% in those aged 85 years or older. More recently, Thomas et al. (2004) showed a change of only 36% to 38% in the prevalence of knee pain between individuals aged 50–59 years and 80 or more years, respectively.

Although knee pain is common in older persons, there have been few community-based studies of the etiology of symptoms in this population. In later life, knee pain is frequently a symptom of degenerative bone diseases such as OA. Studies have shown that radiographic changes in the knee are significantly associated with pain and, in those with OA, pain is a marker for more severe disease (Hochberg et al. 1989). Others, however, have shown a poor correlation between knee pain and radiological evidence of disease (Hannan et al. 2000). Risk markers for OA include older age (Felson 1988), female gender (Odding et al. 1996), and obesity (Hartz et al. 1986), all of which are also associated with knee pain.

FOOT PAIN

Foot pain is perceived to be a common problem among older persons, although there are few epidemiological studies of foot pain in the community. Several studies have focused on foot disorders, many of which are associated with degenerative diseases and with diseases characterized by poor peripheral vascularization (Helfand 2004), but few have studied foot pain per se. In one recent study, Garrow (2002) examined the 1-month period prevalence of foot pain in persons of all ages in the United Kingdom. Prevalence increased with age and then declined in later life: prevalence in those aged 75–80 years was 20% in men and 27% in women. Other authors have noted little change in the occurrence of foot pain at older ages: Thomas et al. (2004) demonstrated the 1-month prevalence to be 22% in individuals aged 50–59 years and 20% in those aged 80 years or more.

Foot pain is associated with poor mobility (Leveille et al. 1998; Chen et al. 2003) and, particularly in older persons, with an increased risk of falling (Budiman-Mak et al. 1991). It commonly occurs in association with pain in the hip and knee (Chen et al. 2003), and in women, severe foot pain has been associated with OA in the hand and knee (Leveille et al. 1998). Studies have shown that the prevalence of foot disorders is high in older persons (Benvenuti et al. 1995; Balint et al. 2003; Dunn et al. 2004; Helfand 2004), although Leveille et al. (1998) found little association between foot pain and disorders such as bunions and hammer toes. These authors also reported that it was foot pain per se rather than other foot disorders that significantly predicted disability and poor mobility.

NON-MUSCULOSKELETAL PAIN

HEADACHE

Scher et al. (1999) provided a comprehensive review of the epidemiological literature on headache and migraine. Based on a meta-analysis of 29 studies (headache) and 18 studies (migraine), these authors demonstrated a greater prevalence of both conditions in women. In men, the prevalence of both headache and migraine remained relatively constant throughout life, whereas in women it increased to middle age, then decreased in later life (Scher et al. 1999).

As part of the Italian Longitudinal Study of Aging, Franceschi et al. (1997) studied the prevalence of headache in individuals aged 65–84 years, finding that 13% of men and 24% of women reported a history of troublesome headaches in the past year that were "sufficiently long and/or painful to interfere with activities of daily living," while 3.6% of men and 8.8% of women experienced current symptoms. Boardman et al. (2003), in persons aged 66 or more years, reported the 3-month prevalence of headache to be 41% in men and 50% in women. Thomas et al. (2004) reported a decrease in the prevalence of head pain with increasing age, from 26% in persons aged 60–69 years to 17% in those aged 80 years or more. However, the proportion of persons with pain who reported that it interfered with their daily lives increased from 70% in the first age group to 83% in the second.

Migraine prevalence is, in general, lower than that of non-migrainous headaches. Again, age and case definition explain a considerable amount of the variation in different prevalence estimates. Stewart et al. (1995) calculated that two-thirds of all variance could be accounted for by case definition and demographic factors. Prevalence of migraine increases with age, more markedly so in females, and then decreases in later life (Rasmussen 1995; Sheffield 1998; Scher et al. 1999). Consequently, the prevalence of migraine in older persons is relatively low. Franceschi et al. (1997) reported that 5.4% of women and 1.8% of men aged 65–84 years had experienced migraine symptoms in the previous year.

There is little epidemiological work examining the etiology of headache in older populations. In persons of all ages, Zwart et al. (2003) demonstrated a significant association between headache and the occurrence of depression and anxiety. Similarly, Fearon and Hotopf (2001) showed that the occurrence of headaches and depression in childhood and a family history of mental illness were associated with the occurrence of headaches in adulthood, and other authors have demonstrated the role of genetic factors in migraine (Russell and Olesen 1995). In persons aged 65–84 years, Franceschi et al. (1997) demonstrated an association between headache, younger age, and female gender, but they also pointed out the important role of other illnesses, such as diabetes.

ABDOMINAL PAIN

Most epidemiological studies of abdominal pain consider its occurrence as a symptom of functional gastrointestinal disorders (Halder et al. 2002). Common presenting symptoms of these disorders include abdominal pain and discomfort and altered bowel habits, and frequently no organic cause can be found (Talley et al. 1991). In a large population sample of persons aged 18 years and older, 18% reported functional abdominal pain symptoms in the previous 12 months, but less than two-thirds of these cases were explained by findings of organic disease (Koloski et al. 2002).

Talley et al. (1991) reported that in individuals aged 30–64 years in the United States, the prevalence of abdominal pain ("more than six times in the past year") was 26%, although others have produced lower prevalence estimates. In a large population-based survey in the United Kingdom, Halder et al. (2002) reported a 1-month period prevalence of 10% in individuals aged 18–65 years. Studies show a greater prevalence in females (Halder et al. 2002; Sandler et al. 2000) and a decrease in prevalence with age (Sandler et al. 2000).

In older age groups, abdominal pain remains significant. In the United Kingdom, Chaplin et al. (2000) reported the 1-year prevalence of abdominal pain to be 25% in a primary care sample of individuals aged 65 years and older, and Thomas et al. (2004) reported the 1-month prevalence in those aged 80 years and older to be 9.7%. In the United States, Sandler et al. (2000) demonstrated that the 1-month prevalence of abdominal pain or discomfort in individuals aged 60 years and older was 7.1% in men and 20% in women. Further, Halder et al. (2002) demonstrated that in individuals aged 50–65 years, 4.3% of individuals who were initially free of abdominal pain reported symptoms 12 months subsequently.

Abdominal pain is a common presenting feature of many, but not all, gastrointestinal disorders (Thompson et al. 1999), and it is a key feature of irritable bowel syndrome and functional abdominal pain syndrome. Nevertheless, there is a paucity of data concerning the etiology of abdominal pain in older persons. Halder et al. (2002) demonstrated that, in persons aged 18–65 years who were free of abdominal pain, high levels of general psychological distress and adverse illness behavior significantly and independently predicted the new onset of symptoms over a 12-month period. Others, however, have failed to show a relationship between psychiatric variables and the occurrence of abdominal pain (Von Korff et al. 1993) or other gastrointestinal symptoms (Talley et al. 2001).

CHRONIC WIDESPREAD PAIN

In 1990, as part of their classification criteria for fibromyalgia, the American College of Rheumatology (ACR) defined chronic widespread pain (CWP) as pain lasting more than 3 months on both the left and right sides of the body, both above and below the waist, and in the anterior chest, cervical, thoracic, or lumbar spine (Wolfe et al. 1990). Since then these criteria have been frequently adopted for epidemiological study. In contrast, the classification of fibromyalgia requires the presence of CWP *plus* palpable tenderness at 11 or more of 18 specific tender point sites.

Some have argued that one need not truly have CWP to be classified as such using the ACR definition (Macfarlane et al. 1996a). For example, a person with LBP and localized pain in the left hand and right foot (for whatever reason) would meet the ACR criteria, which essentially only require pain in the spine or sternum and in two contralateral body quadrants. Thus, CWP may be one of two things: (1) pain that is genuinely widespread throughout the body, often considered to be of rheumatological origin or (2) pain that appears at several (or many) different localized sites throughout the body.

Population prevalence estimates of CWP appear to be remarkably stable, with a number of studies providing estimates ranging between 10% (Wolfe et al. 1995) and 14% (Schochat and Raspe 2003), although White et al. (1999) reported a slightly lower prevalence of 7.3%. Also, studies are consistent in demonstrating that prevalence is higher in females than in males (Croft et al. 1993; Wolfe et al. 1995; Bergman et al. 2001). Because of the additional tender point criteria, the occurrence of fibromyalgia is lower than that of CWP (although all fibromyalgia patients, by definition, also have CWP). Wolfe et al. (1995) demonstrated the prevalence of fibromyalgia to be 3.4% in women and 0.5% in men, in persons of all ages. In older persons (at least 80 years old), these authors reported a prevalence of 5.9% in women and 1.1% in men.

Few studies have examined the prevalence of widespread pain specifically in older persons. Studies in populations of all ages show that prevalence peaks in the seventh decade, after which it decreases (Wolfe et al.

1995; Bergman et al. 2001; Thomas et al. 2004). Wolfe et al. (1995) reported that prevalence peaks at approximately 14% in men and 23% in women aged 60–69 years, then decreases in later life to 8.5% and 15% in men and women aged 80 years or older, respectively. Thomas et al. (2004) reported a similar pattern, noting a prevalence of 6.6% in men and 14% in women aged 80 years and older. Other authors have shown that the onset of CWP is also common in older age groups. McBeth et al. (2001a) demonstrated that among 390 individuals aged 50–64 years who were free of CWP, 7.4% reported symptoms 12 months subsequently.

As with other pain conditions, although there is a literature of the etiology of symptoms, very little focuses specifically on pain in older age groups. However, studies in persons of all ages have highlighted the role not only of a number of postural and mechanical factors (McBeth et al. 2003a; Harkness et al. 2004), but also of psychological distress (Macfarlane et al. 1996a), depression and anxiety (Croft et al. 1993; Benjamin et al. 2000), workplace psychosocial factors (Harkness et al. 2004), and various features of somatization (McBeth et al. 2001a).

In reporting data about multiple sites (Table I), Urwin et al. (1998) showed that 31% of women and 19% of men aged 75 years and older reported pain in three or more areas. It may be the case, therefore, that older persons with multi-site localized pain may be more likely to be classified as having CWP. Certainly, regional pains are important markers for the possible future occurrence of CWP. McBeth et al. (2001a) demonstrated that in a group of individuals initially free of CWP, the occurrence of CWP 12 months subsequently was four times greater in the those who, at baseline, reported regional pain, compared to those who reported no pain.

DISCUSSION

There are marked changes in the prevalence of pain with age. Andersson et al. (1993) present three models of age-related change in the prevalence of pain. The first is pain increasing with age until approximately the sixth decade, then decreasing in later life. This pain (such as may be located in the low back, shoulder, or arm) typically has a mechanical etiological component, and is possibly associated with the occupational environment, as evidenced by the decrease in prevalence beyond normal working age. The second model is pain increasing with age (such as pain in the hip, knee, or foot), which has a mechanical etiological component but also is associated with increasing prevalence of degenerative disease, particularly in older persons. The third model is age-independent pain (such as in the chest, upper back, stomach, and head) that lacks a mechanical etiological component; risk factors for such pain may be constant throughout life, may act only over the short term, and have no cumulative effect over time.

Providing evidence for a fourth model, some studies have shown clear decreases in the prevalence of various pain conditions at older ages: abdominal pain (Sandler et al. 2000), non-cardiac chest pain (Eslick et al. 2003), and orofacial pain (Macfarlane et al. 2002). For all pain symptoms, it is not clear whether these changes are due to the age-related changes in pain and pain perception per se, or due to changes in pain reporting.

It has been suggested that older persons may play down the occurrence of pain due to the occurrence of other significant life events, such as loss of independence or the death of a spouse (Helme and Gibson 1999). However, Bradbeer et al. (2003) demonstrated that in persons aged 65 years and older, widow(er)hood was associated with a three-fold increase in the occurrence of pain.

Several authors have discussed the difficulties of examining the epidemiology of pain in older samples and have suggested that the prevalence of pain in the community setting may be underestimated. Helme and Gibson (1999) note the possible unreliability of memory in older age groups and discuss how this may affect the collection of data. These authors also point out that studies that ask subjects to recollect "any" pain and then, subsequently, to identify the location of this pain may yield different estimates of pain occurrence than those that ask directly about pain in specific sites of the body. Any problems that thus arise will be augmented in a population with cognitive decline. However, Thomas et al. (2004) argue that in a community sample the proportion of older people who are unable to communicate their pain effectively due to cognitive decline is probably very small.

It is possible that the reporting of pain in older persons is different due to alterations in neurophysiology (Chakour et al. 1996; Gibson and Farrell 2004) or an increase in stoicism (Helme and Gibson 1999). It has been suggested that pain is more expected in an older population through the increased occurrence of illness and disease. With an increase in the number of symptoms, both painful and nonpainful, an individual may select which symptoms to report. Thus, population-based studies may be subject to preferential pain reporting, where older persons may under-report LBP, for example, because of more severe and bothersome pain in the hip or knee.

An older population is, by definition, highly selected. Survival to older ages may be an indication of less (pain-causing) disease. In a large prospective cohort study, Macfarlane et al. (2001) demonstrated that, of 6500 persons aged 18–75 years, those with regional and widespread pain symptoms experienced increased mortality over the subsequent eight years, compared to pain-free individuals. Further, these excess deaths were predominantly due to cancer (McBeth et al. 2003b). However, other studies from Sweden and Scotland examining regional pains have not confirmed these findings, noting some effect of pain symptoms on mortality, but not specifically in the case of cancer (Kareholt and Brattberg 1998; Smith et al. 2003).

Few authors have focused specifically on the epidemiology of pain in older persons. Recognizing the need for more targeted studies, Thomas et al. (2004) examined the prevalence and impact of pain in older age groups (50 years and above). In the oldest age group under study (80 years and above), these authors demonstrated that pain prevalence varied considerably with site, from 7.2% in the head to 38% in the knee. They went on to show that most persons experiencing pain reported interference with their normal daily activities.

Some have hypothesized that in determining the impact of pain on a individual, the *number* of sites of pain may be more important than the pain's precise location(s) (Smith et al. 2004). It is possible, however, that individuals under-report pain at some sites, because of a predominant pain at another site, although it should be noted that this problem is not exclusive to the study of pain in older persons. We have considered CWP as a separate entity, although it may be argued that it is an amalgam of several regional pain symptoms. In fact, it has been proposed that regional pain symptoms sit midway along a pain continuum (Macfarlane 1999). At one end of the continuum pains are localized and frequently acute; at the other, pains are widespread and can persist for many years. McBeth et al. (2001b) demonstrated that more than half of persons who report CWP still report symptoms 12 months subsequently, and others have shown that approximately one-third of individuals still report symptoms 2 and 7 years later (Macfarlane et al. 1996b; Papageorgiou et al. 2002).

In summary, regional and widespread pain conditions are common in older persons, although their measurement in the community is difficult and may be underestimated. Little work has focused specifically on the epidemiology of pain at older ages, although, as in persons of all ages, pain is more prevalent in women than men, and the evidence suggests that it results from a combination of constitutional, lifestyle, mechanical, and psychosocial factors. Particularly in older persons, pain may be a symptom of underlying disease such as arthritis, and this pathology may often provide the best indicator of pain prognosis.

REFERENCES

Andersson HI, Ejlertsson G, Leden I, Rosenberg C. Chronic pain in a geographically defined general population: studies of differences in age, gender, social class, and pain localization. *Clin J Pain* 1993; 9(3):174–182.

Balint GP, Korda J, Hangody L, Balint PV. Regional musculoskeletal conditions: foot and ankle disorders. *Best Pract Res Clin Rheumatol* 2003; 17(1):87–111.

Bellamy N, Sothern RB, Campbell J, Buchanan WW. Circadian rhythm in pain, stiffness, and manual dexterity in rheumatoid arthritis: relation between discomfort and disability. *Ann Rheum Dis* 1991; 50(4):243–248.

Bellamy N, Sothern RB, Campbell J, Buchanan WW. Rhythmic variations in pain, stiffness, and manual dexterity in hand osteoarthritis. *Ann Rheum Dis* 2002; 61(12):1075–1080.

Benjamin S, Morris S, McBeth J, Macfarlane GJ, Silman AJ. The association between chronic widespread pain and mental disorder: a population-based study. *Arthritis Rheum* 2000; 43:561–567.

Benvenuti F, Ferrucci L, Guralnik JM, Gangemi S, Baroni A. Foot pain and disability in older persons: an epidemiologic survey. *J Am Geriatr Soc* 1995; 43(5):479–484.

Bergman S, Herrstrom P, Hogstrom, K, et al. Chronic musculoskeletal pain, prevalence rates, and sociodemographic associations in a Swedish population study. *J Rheumatol* 2001; 28(6):1369–1377.

Birrell F, Croft PR, Cooper C, et al. Health impact of pain in the hip region with and without radiographic evidence of osteoarthritis: a study of new attenders to primary care. PCR Hip Study Group. *Ann Rheum Dis* 2000a; 59(11):857–863.

Birrell F, Croft PR, Cooper, C, et al. Radiographic change is common in new presenters in primary care with hip pain. PCR Hip Study Group. *Rheumatology (Oxford)* 2000b; 39(7):772–775.

Birrell F, Afzal C, Nahit ES, et al. Predictors of hip joint replacement in new attenders in primary care with hip pain. *Br J Gen Pract* 2003; 53(486):26–30.

Boardman HF, Thomas E, Croft PR, Millson DS. Epidemiology of headache in an English district. *Cephalalgia* 2003; 23(2):129–137.

Bradbeer M, Helme RD, Yong HH, Kendig HL, Gibson SJ. Widowhood and other demographic associations of pain in independent older people. *Clin J Pain* 2003; 19(4):247–254.

Budiman-Mak E, Conrad KJ, Roach KE. The Foot Function Index: a measure of foot pain and disability. *J Clin Epidemiol* 1991; 44(6):561–570.

Chakour MC, Gibson SJ, Bradbeer M, Helme RD. The effect of age on A delta- and C-fibre thermal pain perception. *Pain* 1996; 64(1):143–152.

Chaplin A, Curless R, Thomson R, Barton R. Prevalence of lower gastrointestinal symptoms and associated consultation behaviour in a British elderly population determined by face-to-face interview. *Br J Gen Pract* 2000; 50(459):798–802.

Chen J, Devine A, Dick IM, Dhaliwal SS, Prince RL. Prevalence of lower extremity pain and its association with functionality and quality of life in elderly women in Australia. *J Rheumatol* 2003; 30(12):2689–2693.

Christmas C, Crespo CJ, Franckowiak SC, et al. How common is hip pain among older adults? Results from the Third National Health and Nutrition Examination Survey. *J Fam Pract* 2002; 51(4):345–348.

Coari G, Paoletti F, Iagnocco A. Shoulder involvement in rheumatic diseases. Sonographic findings. *J Rheumatol* 1999; 26(3):668–673.

Croft PR, Rigby AS. Socioeconomic influences on back problems in the community in Britain. *J Epidemiol Community Health* 1994; 48:166–170.

Croft PR, Rigby AS, Boswell R, Schollum J, Silman AJ. The prevalence of chronic widespread pain in the general population. *J Rheumatol* 1993; 20(4):710–713.

de Vet HC, Heymans MW, Dunn KM, et al. Episodes of low back pain: a proposal for uniform definitions to be used in research. *Spine* 2002; 27(21):2409–2416.

Dionne CE. Low back pain. In: Crombie IK, Croft PR, Linton SJ, LeResche L, Von Korff M (Eds). *Epidemiology of Pain.* Seattle: IASP Press, 1999, pp 283–297.

Dunn JE, Link CL, Felson DT, et al. Prevalence of foot and ankle conditions in a multiethnic community sample of older adults. *Am J Epidemiol* 2004; 159(5):491–498.

Eslick GD, Jones MP, Talley NJ. Non-cardiac chest pain: prevalence, risk factors, impact and consulting—a population-based study. *Aliment Pharmacol Ther* 2003; 17(9):1115–1124.

Fearon P, Hotopf M. Relation between headache in childhood and physical and psychiatric symptoms in adulthood: national birth cohort study. *BMJ* 2001; 322(7295):1145.

Felson DT. Epidemiology of hip and knee osteoarthritis. *Epidemiol Rev* 1988; 10:1–22.

Franceschi M, Colombo B, Rossi P, Canal N. Headache in a population-based elderly cohort. An ancillary study to the Italian Longitudinal Study of Aging (ILSA). *Headache* 1997; 37(2):79–82.

Frankel S, Eachus J, Pearson N, et al. Population requirement for primary hip-replacement surgery: a cross-sectional study. *Lancet* 1999; 353(9161):1304–1309.

Fredriksson K, Alfredsson L, Koster M, et al. Risk factors for neck and upper limb disorders: results from 24 years of follow up. *Occup Environ Med* 1999; 56:59–66.

Garrow AP. *Foot Pain and Disability in the Adult Population.* PhD thesis, University of Manchester, 2002.

Gibson SJ, Farrell M. A review of age differences in the neurophysiology of nociception and the perceptual experience of pain. *Clin J Pain* 2004; 20(4):227–239.

Halder SL, McBeth J, Silman AJ, Thompson DG, Macfarlane G. J. Psychosocial risk factors for the onset of abdominal pain. Results from a large prospective population-based study. *Int J Epidemiol* 2002; 31(6):1219–1225.

Hannan MT, Felson DT, Pincus T. Analysis of the discordance between radiographic changes and knee pain in osteoarthritis of the knee. *J Rheumatol* 2000; 27(6):1513–1517.

Harkness EF, Macfarlane GJ, Nahit ES, Silman AJ, McBeth J. Mechanical and psychosocial factors predict new onset shoulder pain: a prospective cohort study of newly employed workers. *Occup Environ Med* 2003a; 60(11):850–857.

Harkness EF, Macfarlane GJ, Nahit ES, Silman AJ, McBeth J. Risk factors for new-onset low back pain amongst cohorts of newly employed workers. *Rheumatology (Oxford)* 2003b; 42(8):959–968.

Harkness EF, Macfarlane GJ, Nahit ES, Silman AJ, McBeth J. Mechanical injury and psycho-social factors in the work place predict the onset of widespread body pain: a two-year prospective study among cohorts of newly employed workers. *Arthritis Rheum* 2004; 50(5):1655–1664.

Hartz AJ, Fischer ME, Bril G, et al. The association of obesity with joint pain and osteoarthritis in the HANES data. *J Chron Dis* 1986; 39(4):311–319.

Helfand AE. Foot problems in older patients: a focused podogeriatric assessment study in ambulatory care. *J Am Podiatr Med Assoc* 2004; 94(3):293–304.

Helme RD, Gibson SJ. Pain in older people. In: Crombie IK, Croft PR, Linton SJ, LeResche L, Von Korff M (Ed). *Epidemiology of Pain.* Seattle: IASP Press, 1999, pp 103–112.

Hillman M, Wright A, Rajaratnam G, Tennant A, Chamberlain MA. Prevalence of low back pain in the community: implications for service provision in Bradford, UK. *J Epidemiol Community Health* 1996; 50:347–352.

Hochberg MC, Lawrence RC, Everett DF, Cornoni-Huntley J. Epidemiologic associations of pain in osteoarthritis of the knee: data from the National Health and Nutrition Examination Survey and the National Health and Nutrition Examination-I Epidemiologic Follow-up Survey. *Semin Arthritis Rheum* 1989; 18(4 Suppl 2):4–9.

Hoogendoorn WE, Bongers PM, De Vet, HCW, et al. Flexion and rotation of the trunk and lifting at work are risk factors for low back pain: results of a prospective cohort study. *Spine* 2000; (25)23:3087–3092.

Hoogendoorn WE, Bongers PM, de Vet, HC, et al. Psychosocial work characteristics and psychological strain in relation to low-back pain. *Scand J Work Environ Health* 2001; 27(4):258–267.

Hunt IM, Silman AJ, Benjamin S, McBeth J, Macfarlane GJ. The prevalence and associated features of chronic widespread pain in the community using the 'Manchester' definition of chronic widespread pain. *Rheumatology (Oxford)* 1999; 38(3):275–279.

Jinks C, Jordan K, Croft PR. Measuring the population impact of knee pain and disability with the Western Ontario and McMaster Universities Osteoarthritis Index (WOMAC). *Pain* 2002; 100(1–2):55–64.

Josephson M, Hagberg M, Hjelm EW. Self-reported physical exertion in geriatric care. A risk indicator for low back symptoms? *Spine* 1996; 21(23):2781–2785.

Kareholt I, Brattberg G. Pain and mortality risk among elderly persons in Sweden. *Pain* 1998; 77:271–278.

Koloski NA, Talley NJ, Boyce PM. Epidemiology and health care seeking in the functional GI disorders: a population-based study. *Am J Gastroenterol* 2002; 97(9):2290–2299.

Latza U, Karmaus W, Sturmer T, et al. Cohort study of occupational risk factors of low back pain in construction workers. *Occup Environ Med* 2000; 57:28–34.

Leveille SG, Guralnik JM, Ferrucci L, et al. Foot pain and disability in older women. *Am J Epidemiol* 1998; 148(7):657–665.

Macfarlane GJ. Generalized pain, fibromyalgia and regional pain: an epidemiological view. *Best Pract Res Clin Rheumatol* 1999; 13(3):403–414.

Macfarlane GJ, Croft PR, Schollum J, Silman AJ. Widespread pain: is an improved classification possible? *J Rheumatol* 1996a; 23(9):1628–1632.

Macfarlane GJ, Thomas E, Papageorgiou AC, et al. The natural history of chronic pain in the community: a better prognosis than in the clinic? *J Rheumatol* 1996b; 23:1617–1620.

Macfarlane GJ, Thomas E, Papageorgiou AC, et al. Employment and physical work activities as predictors of future low back pain. *Spine* 1997; 22(10):1143–1149.

Macfarlane GJ, Hunt IM, Silman AJ. Role of mechanical and psychosocial factors in the onset of forearm pain: prospective population based study. *Br Med J* 2000; 321(7262):676–679.

Macfarlane GJ, McBeth J, Silman AJ. Widespread body pain and mortality: prospective population based study. *Br Med J* 2001; 323(7314):662–665.

Macfarlane TV, Blinkhorn AS, Davies RM, Kincey J, Worthington HV. Orofacial pain in the community: prevalence and associated impact. *Community Dent Oral Epidemiol* 2002; 30(1):52–60.

McAlindon TE, Cooper C, Kirwan JR, Dieppe PA. Knee pain and disability in the community. *Br J Rheumatol* 1992; 31(3):189–192.

McBeth J, Macfarlane GJ, Benjamin S, Silman AJ. Features of somatization predict the onset of chronic widespread pain: results of a large population-based study. *Arthritis Rheum* 2001a; 44(4):940–946.

McBeth J, Macfarlane GJ, Hunt IM, Silman AJ. Risk factors for persistent chronic widespread pain: a community-based study. *Rheumatology (Oxford)* 2001b; 40(1):95–101.

McBeth J, Harkness EF, Silman AJ, Macfarlane GJ. The role of workplace low-level mechanical trauma, posture and environment in the onset of chronic widespread pain. *Rheumatology (Oxford)* 2003a; 42(12):1486–1494.

McBeth J, Silman AJ, Macfarlane GJ. Association of widespread body pain with an increased risk of cancer and reduced cancer survival: a prospective, population-based study. *Arthritis Rheum* 2003b; 48(6):1686–1692.

Miranda H, Viikari-Juntura E, Martikainen R, Takala EP, Riihimaki H. A prospective study of work related factors and physical exercise as predictors of shoulder pain. *Occup Environ Med* 2001; 58(8):528–534.

Odding E, Valkenburg HA, Algra D, et al. The association of abnormalities on physical examination of the hip and knee with locomotor disability in the Rotterdam Study. *Br J Rheumatol* 1996; 35(9):884–890.

Olofsson Y, Book C, Jacobsson LT. Shoulder joint involvement in patients with newly diagnosed rheumatoid arthritis. Prevalence and associations. *Scand J Rheumatol* 2003; 32(1):25–32.

Papageorgiou AC, Croft PR, Ferry S, Jayson MIV, Silman AJ. Estimating the prevalence of low back pain in the general population. Evidence from the South Manchester Back Pain Survey. *Spine* 1995; 20(17):1889–1894.

Papageorgiou AC, Macfarlane GJ, Thomas E, et al. Psychosocial factors in the workplace—do they predict new episodes of low back pain? Evidence from the South Manchester Back Pain Study. *Spine* 1997; 22(10):1137–1142.

Papageorgiou AC, Croft PR, Thomas E, et al. Psychosocial risks for low back pain: are these related to work? *Ann Rheum Dis* 1998; 57(8):500–502.

Papageorgiou AC, Silman AJ, Macfarlane GJ. Chronic widespread pain in the population: a seven year follow up study. *Ann Rheum Dis* 2002; 61(12):1071–1074.

Pope DP, Croft PR, Pritchard CM, Silman AJ. Prevalence of shoulder pain in the community: the influence of case definition. *Ann Rheum Dis* 1997; 56(5):308–312.

Pope DP, Hunt IM, Birrell, FN, Silman AJ, Macfarlane GJ. Hip pain onset in relation to cumulative workplace and leisure time mechanical load: a population based case-control study. *Ann Rheum Dis* 2003; 62(4):322–326.

Power C, Frank J, Hertzman C, Schierhout G, Li L. Predictors of low back pain onset in a prospective British study. *Am J Public Health* 2001; 91(10):1671–1678.

Rasmussen BK. Epidemiology of headache. *Cephalalgia* 1995; 15(1):45–68.

Russell MB, Olesen J. Increased familial risk and evidence of genetic factor in migraine. *Br Med J* 1995; 311(7004):541–544.

Sandler RS, Stewart WF, Liberman JN, Ricci JA, Zorich NL. Abdominal pain, bloating, and diarrhea in the United States: prevalence and impact. *Dig Dis Sci* 2000; 45(6):1166–1171.

Scher A, Stewart WF, Lipton RB. Migraine and headache: a meta-analytic approach. In: Crombie IK, Croft PR, Linton SJ, LeResche L, Von Korff M (Eds). *Epidemiology of Pain*. Seattle: IASP Press, 1999, pp 159–170.

Schochat T, Raspe H. Elements of fibromyalgia in an open population. *Rheumatology (Oxford)* 2003; 42(7):829–835.

Sheffield RE. Migraine prevalence: a literature review. *Headache* 1998; 38(8):595–601.

Smith BH, Elliott AM, Hannaford PC. Pain and subsequent mortality and cancer among women in the Royal College of General Practitioners Oral Contraception Study. *Br J Gen Pract* 2003; 53(486):45–46.

Smith BH, Elliott AM, Hannaford PC. Royal College of General Practitioners' Oral Contraception Study. Is chronic pain a distinct diagnosis in primary care? Evidence arising from the Royal College of General Practitioners' Oral Contraception study. *Fam Pract* 2004; 21(1):66–74.

Stewart WF, Simon D, Shechter A, Lipton RB. Population variation in migraine prevalence: a meta-analysis. *J Clin Epidemiol* 1995; 48(2):269–280.

Talley NJ, Zinmeister AR, Van Dyke C. Epidemiology of colonic symptoms and the irritable bowel syndrome. *Gastroenterology* 1991; 101:927.

Talley NJ, Howell S, Poulton R. The irritable bowel syndrome and psychiatric disorders in the community: is there a link? *Am J Gastroenterol* 2001; 96(4):1072–1079.

Thomas E, Silman AJ, Papageorgiou AC, Macfarlane GJ, Croft PR. Association between measures of spinal mobility and low back pain. An analysis of new attenders in primary care. *Spine* 1998; 23(3):343–347.

Thomas E, Peat G, Harris L, Wilkie R, Croft PR. The prevalence of pain and pain interference in a general population of older adults: cross-sectional findings from the North Staffordshire Osteoarthritis Project (NorStOP). *Pain* 2004; 110(1–2):361–368.

Thompson WG, Longstreth GF, Drossman DA, et al. Functional bowel disorders and functional abdominal pain. *Gut* 1999; 45(Suppl 2):II43–II47.

Urwin M, Symmons D, Allison T, et al. Estimating the burden of musculoskeletal disorders in the community: the comparative prevalence of symptoms at different anatomical sites, and the relation to social deprivation. *Ann Rheum Dis* 1998; 57:649–655.

van der Windt DA, Croft PR. Shoulder pain. In: Crombie IK, Croft PR, Linton SJ, LeResche L, Von Korff M (Eds). *Epidemiology of Pain*. Seattle: IASP Press, 1999, pp 257–281.

van Schaardenburg D, Van den Brande KJ, Ligthart GJ, Breedveld FC, Hazes JM. Musculosk-
eletal disorders and disability in persons aged 85 and over: a community survey. *Ann Rheum Dis* 1994; 53(12):807–811.

Vogt MT, Simonsick EM, Harris TB, et al. Neck and shoulder pain in 70- to 79-year-old men and women: findings from the Health, Aging and Body Composition Study. *Spine J* 2003; 3(6):435–441.

Von Korff M, Le Resche L, Dworkin SF. First onset of common pain symptoms: a prospective study of depression as a risk factor. *Pain* 1993; 55:251–258.

Weiner DK, Haggerty CL, Kritchevsky SB, et al. How does low back pain impact physical function in independent, well-functioning older adults? Evidence from the Health ABC Cohort and implications for the future. *Pain Med* 2003; 4(4):311–320.

White KP, Speechley M, Harth M, Ostbye T. The London Fibromyalgia Epidemiology Study: the prevalence of fibromyalgia syndrome in London, Ontario. *J Rheumatol* 1999; 26(7):1570–1576.

Wolfe F, Smythe HA, Yunus MB, et al. The American College of Rheumatology 1990 criteria for the classification of fibromyalgia. *Arthritis Rheum* 1990; 33(2):160–172.

Wolfe F, Ross K, Anderson J, Russell IJ, Hebert L. The prevalence and characteristics of fibromyalgia in the general population. *Arthritis Rheum* 1995; 38(1):19–28.

Zwart JA, Dyb G, Hagen K, et al. Depression and anxiety disorders associated with headache frequency. The Nord-Trondelag Health Study. *Eur J Neurol* 2003; 10(2):147–152.

Correspondence to: Prof. Gary J. Macfarlane, PhD, Epidemiology Group, Department of Public Health, School of Medicine, Polwarth Building, University
of Aberdeen, Foresterhill, Aberdeen, AB25 2ZD, United Kingdom. Email:
g.j.macfarlane@abdn.ac.uk.

Part II

Age Differences in Pain

Pain in Older Persons, Progress in Pain Research and Management, Vol. 35, edited by Stephen J. Gibson and Debra K. Weiner, IASP Press, Seattle, © 2005.

2

The Neurobiology of Aging, Nociception, and Pain: An Integration of Animal and Human Experimental Evidence

Lucia Gagliese[a,b,c] and Michael J. Farrell[d,e]

[a]School of Kinesiology and Health Science, York University, Toronto, Ontario, Canada; [b]Department of Anaesthesia and Pain Management, University Health Network, Toronto General Hospital, Toronto, Ontario, Canada; [c]Departments of Anaesthesia and Psychiatry, University of Toronto, Toronto, Ontario, Canada; [d]Howard Florey Institute and Centre for Neuroscience, University of Melbourne, Melbourne, Victoria, Australia; [e]National Ageing Research Institute, Parkville, Victoria, Australia

The neurobiology of pain involves complex interactions of peripheral and central factors. Similarly, the neurobiology of aging involves multiple, complex changes and interactions of peripheral and central substrates. Many of these changes are not uniform across systems, and their unique and interactive effects are not always clear. In addition, the functional and behavioral consequences of these changes are not easy to predict. In studying the neurobiology of aging as it relates to nociception, pain, and recovery from injury, we may require a network and remodeling theoretical conceptualization. That is, the various interconnected systems (including, but not limited to, the nervous, musculoskeletal, immune, and neuroendocrine systems) must be considered together to arrive at an integrated understanding. This conceptualization is consistent with network approaches to both pain (Melzack 1996) and aging (Franceschi et al. 2000).

This chapter examines age effects on pain processing and discusses the morphological and biochemical changes that may be involved in these age-related effects. Two aspects of pain processing warrant attention in the context of aging effects. The first is the influence of aging on nociception, antinociception, and pain under physiological conditions. That is, how does normal aging affect the processing of brief, noxious stimuli that do not cause ongoing damage? The second area of inquiry is the interaction of aging and the processing of pain associated with pathology. Here the focus is on the behavioral and neurobiological response of the aging nervous system to insult, both immediately and over time. Because clinical pain in humans is largely a consequence of tissue inflammation or nerve injury, there is considerable interest in factors that are likely to modulate pain plasticity, not least of which is the impact of aging. The richest vein of information comes from animal models of nociception, and this chapter focuses primarily on the results of animal experimentation. When possible, data from human experimentation and clinical studies are juxtaposed with the animal literature in order to identify consistent or divergent patterns across species.

NORMAL AGING, NOCICEPTION, AND PAIN SENSITIVITY

ANIMAL MODELS OF PHASIC NOCICEPTIVE STIMULATION

Most studies of age differences in nociception under physiological conditions have used models of transient pain. The most commonly used model is the rodent tail-flick test, a measure of simple reflexive behavior that involves exposure of the tail to a source of heat. The time from heat onset to a flick of the tail away from the stimulation is taken as a measure of nociceptive sensitivity (Dubner and Ren 1999). Although not all studies agree, the majority have not found age differences on this test (see Gagliese and Melzack 2000 for a detailed review). These findings are consistent with the lack of age differences documented in the performance of many simple reflexive tasks (Wallace et al. 1980). Tests of organized unlearned behaviors require the animal to perform a complex, supraspinally mediated behavior in response to painful stimulation (Dubner and Ren 1999). Generally, with increasing age, the intensity or duration of stimulation required to elicit the response of interest increases on the hot-plate, vocalization, and jump-flinch tests (see Gagliese and Melzack 2000 for a detailed review). Although the potential role of age differences in motoric abilities remains to be clarified, it appears that older animals may be less responsive than younger animals on more highly organized tests of nociception. Similar patterns have been observed in other domains; reflexive behaviors are less likely than complex behaviors to be impaired with aging (Campbell et al. 1980).

EXPERIMENTAL PAIN IN HUMANS

Human equivalents of nociception-related reflexes and organized behaviors in the rat are not immediately apparent. The closest human facsimile of animal tests of nociception is the nociceptive flexion reflex (NFR). The NFR is a time-locked change in the EMG of a proximal muscle subsequent to a brief, noxious stimulus at a distal site (Willer 1977). The threshold for the NFR approximates, but usually exceeds, the pain threshold. In humans, the threshold for eliciting an NFR response does not appear to change as a function of age (Gibson et al. 2002). Stimuli in excess of the NFR threshold are required to elicit a reliably observable withdrawal response. Thus, an NFR of a magnitude likely to replicate the degree of movement represented by a tail flick in the rat would be associated with frank pain in a human subject. While it is incautious to draw too fine an association between human and animal experiences, nociceptive reflexes and complex behaviors in the rat may translate to suprathreshold segments of the pain-related stimulus/response function in humans. The bulk of psychophysical studies under physiological conditions in humans have focused on pain threshold, and they generally support an age-related decrease in acuity for pain (see Chapter 3). However, the cognitively demanding and attention-dependent detection of "just noticeable" pain in humans does not have an equivalent in animal models. Empirical data for age effects on suprathreshold ratings in humans are scarce, being confined to a single study using thermal stimuli (Harkins et al. 1986). The absence of an aging effect in this study is consistent with the animal literature. Thus, while the animal and human data for nociception and pain, respectively, have developed along different paths, there appears to be convergence in the isolated instance where meaningful comparisons can be made.

NEUROBIOLOGY OF NORMAL AGING AND NOCICEPTION

Normal aging is associated with multiple, non-uniform changes throughout the peripheral and central nervous system that may each contribute to age differences in nociception. Although there remain sizable gaps in our knowledge, we will examine animal and human data to characterize age-related changes in the substrates of nociception and to posit functional consequences of those changes.

The peripheral nerves of both older animals and humans are notable for selective loss of myelinated fibers (O'Sullivan and Swallow 1968; Ochoa and Mair 1969; Verdu et al. 2000) and signs of spontaneous damage including axonal involution and Wallerian degeneration (Knox et al. 1989; Drac et al. 1991). Furthermore, the pattern of neuropeptide expression of substance P, calcitonin gene-related peptide (CGRP), and somatostatin in older rats has been likened to the effects of axonal injury in young animals (Bergman et al. 1996a,b). The profile of neuropeptides in older rats may be a consequence of age-related changes in neurotrophic processes (Ulfhake et al. 2002). However, the association between age-related changes in the expression of neurotrophin (trk) receptors, levels of neuropeptides, and attenuation of cutaneous sensation is most notable for larger Aα and Aβ fibers (Bergman et al. 1996b). Despite this caveat, it seems probable that smaller myelinated nociceptive fibers are also subject to the effects of aging. Given that there is functional reserve in the nervous system, the impact of decreased Aδ-fiber numbers may be most apparent at the margins of functional performance. Indeed, it has been suggested that peripheral changes are unlikely to make a substantial contribution to aging effects in animal models of nociception (Iwata et al. 2002). Psychophysical evaluation of human pain perception allows for the identification of relatively subtle effects, and it may be that age-related changes in peripheral morphology are more likely to find expression in measures of the pain threshold. It has been noted that Aδ-fiber blockade has less effect on pain thresholds in older than in younger subjects, suggesting a diminished contribution from this fiber type in the elderly (Chakour et al. 1996). In addition, the reaction time of older people to laser stimulation, primarily a test of the integrity of Aδ primary afferents, may be up to twice that of younger subjects (Chakour et al. 1996; Harkins et al. 1996). It is possible that spatial summation and spatial acuity/localization of noxious stimuli near the pain threshold may also be impaired in older subjects, but this hypothesis remains to be tested. Of the neurobiological changes observed in the nerves of older rats, the impairment of regenerative processes may have the most significant functional consequences. It is very likely that these changes have implications for pain processing under pathological conditions, such as nerve injury and disease.

The morphological and biochemical changes that typify aging peripheral nerves can also be identified in the dorsal horn. Axonal involution, decreased myelin, and diminished levels of CGRP, substance P, and somatostatin have all been described in tissues sampled from the dorsal horns of either older animals or human post mortem material (Prineas and Spencer 1975; Bergman et al. 1996b; Ko et al. 1997; Hukkanen et al. 2002). The aging dorsal horn, in particular lamina I, exhibits changes that suggest degeneration of descending modulatory circuits. There is strong evidence that serotonin (5HT) and norepinephrine (NE) levels decrease with advancing age (Ko et al. 1997; Furst 1999; Iwata et al. 2002). These degenerative changes may contribute to the impaired descending inhibitory mechanisms reported in older animals and human subjects (Hamm and Knisely 1985, 1986; Bodnar et al. 1988; Knisely and Hamm 1989; Washington et al. 2000) and may also underlie the age-related decrease in pain tolerance (Collins and Stone 1966; Woodrow et al. 1972; Walsh et al. 1989; Edwards and Fillingim 2001), pointing toward impairment of endogenous inhibitory mechanisms in older people. The implications of these converging lines of evidence should not be understated. The countervailing influence of these ascending and descending inputs is of critical importance to the neuroplasticity of dorsal horn neurons subsequent to injury and disease. An imbalance between excitation and inhibition, notably impaired inhibition with advancing age, could significantly change the expression of pain associated with inflammatory and neuropathic conditions (Gagliese and Melzack 2000; Iwata et al. 2004).

Pain, as opposed to nociception, is created in the brain (Melzack 1996). Age-related change in the human brain is both sizable and ubiquitous (Anderton 2002), but the implication of these changes for pain processing remains a matter for conjecture. A single report of electrophysiological recordings from the nucleus basalis magnocellularis in anesthetized rats has identified cells with nocispecific response properties that are attenuated in older animals (Zhang et al. 2002). However, the extensive receptive fields and extremely intense stimuli required to elicit responses in a region homologous to the human putamen and globus pallidus leaves some doubt about the role of these cells in perceptual processes. It seems more likely that pain-related motoric responses would be sensitive to age-related change in the striatum, and this effect may constitute a partial explanation for aging effects on complex animal behaviors motivated by noxious stimulation. However, studies in humans suggest that dopaminergic pathways are implicated in regulation of intense pain arising from some modalities of stimulation (Hagelberg et al. 2004), raising the possibility of differential aging effects on pain-modulating circuits. In the human, event-related encephalographic measures of responses to painful stimuli are slower and of decreased amplitude in older people, suggesting an attenuation of pain-related cortical processes in the elderly (Gibson et al. 1991). Further exploration of age-related effects on supraspinal pain processing may benefit from the application of functional brain imaging techniques including positron emission tomography and functional magnetic resonance imaging.

In summary, the general indications from studies of the effects of aging on the neurobiological substrates of nociception are that change is widespread but not uniformly expressed. It seems probable that considerable functional capacity for nociceptive processes would be preserved in the aging nervous system under physiological conditions. However, disproportionate loss of reserve in one domain of countervailing modulatory circuits (i.e., excitatory versus inhibitory) could have functional consequences, particularly under conditions where the nociceptive system is substantially perturbed. In order to examine this possibility, we now turn to a discussion of responses to pathological insult.

AGING AND MODELS OF INFLAMMATION AND TISSUE INJURY

The second approach to the study of the neurobiology of pain and aging is to assess behavioral, neurophysiological, and neuroanatomical responses to injury. These models may be more directly comparable to the human clinical situation than the models of nociception described earlier. Age differences in responses on models of visceral pain, acute tissue injury and inflammation, and neuropathic pain have been examined.

ANIMAL MODELS OF VISCERAL PAIN

The writhing test has been used to assess age differences in visceral pain. In this model, 0.6% acetic acid is injected into the abdomen, and the number and/or intensity of writhing (or stretching) behaviors is taken as a measure of pain. It has been suggested that the response on this test reflects both inflammation and hyperalgesia. There are two reports suggesting that mid-life and older animals make fewer writhing responses than younger animals (Serrano et al. 2002; Todorovic et al. 2003). Interestingly, taurine (an essential amino acid with effects on multiple neurotransmitter systems) has significant antinociceptive properties in young animals but not in older ones, possibly implicating age-related declines in the integrity of neurotransmitter systems important to nociception (Serrano et al. 2002).

THE HUMAN EXPERIENCE OF VISCERAL PAIN

Human models of pain associated with visceral pathology are not available; however, older people are less sensitive than younger people to experimentally applied noxious visceral stimuli (i.e., balloon distension of the esophagus or colon) (Lasch et al. 1997; Lagier et al. 1999). In addition, the prevalence of pain associated with visceral pathology appears to decrease with advancing age (see Chapter 4). Although limited, evidence from both human and animal studies supports an age-related decline in visceral pain sensitivity. The mechanisms for these differences remain to be fully elucidated (Moore and Clinch 2004).

ANIMAL MODELS OF TISSUE INJURY/INFLAMMATION

One of the most widely used models of tissue injury and inflammation is the formalin test (Dubner and Ren 1999). In this test, diluted formalin is injected subcutaneously into the hindpaw, and nociceptive behaviors, such as licking and elevation of the paw, are scored for one hour following the injection (Dubuisson and Dennis 1977). To our knowledge, only one study has assessed age differences in spontaneous behavioral responses on this model. Gagliese and Melzack (1999) presented both cross-sectional and longitudinal data which showed that the relationship between age and pain behaviors subsequent to formalin injection may be curvilinear. Specifically, formalin test scores increased through early adulthood (3 months), peaked at mid-life (18 months) and decreased thereafter (24 months). Consistent with these results, Zhang et al. (2004) recently reported that 18-month-old rats exhibit greater thermal hyperalgesia than 3-month-old rats following injection of complete Freund's adjuvant (CFA) into the hindpaw. In this study, paw inflammation was greater in mid-life rats than in young rats, highlighting the potential importance of age-related changes in inflammatory and hypothalamic-pituitary-adrenal axis responses to stressors. Although further evidence is required, it appears that there may be age-related changes in the behavioral and inflammatory response to tissue injury, and that these changes may peak at mid-life.

Age differences in the neurochemical consequences of tissue injury associated with inflammation have been reported. Following formalin injection, C-fos-positive cells, a marker of the excitation of second-order neurons activated by noxious stimulation (Hunt et al. 1987), were more numerous in the superficial laminae of both the medullary dorsal horn (MDH) and the C1 section of the spinal cord of older rats compared to younger rats (Iwata et al. 1995). Aberrant serotonergic fibers and varicosities, consistent with degeneration of this system, were more numerous in the old rats. Following hindpaw injection of CFA, 18-month-old rats showed decreased activity of serotonergic fibers as compared to 3-month-old rats (Zhang et al. 2004). Iwata et al. (1995) proposed that the age-related degeneration of endogenous descending pain inhibition systems may be associated with facilitation of responses at the spinal level. Consistent with this finding, serotonergic decreases were associated with increased dynorphin levels in the spinal cord (Zhang et al. 2004). It may be postulated that this facilitation, or disinhibition, would be greatest once the degeneration has begun (possibly at mid-life), but before compensatory mechanisms have restored homeostasis. If this is true, there would be a relatively short period of time during which behavioral responses to tissue injury would be exaggerated. Subsequent to this period of disinhibition, compensatory mechanisms would be established, and the behavioral response to inflammation would return to pre-disinhibition levels (possibly by 24 months of age). More data are needed before conclusions can be drawn.

INFLAMMATORY PAIN STATES IN HUMANS

There is considerable impetus for interest in the effects of aging on inflammatory pain states. Musculoskeletal disease is the single most prevalent cause of pain across the age spectrum in humans. Broad age-related trends in the epidemiology of pain are largely a function of levels of inflammatory pain, with other causes coming a distant second (Helme and Gibson 2001). Consequently, any debate about the peak of prevalence of pain in middle age versus old age resonates with age-related changes in the manifestation of the formalin test in rats. The nuances of the epidemiology of pain are eloquently discussed in Chapter 1. Age differences in the intensity and qualities of musculoskeletal pain are unclear, with reports of increases, decreases, and no change across age groups (Gagliese et al. 1999). Importantly, the gaps in our current understanding of the interaction of aging and inflammatory pain states are unacceptable. The burden of persistent pain and disability associated with the occurrence and medical treatment of musculoskeletal disease in the middle-aged and elderly may ultimately admit to a disease-based cure. In the interim, the research community should be encouraged to undertake parallel investigations of pain, aging, and inflammatory disorders as a matter of priority. The potential role of age differences in inflammatory responses to recovery from injury will be discussed separately.

AGING AND THE RESPONSE TO NERVE INJURY

ANIMAL MODELS OF NEUROPATHIC PAIN

The prevalence of neuropathies increases with age, both in humans (Gregg et al. 2004) and in rats (Majeed 1992). The algesic qualities of spontaneous neuropathies in old rats have not been described. There has been increasing attention to age differences in the behavioral and neurophysiological consequences of nerve damage, including surgical transection or ligation of nerves. Increasing age has been associated with slower regeneration of crushed (Van der Zee et al. 1991) or resutured (Choi et al. 1995) nerves. While age differences in the intensity of thermal hyperalgesia remain unclear, several studies have reported that both the onset and recovery from hyperalgesia may be delayed in older animals (Novak et al. 1999; Stuesse et al. 2001; Crisp et al. 2003). The data regarding tactile allodynia are less clear, with no consistent patterns of age differences apparent in its intensity, onset, or resolution (Ramer and Bisby 1998). These inconsistencies may be due to differences in the model of nerve injury employed (Kim et al. 1995). Interestingly, in a study directly comparing the chronic constriction injury (CCI) and partial sciatic nerve ligation (PSNL) models, aged animals developed more vigorous and longer-lasting thermal hyperalgesia after PSNL than after CCI (Crisp et al. 2003). This difference may be due to the greater inflammatory response associated with CCI. These results highlight the importance of the type and extent of injury when assessing age-related differences.

The development and maintenance of hyperalgesia depend on complex plastic changes in peripheral and central substrates after nerve damage. Afferent impulses signaling the damage are carried to the dorsal horn by slowly conducting, unmyelinated C fibers (Bennett 2000). C fibers release glutamate, which acts at three receptor types: metabotropic, kainate/AMPA, and *N*-methyl-D-aspartate (NMDA) (Bennett 2000). Activation of the NMDA receptor, through a complex cascade of intracellular events, results in dorsal horn neuron hyperexcitability, or central sensitization, including increased spontaneous activity, decreased threshold, increased response to afferent input, prolonged afterdischarge to repeated stimulation, and an expansion of receptive fields (Doubell et al. 1999). Central sensitization also may trigger pathological reorganization of neural circuitry, thus contributing to the development of chronic pain (Doubell et al. 1999). Through these processes, injury may have profound effects on the central nervous system (CNS) that long outlast the injury.

The NMDA receptor is ubiquitous throughout the CNS. In the brain, NMDA-receptor function and binding decline with increasing age, although the extent of decline is highly variable in different regions (Tamaru et al. 1991; Magnusson 1998). Growing evidence indicates that age-associated neurodegeneration may be mediated by glutaminergic activity at the NMDA receptor (Troulinaki and Tavernarakis 2005) and that older rats may be more susceptible than younger rats to NMDA-receptor-mediated excitotoxicity (Vatassery et al. 1998; Segovia et al. 2001). Unfortunately, age differences in NMDA-receptor properties have not been studied in the spinal cord. Given the variability in the changes throughout the brain, it is impossible to draw firm conclusions regarding the spinal cord. Interestingly, plastic changes in the spinal cord associated with "wind-up," in which repeated nociceptive events result in a state of sensitization, are dependent on NMDA-receptor activity. Evidence that wind-up may be more prolonged in older than in younger rats (Kanda et al. 2001) suggests that age differences at the NMDA-receptor level may be involved in the prolonged hyperalgesia documented in older animals.

In addition to NMDA-receptor activity, other important neurochemical and neurohistological consequences of nerve injury also may be age-related and may contribute to the differences described above. In the periphery, recovery of microvascular blood flow to the hind footpad is faster in young than older rats (Khalil and Khodr 2001). The amount of somatostatin transported from the cell body to the area proximal to the ligation decreases with age, but the rate of transport of somatostatin is lower in 18-month-old rats than in both 12- and 25-month-old rats, which do not differ from each other (Maclean et al. 1988). There is less axonal atrophy but greater nuclear eccentricity and focal intramyelinic edema in mid-life rats than in young rats following sciatic nerve transection (Kerezoudi et al. 1995). In addition, there is an almost three-fold greater increase in free radical activity in the sciatic nerve of older compared to younger rats 2 weeks after CCI (Khalil and Khodr 2001). In the L4–L5 spinal cord, astrocytic activation is less robust but remains elevated for a longer period of time in older than in young rats following CCI (Stuesse et al. 2001). In the superficial laminae of the dorsal horns, CCI-associated substance P activity is greater in mid-life rats than in young or old rats, but it returns to preinjury levels more rapidly in young rats (Cruce et al. 2001). At the level of the dorsal root ganglia (DRG), there is greater sympathetic sprouting in the DRG of 16-month-old than 3-month-old rats following CCI (Ramer and Bisby 1998). A consistent pattern has been documented in the gracile nuclei. More dystrophic CGRP-immunoreactive axons are found in 16-month-old than in 3-month-old rats (Ma and Bisby 1998). Furthermore, following sciatic nerve axotomy, the gracile nuclei of older rats, as compared to younger rats, develop more axonal abnormalities and fewer delicate axonal sprouts and show blunted expression of neuronal nitric oxide synthase (Ohara et al. 1994, 1995; Ma et al. 2000). Taken together, there appear to be age differences in various components of the response to nerve injury. Although it is likely that their interaction, including changes not yet documented, is responsible for the lengthier recovery seen with age, several studies have failed to find a correlation between the extent of the various neurochemical changes and behavioral responses (Bergman et al. 1996b; Cruce et al. 2001; Stuesse et al. 2001). This inconclusiveness may reflect the nonlinear, interactive nature of physiological and behavioral changes over the life course and shows the need for further study.

The importance of multiple interactions among multiple levels is further supported by studies of age differences in neuroanatomy. Although some reports are contradictory (Thomas et al. 1980; La Forte et al. 1991), most of the data suggest that the number and size of sensory nerve cells in the lumbar DRG increase through early adulthood, peak at mid-life (13–18 months), and decrease thereafter (Rao and Krinke 1983; Kazui and Fujisawa 1988; Cecchini et al. 1995). Devor (1991) proposed that, in old rats, spontaneous involution, i.e., cell loss, of DRG cells may have the same consequences as nerve injury. Specifically, spontaneous involution may be associated with increased ongoing spontaneous DRG activity and cross-excitation. Consistent with this hypothesis, the pattern of neuropeptide changes in the DRG of old rats with spontaneous hindlimb neuropathies is similar to that of younger rats following sensory nerve injury (Bergman et al. 1996a, 1999). In addition, following thermal nociceptive stimulation of the hindpaw, nociceptive-specific and wide-dynamic-range neurons in the dorsal horn of older rats show larger receptive fields and more background activity and afterdischarges than comparable neurons in younger rats (Iwata et al. 2002). Evidence that sympathetic innervation of the DRG increases in mid-life (Ramer and Bisby 1998) further adds to the complexity of the neuroanatomical changes, which may contribute to increased susceptibility to neuropathies and poorer recovery from nerve injury with age (Devor 1991). Research is urgently needed to identify the full spectrum of changes that underlie the age differences in the response to nerve injury, providing the basis for new interventions to enhance the recovery of elderly patients from neuropathic pain.

NEUROPATHIC PAIN IN HUMANS

Similar to the animal data, the persistence of signs and symptoms associated with neuropathic pain in humans is strongly related to age. From an epidemiological perspective, the incidence of postherpetic neuralgia (PHN) is an archetypal demonstration of an age-related disorder (see Chapter 17). The risk of PHN following an acute herpes zoster infection increases markedly with advancing age in an analogous trajectory to the experimental situation in animals (Portenoy et al. 1986). However, the clinical expression of neuropathic pain in humans is notable for heterogeneity (Morris et al. 1995), in contrast to the apparent interaction between age, modality-specific change, and type of lesion encountered in animal models. Limited evidence from experimental models in studies of healthy humans is also in line with an interaction between aging and plasticity of pain responses. Temporal summation of successive painful stimuli in humans, analogous to the summation of nociceptive reflexes in the rat and the presumed effect of wind-up, occurs at much lower frequencies in older subjects (Gibson et al. 2002). Furthermore, persistence of secondary mechanical hyperalgesia subsequent to topical application of capsaicin characterizes older subjects' responses, despite the absence of any age-related changes in the peak amplitude and duration of primary thermal hyperalgesia (Zheng et al. 2000). Taken together, it would appear that the capacity of the nociceptive system to upregulate subsequent to neural damage and increased afferent input does not differ significantly as a function of age. The major difference between young and old appears to be the impaired ability of the nociceptive system in older animals and humans to downregulate, leading to prolonged recovery after perturbation.

INFLAMMATION, WOUND HEALING, AND PAIN BEHAVIORS

Age differences in inflammation may also be important in recovery from tissue and nerve injury. Inflammatory processes are important not just in models such as the formalin test that are predominately associated with inflammation, but also in models of visceral and neuropathic pain. The significance of inflammation is highlighted in the study described earlier (Crisp et al. 2003) which compared the consequences of two types of nerve injury; the one with a larger inflammatory component (CCI) was associated with a less robust pattern of response than the one with the lesser inflammatory component (PSNL). Normal aging is associated with increased baseline inflammatory activity, especially increased levels of circulating cytokines, in particular interleukin-6 (IL-6) and tumor necrosis factor (TNF) (Krabbe et al. 2004). Injury and subsequent wound healing are associated with increased and prolonged inflammatory responses with age (Ashcroft et al. 2002). Interestingly, IL-6 and TNF are both involved in the generation and maintenance of hyperalgesia (Watkins et al. 2003; Sommer and Kress 2004). Of particular interest, they both may increase the susceptibility of sensory neurons to noxious heat (Sommer and Kress 2004). Therefore, it is possible that increased activity of proinflammatory cytokines, such as IL-6 and TNF, also contribute to prolonged resolution of thermal hyperalgesia with age. Undoubtedly, future research will reveal that prolonged hyperalgesia and slower recovery with age are the end product of multiple interacting changes in the response to injury.

AGE DIFFERENCES IN ANTINOCICEPTION AND PAIN INHIBITION

To this point, we have been examining age differences in the experience of pain and nociception. Another fruitful approach has been to consider age differences in antinociception and endogenous pain inhibition. Age-related differences in the opioidergic system and in the response to opioid agonists and antagonists have received the most empirical attention. There is a general decline in this system with age. The concentration of opioid receptors in the cortex, striatum, and hypothalamus decreases with age (Amenta et al. 1991), but the binding affinity of the ligand for its sites within the brain is not age-related (Hess et al. 1981). The concentration of endogenous opioids in the dorsal horn at the cervical and thoracic levels, but not at the lumbar level of the spinal cord may decrease with age (Missale et al. 1983). Opioid receptor density in the spinal cord does not change with age (Hoskins et al. 1998), but levels of circulating β-endorphin decrease with age (Gambert et al. 1980; Dupont et al. 1981).

Interestingly, in animal models, advancing age may be associated with decreased sensitivity to opioid agonists (Islam et al. 1993; Crisp et al. 1994a,b). This finding has been attributed to degeneration of the endogenous pain-inhibition systems (Kramer and Bodnar 1986; Crisp et al. 1994a) and to age differences in the pharmacodynamics and pharmacokinetics of opioid agonists (Islam et al. 1993; Crisp et al. 1994a; Jourdan et al. 2002). Importantly, these studies have suggested that sex, test of nociception, and class of opioid drug may be critical factors. For instance, older female rats show less opioid analgesia than young female rats on the tail-flick (Islam et al. 1993) and jump tests (Kramer and Bodnar 1986), whereas older male rats show greater opioid analgesia than younger male rats on the hot-plate (Chan and Lai 1982) and vocalization tests (Saunders et al. 1974). In different studies, older male rats have shown both increased (Smith and Gray 2001) and decreased opioid analgesia compared to younger male rats on the tail-flick test (Islam et al. 1993). The majority of the available studies have tested the effects of drugs active at the μ-opioid receptor. There are some interesting data suggesting that age-related differences in κ-opioid analgesia may be sex-related. Sternberg et al. (2004) recently reported that κ-opioid analgesia was greater in young male mice than both young and older female mice, who did not differ from each other (but see Smith and Gray 2001). Interestingly, NMDA-receptor antagonism reduced the analgesia in young male and older female mice but not in young female mice (Sternberg et al. 2004). This finding suggests not only that κ-opioid analgesia is mediated by NMDA-receptor activation in males and older females, but also that young, hormonally intact females are using a unique analgesic mechanism, possibly mediated by ovarian hormones, which is not available to males or older females. These sex and opioid class-specific patterns require further investigation, but they highlight the importance of the aging neuroendocrine system in pain and nociception. It is important to note that humans show the opposite pattern; elderly people are more sensitive than younger people to the effects of opioids (Macintyre and Jarvis 1995; Gagliese et al. 2000), and while gender differences remain unclear, women appear to be more sensitive than men to the effects of κ opioids (Gear et al. 1996). Several reasons have been proposed, including cross-species differences in the metabolism of opioids (Van Crugten et al. 1997) and the diversity of pain models tested. Further research is needed to clarify this issue. In particular, data are urgently needed regarding the analgesic response in models of tissue or nerve injury.

AGE DIFFERENCES IN STRESS-INDUCED ANALGESIA

Stressful events increase the activity of endogenous pain inhibition systems and induce a transient state of hypoalgesia, an effect known as stress-induced analgesia. Different types of stressors induce analgesia mediated by various endogenous inhibitory systems including hormonal, opioid, and other neural systems (Mayer and Watkins 1984). As mentioned previously, there appears to be a general decline in both neural opioid and non-opioid inhibitory systems that parallels declines in CNS function with age (Hamm and Knisely 1985, 1986). On the other hand, there appears to be an increase or no difference with age in the analgesia induced by stressors that activate hormonally mediated inhibitory systems, specifically the hypothalamic-pituitary-adrenal (HPA) axis response to stress. This pattern is consistent with an age-related decline in neural systems (see above) and with an age-related dysregulation of the HPA-axis response to stressors. Specifically, with increasing age, the ability to recover from a stressor is impaired, possibly due to decreased sensitivity of negative feedback systems (Sapolsky et al. 1983). As such, the stress response lasts longer, and the analgesia induced by this response is greater in old rats than younger rats. Consistent with this, old rats chronically treated with acetyl-L-carnitine, which increases control of HPA-axis responses, did not differ from untreated young and mid-life rats in the extent of hormonally mediated stress-induced analgesia (Ghirardi et al. 1994). HPA-axis dysregulation may also underlie impaired adaptation to chronic stress among mid-life rats (Girardot and Holloway 1985), although this effect has not always been shown (Pinto-Ribeiro et al. 2004). While more work is needed to elucidate the relationship between aging, HPA-axis responses, and stress-induced analgesia, the available data are consistent with the hypothesis that with age comes a decline in neurally mediated systems of pain inhibition and a dysregulation of the HPA axis.

The HPA-axis response to stressors is intimately connected to the immune system through proinflammatory cytokines. It has been suggested that impaired ability to cope with and recover from stressors, including tissue and nerve injury, coupled with a progressive increase in proinflammatory status, underlies many of the pathophysiological changes seen with aging (Franceschi et al. 2000). According to this approach, as the deleterious effects of stress and elevated inflammatory status accumulate over time, the ability to adapt and recover decreases. These changes, in addition to, and in interaction with, age-related changes in the peripheral, autonomic, and central nervous system substrates of nociception and pain behavior, may provide a framework for understanding the age differences documented in various animal models of pain.

CONCLUSION

This chapter has presented an overview of age differences in nociception and pain in both animals and humans. Throughout, we have highlighted cross-species differences and similarities and have advocated more research to fill the many gaps in our knowledge. In summary, the available data suggest that the effects of aging on pain processing under physiological conditions are far from robust, emerging only inconsistently. When differences do emerge, there appear to be age-related decreases in sensitivity to experimentally applied transient noxious stimuli. The interaction of aging with the neurobiology of pain is most pronounced under conditions that model clinical pain states. In both human and animal models, advancing age is associated with lower sensitivity to stimulation associated with inflammatory processes. Interestingly, following nerve injury, the capacity of the aging nervous system to restore normative response patterns after upregulation appears to be particularly impaired. Although not yet documented in the clinical setting, prolonged periods of sensitization could place older people at greater risk of persistent pain following injury or the onset of disease. These age-related patterns can best be interpreted from a life course perspective that includes a network and remodeling conceptualization of multiple, multilevel interactions among substrates in the determination of an outcome. To this end, we have attempted to integrate the disparate lines of research which, taken together, suggest that the neurobiology of aging as it applies to pain is dependent on interactions of the peripheral, autonomic, and central nervous systems with the immune, endocrine, and musculoskeletal systems. This framework can guide future studies into various components of the network in order to increase our knowledge of pain and aging and to better equip us to provide effective and safe pain management to suffering people across the adult lifespan.

REFERENCES

Amenta F, Zaccheo D, Collier WL. Neurotransmitters, neuroreceptors and aging. *Mech Ageing Dev* 1991; 61:249–273.

Anderton BH. Ageing of the brain. *Mech Ageing Dev* 2002; 123(7):811–817.

Ashcroft GS, Mills SJ, Ashworth JJ. Ageing and wound healing. *Biogerontology* 2002; 3(6):337–345.

Bennett GJ. Update on the neurophysiology of pain transmission and modulation: focus on the NMDA-receptor. *J Pain Symptom Manage* 2000; 19(1 Suppl):S2–6.

Bergman E, Johnson H, Zhang X, et al. Neuropeptides and neurotrophin receptor mRNAs in primary sensory neurons of aged rats. *J Comp Neurol* 1996a; 375:303–319.

Bergman E, Johnson H, Zhang X, et al. Neuropeptides and neurotrophin receptor mRNAs in primary sensory neurons of aged rats. *J Comp Neurol* 1996b; 375(2):303–319.

Bergman E, Carlsson K, Liljeborg A, et al. Neuropeptides, nitric oxide synthase and GAP-43 in B4-binding and RT97 immunoreactive primary sensory neurons: normal distribution pattern and changes after peripheral nerve transection and aging. *Brain Res* 1999; 832(1–2):63–83.

Bodnar RJ, Romero MT, Kramer E. Organismic variables and pain inhibition: roles of gender and aging. *Brain Res Bull* 1988; 21:947–953.

Campbell BA, Krauter EE, Wallace JE. Animal models of aging: Sensory-motor and cognitive function in the age rat. In: Stein DG. *The Psychobiology of Aging: Problems and Perspectives*. Amsterdam: Elsevier, 1980, pp 201–226.

Cecchini T, Cuppini R, Ciaroni S, et al. Changes in the number of primary sensory neurons in normal and vitamin-E-deficient rats during aging. *Somatosens Mot Res* 1995; 12:317–327.

Chakour MC, Gibson SJ, Bradbeer M, et al. The effect of age on A delta- and C-fibre thermal pain perception. *Pain* 1996; 64:143–152.

Chan SHH, Lai YY. Effects of aging on pain responses and analgesic efficacy of morphine and clonidine in rats. *Exp Neurol* 1982; 75:112–119.

Choi SJ, Harii K, Lee MJ, et al. Electrophysiological, morphological, and morphometric effects of aging on nerve regeneration in rats. *Scand J Plast Reconstr Hand Surg* 1995; 29:133–140.

Collins LG, Stone LA. Pain sensitivity, age and activity level in chronic schizophrenics and in normals. *Br J Psychiatry* 1966; 112:33–35.

Crisp T, Stafinsky JL, Hoskins DL, et al. Effects of aging on spinal opioid-induced antinociception. *Neurobiol Aging* 1994a; 15:169–174.

Crisp T, Stafinsky JL, Hoskins DL, et al. Age-related changes in the spinal antinociceptive effects of DAGO, DPDPE and beta-endorphin in the rat. *Brain Res* 1994b; 643:282–286.

Crisp T, Giles JR, Cruce WL, et al. The effects of aging on thermal hyperalgesia and tactile-evoked allodynia using two models of peripheral mononeuropathy in the rat. *Neurosci Lett* 2003; 339(2):103–106.

Cruce WL, Lovell JA, Crisp T, et al. Effect of aging on the substance P receptor, NK-1, in the spinal cord of rats with peripheral nerve injury. *Somatosens Mot Res* 2001; 18(1):66–75.

Devor M. Chronic pain in the aged: possible relation between neurogenesis, involution and pathophysiology in adult sensory ganglia. *J Basic Clin Physiol Pharmacol* 1991; 2:1–15.

Doubell TP, Mannion RJ, Woolf CJ. The dorsal horn: state-dependent sensory processing, plasticity and the generation of pain. In: Wall PD, Melzack R (Eds). *Textbook of Pain*. Edinburgh: Churchill Livingstone, 1999, pp 165–181.

Drac H, Babiuch M, Wisniewska W. Morphological and biochemical changes in peripheral nerves with aging. *Neuropatol Pol* 1991; 29(1–2):49–67.

Dubner R, Ren K. Assessing transient and persistent pain in animals. In: Wall PD, Melzack R (Eds). *Textbook of Pain*. Edinburgh: Churchill Livingstone, 1999, pp 359–369.

Dubuisson D, Dennis SG. The formalin test: a quantitative study of the analgesic effects of morphine, meperidine and brain-stem stimulation in rats and cats. *Pain* 1977; 4:161–174.

Dupont A, Savard P, Merand Y, et al. Age-related changes in central nervous system enkephalins and substance P. *Life Sci* 1981; 29:2317–2322.

Edwards RR, Fillingim RB. Age-associated differences in responses to noxious stimuli. *J Gerontol A Biol Sci Med Sci* 2001; 56(3):180–185.

Franceschi C, Valensin S, Bonafe M, et al. The network and the remodeling theories of aging: historical background and new perspectives. *Exp Gerontol* 2000; 35(6–7):879–896.

Furst S. Transmitters involved in antinociception in the spinal cord. *Brain Res Bull* 1999; 48(2):129–141.

Gagliese L, Melzack R. Age differences in the response to the formalin test in rats. *Neurobiol Aging* 1999; 20:699–707.

Gagliese L, Melzack R. Age differences in nociception and pain behaviours in the rat. *Neurosci Biobehav Rev* 2000; 24:843–854.

Gagliese L, Katz J, Melzack R. Pain in the elderly. In: Wall PD, Melzack R (Eds). *Textbook of Pain*. Edinburgh: Churchill Livingstone, 1999, pp 991–1006.

Gagliese L, Jackson M, Ritvo P, et al. Age is not an impediment to effective use of patient controlled analgesia by surgical patients. *Anesthesiology* 2000; 93:601–610.

Gambert SR, Garthwaite TL, Pontzer CH, et al. Age-related changes in central nervous system beta-endorphin and ACTH. *Neuroendocrinology* 1980; 31:252–255.

Gear RW, Miaskowski C, Gordon NC, et al. Kappa-opioids produce significantly greater analgesia in women than in men. *Nature Med* 1996; 2:1248–1250.

Ghirardi O, Caprioli A, Ramacci MT, et al. Effect of long-term acetyl-l-carnitine on stress-induced analgesia in the aging rat. *Exp Gerontol* 1994; 29:569–574.

Gibson SJ, Gorman MM, Helme RD. Assessment of pain in the elderly using event-related cerebral potentials. In: Bond MR, Charlton JE, Woolf CJ. *Proceedings of the VIth World Congress on Pain*. New York: Elsevier, 1991, pp 527–533.

Gibson SJ, Chang WC, Farrell MJ. Age interacts with frequency in the temporal summation of painful electrical stimuli. *Abstracts: 10th World Congress on Pain*. Seattle: IASP Press, 2002, p 302.

Girardot MN, Holloway FA. Effect of age and long-term stress experience on adaptation to stress analgesia in mature rats: role of opioids. *Behav Neurosci* 1985; 99:411–422.

Gregg EW, Sorlie P, Paulose-Ram R, et al. Prevalence of lower-extremity disease in the US adult population ≥40 years of age with and without diabetes: 1999–2000 national health and nutrition examination survey. *Diabetes Care* 2004; 27(7):1591–1597.

Hagelberg N, Jaaskelainen SK, Martikainen IK, et al. Striatal dopamine D2 receptors in modulation of pain in humans: a review. *Eur J Pharmacol* 2004; 500:187–192.

Hamm RJ, Knisely JS. Environmentally induced analgesia: an age-related decline in an endogenous opioid system. *J Gerontol* 1985; 40:268–274.

Hamm RJ, Knisely JS. Environmentally induced analgesia: age-related decline in a neurally mediated, nonopioid system. *Psychol Aging* 1986; 1:195–201.

Harkins SW, Price DD, Martelli M. Effects of age on pain perception: thermonociception. *J Gerontol* 1986; 41:58–63.

Harkins SW, Davis MD, Bush FM, et al. Suppression of first pain and slow temporal summation of second pain in relation to age. *J Gerontol Med Sci* 1996; 51A:M260–M265.

Helme RD, Gibson SJ. The epidemiology of pain in elderly people. *Clin Geriatr Med* 2001; 17(3):417–431.

Hess GD, Joseph JA, Roth GS. Effect of age on sensitivity to pain and brain opiate receptors. *Neurobiol Aging* 1981; 2:49–55.

Hoskins DL, Gordon TL, Crisp T. The effects of aging on mu and delta opioid receptors in the spinal cord of Fischer-344 rats. *Brain Res* 1998; 791(1–2):299–302.

Hukkanen M, Platts LA, Corbett SA, et al. Reciprocal age-related changes in GAP-43/B-50, substance P and calcitonin gene-related peptide (CGRP) expression in rat primary sensory neurones and their terminals in the dorsal horn of the spinal cord and subintima of the knee synovium. *Neurosci Res* 2002; 42(4):251–260.

Hunt SP, Pini A, Evan G. Induction of c-fos-like protein in spinal cord neurons following sensory stimulation. *Nature* 1987; 328:632–634.

Islam AK, Cooper ML, Bodnar RJ. Interactions among aging, gender and gonadectomy effects upon morphine antinociception in rats. *Physiol Behav* 1993; 54:45–53.

Iwata K, Kanda K, Tsuboi Y, et al. Fos induction in the medullary dorsal horn and C1 segment of the spinal cord by acute inflammation in aged rats. *Brain Res* 1995; 678:127–139.

Iwata K, Fukuoka T, Kondo E, et al. Plastic changes in nociceptive transmission of the rat spinal cord with advancing age. *J Neurophysiol* 2002; 87(2):1086–1093.

Iwata K, Tsuboi Y, Shima A, et al. Central neuronal changes after nerve injury: neuroplastic influences of injury and aging. *J Orofac Pain* 2004; 18(4):293–298.

Jourdan D, Pickering G, Marchand F, et al. Impact of ageing on the antinociceptive effect of reference analgesics in the Lou/c rat. *Br J Pharmacol* 2002; 137(6):813–820.

Kanda K, Sato H, Kemuriyama T, et al. Temporal facilitation of the flexor reflex induced by C-fiber activity: comparison between adult and aged rats. *Neurosci Lett* 2001; 304(1–2):49–52.

Kazui H, Fujisawa K. Radiculoneuropathy of ageing rats: a quantitative study. *Neuropathol Appl Neurobiol* 1988; 14:137–156.

Kerezoudi E, King RHM, Muddle JR, et al. Influence of age on the late retrograde effects of sciatic nerve section in the rat. *J Anat* 1995; 187:27–35.

Khalil Z, Khodr B. A role for free radicals and nitric oxide in delayed recovery in aged rats with chronic constriction nerve injury. *Free Radic Biol Med* 2001; 31(4):430–439.

Kim YI, Na HS, Yoon YW, et al. Mechanical allodynia is more strongly manifested in older rats in an experimental model of peripheral neuropathy. *Neurosci Lett* 1995; 199:158–160.

Knisely JS, Hamm RJ. Physostigmine-induced analgesia in young, middle-aged, and senescent rats. *Exp Aging Res* 1989; 15:3–11.

Knox CA, Kokmen E, Dyck PJ. Morphometric alteration of rat myelinated fibers with aging. *J Neuropathol Exp Neurol* 1989; 48(2):119–139.

Ko ML, King MA, Gordon TL, et al. The effects of aging on spinal neurochemistry in the rat. *Brain Res Bull* 1997; 42:95–98.

Krabbe KS, Pedersen M, Bruunsgaard H. Inflammatory mediators in the elderly. *Exp Gerontol* 2004; 39(5):687–699.

Kramer E, Bodnar RJ. Age-related decrements in morphine analgesia: a parametric analysis. *Neurobiol Aging* 1986; 7:185–191.

La Forte RA, Melville S, Chung K, et al. Absence of neurogenesis of adult rat dorsal root ganglion cells. *Somatosens Mot Res* 1991; 8:3–7.

Lagier E, Delvaux M, Vellas B, et al. Influence of age on rectal tone and sensitivity to distension in healthy subjects. *Neurogastroenterol Motil* 1999; 11(2):101–107.

Lasch H, Castell DO, Castell JA. Evidence for diminished visceral pain with aging: Studies using graded intraesophageal balloon distension. *Am J Physiol* 1997; 272:G1–G3.

Ma SX, Cornford ME, Vahabnezhad I, et al. Responses of nitric oxide synthase expression in the gracile nucleus to sciatic nerve injury in young and aged rats. *Brain Res* 2000; 855(1):124–131.

Ma W, Bisby MA. Increase of calcitonin gene-related peptide immunoreactivity in the axonal fibers of the gracile nuclei of adult and aged rats after complete and partial sciatic nerve injuries. *Exp Neurol* 1998; 152(1):137–149.

Macintyre PE, Jarvis DA. Age is the best predictor of postoperative morphine requirements. *Pain* 1995; 64:357–364.

Maclean DB, Eldridge JC, Brodish A. Substance P and somatostatin content and transport in the vagus and sciatic nerves of the aging Fischer 344 rat. *Neurobiol Aging* 1988; 9:273–277.

Magnusson KR. The aging of the NMDA receptor complex. *Front Biosci* 1998; 3:e70–80.

Majeed SK. Survey on spontaneous peripheral neuropathy in aging rats. *Arzneimittelforschung* 1992; 42:986–990.

Mayer DJ, Watkins LR. Multiple endogenous opiate and nonopiate analgesia systems. *Adv Pain Res* 1984; 6:253–276.

Melzack R. Gate control theory: on the evolution of pain concepts. *Pain Forum* 1996; 5:128–138.

Missale C, Govoni S, Castelletti L, et al. Age related changes of enkephalin in rat spinal cord. *Brain Res* 1983; 262:160–162.

Moore AR, Clinch D. Underlying mechanisms of impaired visceral pain perception in older people. *J Am Geriatr Soc* 2004; 52(1):132–136.

Morris GC, Gibson SJ, Helme RD. Capsaicin-induced flare and vasodilatation in patients with post-herpetic neuralgia. *Pain* 1995; 63(1):93–101.

Novak JC, Lovell JA, Stuesse SL, et al. Aging and neuropathic pain. *Brain Res* 1999; 833(2):308–310.

Ochoa J, Mair WG. The normal sural nerve in man. II. Changes in the axons and Schwann cells due to ageing. *Acta Neuropathol* 1969; 13(3):217–239.

Ohara S, Roth KA, Beaudet LN, et al. Transganglionic neuropeptide Y response to sciatic nerve injury in young and aged rats. *J Neuropathol Exp Neurol* 1994; 53:646–662.

Ohara S, Beaudet LN, Schmidt RE. Transganglionic response of GAP-43 in the gracile nucleus to sciatic nerve injury in young and aged rats. *Brain Res* 1995; 705(1–2):325–331.

O'Sullivan DJ, Swallow M. The fibre size and content of the radial and sural nerves. *J Neurol Neurosurg Psychiatry* 1968; 31(5):464–740.

Pinto-Ribeiro F, Almeida A, Pego JM, et al. Chronic unpredictable stress inhibits nociception in male rats. *Neurosci Lett* 2004; 359(1–2):73–76.

Portenoy RK, Duma C, Foley KM. Acute herpetic and postherpetic neuralgia: clinical review and current management. *Ann Neurol* 1986; 20(6):651–664.

Prineas JW, Spencer PS. Pathology of the nerve cell body in disorders of the peripheral nervous system. In: Dyck PJ, Thomas PK, Lambert EH (Eds). *Peripheral Neuropathy*. Philadelphia: Saunders, 1975, pp 253–295.

Ramer MS, Bisby MA. Normal and injury-induced sympathetic innervation of rat dorsal root ganglia increases with age. *J Comp Neurol* 1998; 394(1):38–47.

Rao RS, Krinke G. Changes with age in the number and size of myelinated axons in the rat L4 dorsal spinal root. *Acta Anat* 1983; 117:187–192.

Sapolsky R, Krey L, McEwen B. The adrenocortical stress response in the aged male rat: impairment of recovery from stress. *Exp Gerontol* 1983; 18:55–62.

Saunders DR, Paolino RM, Bousquet WF, et al. Age-related responsiveness of the rat to drugs affecting the central nervous system. *Proc Soc Exp Biol Med* 1974; 147:593–595.

Segovia G, Porras A, Del Arco A, et al. Glutamatergic neurotransmission in aging: a critical perspective. *Mech Ageing Dev* 2001; 122(1):1–29.

Serrano MI, Goicoechea C, Serrano JS, et al. Age-related changes in the antinociception induced by taurine in mice. *Pharmacol Biochem Behav* 2002; 73(4):863–867.

Smith MA, Gray JD. Age-related differences in sensitivity to the antinociceptive effects of opioids in male rats—influence of nociceptive intensity and intrinsic efficacy at the mu receptor. *Psychopharmacology* 2001; 156(4):445–453.

Sommer C, Kress M. Recent findings on how proinflammatory cytokines cause pain: peripheral mechanisms in inflammatory and neuropathic hyperalgesia. *Neurosci Lett* 2004; 361(1–3):184–187.

Sternberg WF, Ritchie J, Mogil JS. Qualitative sex differences in kappa-opioid analgesia in mice are dependent on age. *Neurosci Lett* 2004; 363(2):178–181.

Stuesse SL, Crisp T, McBurney DL, et al. Neuropathic pain in aged rats: behavioral responses and astrocytic activation. *Exp Brain Res* 2001; 137(2):219–227.

Tamaru M, Yoneda Y, Ogita K, et al. Age-related decreases of the N-methyl-D-aspartate receptor complex in the rat cerebral cortex and hippocampus. *Brain Res* 1991; 542(1):83–90.

Thomas PK, King RHM, Sharma AK. Changes with age in the peripheral nerves of the rat. *Acta Neuropathol (Berl)* 1980; 52:1–6.

Todorovic C, Dimitrijevic M, Stanojevic S, et al. Correlation between age-related changes in open field behavior and plaque forming cell response in DA female rats. *Int J Neurosci* 2003; 113(9):1259–1273.

Troulinaki K, Tavernarakis N. Neurodegenerative conditions associated with ageing: a molecular interplay? *Mech Ageing Dev* 2005; 126(1):23–33.

Ulfhake B, Bergman E, Fundin BT. Impairment of peripheral sensory innervation in senescence. *Auton Neurosci* 2002; 96(1):43–49.

Van Crugten JT, Somogyi AA, Nation RL, et al. The effect of old age on the disposition and antinociceptive response of morphine and morphine-6-beta-glucuronide in the rat. *Pain* 1997; 71:199–205.

Van der Zee CEEM, Brakkee JH, Gispen WH. Putative neurotrophic factors and functional recovery from peripheral nerve damage in the rat. *Br J Pharmacol* 1991; 103:1041–1046.

Vatassery GT, Lai JC, Smith WE, et al. Aging is associated with a decrease in synaptosomal glutamate uptake and an increase in the susceptibility of synaptosomal vitamin E to oxidative stress. *Neurochem Res* 1998; 23(2):121–125.

Verdu E, Ceballos D, Vilches JJ, et al. Influence of aging on peripheral nerve function and regeneration. *J Peripher Nerv Syst* 2000; 5(4):191–208.

Wallace JE, Krauter EE, Campbell BA. Motor and reflexive behavior in the aging rat. *J Gerontol* 1980; 35:364–370.

Walsh NE, Schoenfeld L, Ramamurthy S, et al. Normative model for cold pressor test. *Am J Phys Med Rehabil* 1989; 68:6–11.

Washington LL, Gibson SJ, Helme RD. Age-related differences in the endogenous analgesic response to repeated cold water immersion in human volunteers. *Pain* 2000; 89(1):89–96.

Watkins LR, Milligan ED, Maier SF. Glial proinflammatory cytokines mediate exaggerated pain states: implications for clinical pain. *Adv Exp Med Biol* 2003; 521:1–21.

Willer JC. Comparative study of perceived pain and nociceptive flexion reflex in man. *Pain* 1977; 3(1):69–80.

Woodrow KM, Friedman GD, Siegelaub AB, et al. Pain tolerance: differences according to age, sex and race. *Psychosom Med* 1972; 34:548–556.

Zhang RX, Lao L, Qiao JT, et al. Effects of aging on hyperalgesia and spinal dynorphin expression in rats with peripheral inflammation. *Brain Res* 2004; 999(1):135–141.

Zhang YQ, Mei J, Lu SG, et al. Age-related alterations in responses of nucleus basalis magnocellularis neurons to peripheral nociceptive stimuli. *Brain Res* 2002; 948(1–2):47–55.

Zheng Z, Gibson SJ, Khalil Z, et al. Age-related differences in the time course of capsaicin-induced hyperalgesia. *Pain* 2000; 85(1–2):51–58.

Correspondence to: Lucia Gagliese, PhD, Department of Anaesthesia and Pain Management, Toronto General Hospital, 200 Elizabeth Street, Toronto, Ontario, Canada M5G 2C4. Tel: 416-340-4296, Fax: 416-340-4739; email: lucia.gagliese@uhn.on.ca.

Pain in Older Persons, Progress in Pain
Research and Management, Vol. 35, edited
by Stephen J. Gibson and Debra K. Weiner,
IASP Press, Seattle, © 2005.

3

Age-Associated Differences in Pain Perception and Pain Processing

Robert R. Edwards

*Department of Psychiatry and Behavioral Sciences, Johns Hopkins
University School of Medicine, Baltimore, Maryland, USA*

Older age is increasingly recognized as an important risk factor for many chronically painful conditions (Helme and Gibson 2001). While numerous biopsychosocial factors influence the likelihood and experience of pain, changes in the perception of pain and the central and peripheral nervous system structures that subserve the processing of information relating to nociceptive stimulation are clearly important contributors to these effects. Evidence from many psychophysical studies suggests a small, but potentially important, age-related impairment in the detection of superficial, cutaneous pain (e.g., an increase in pain threshold), which may detract from the adaptive, early-warning functions of pain and place older persons at greater risk for more severe injuries. Moreover, the reduced efficacy of endogenous analgesic systems and the greater apparent sensitizability of the aging nervous system's pain-processing pathways may contribute to pain's greater persistence and anatomic spread in the elderly.

It is important to emphasize the duality of pain's impact: on the one hand, persistent pain has substantially deleterious effects, including burdensome health care costs, reduced physical functioning, distress and depression, impaired quality of life, inability to work, social isolation, substantially heightened suicide rates, and increased mortality (Macfarlane et al. 2001; Turk 2002). On the other, the experience of pain has important implications for homeostatic integrity. For example, individuals born without the capacity to experience pain do not lead long, disability-free lives; rather, they are at disproportionate risk for severe injury and early mortality (Mogil et al. 2000). Similar to hunger, pain is an unpleasant affective and sensory experience, but one that contributes to the maintenance of homeostasis and survival. Hence, as with most biosensory systems, the optimal pain-processing system balances the need for sensitive detection with the need for regulation of input, a balance that may be disrupted over the course of the aging process.

PAIN PSYCHOPHYSICS: AN OVERVIEW

A full characterization of the field of pain psychophysics is beyond the scope of this chapter; however, a number of excellent sources are available for interested readers (Gracely 1999; Gracely et al. 2003). Briefly, the assessment of pain perception and pain processing in humans involves the administration of standardized noxious stimuli and the standardized quantification of subjects' responses. One of the original goals of such studies was to evaluate the efficacy of analgesic agents (i.e., a standardized noxious stimulus should be reported as less painful after effective analgesic administration), but more recent developments in the field have often centered around identifying the peripheral and central nervous system processes that mediate both normal and abnormal pain perception. Indeed, several recent editorials have called for a more widespread application of quantitative sensory testing (QST) in the clinical realm in order to evaluate the neural processes underpinning persistent pain conditions and to facilitate a more mechanism-based diagnosis of painful disorders (Woolf and Max 2001; Coghill and Eisenach 2003).

Desirable properties of experimental stimuli include repeatability; rapid, controlled onset and offset; minimal provocation of tissue damage; analgesic dose relationships; and some similarity to natural noxious stimuli that might be experienced in day-to-day life (Gracely 1999). Modalities of noxious stimulation include thermal (both radiant and contact heat), mechanical, electrical, ischemic, and chemical. These various modalities of stimulation differ from one another along many dimensions, including the time course of the pain they produce, the types of fibers stimulated, the depth of stimulated structures, the area of stimulation, the relative weights of the affective and sensory components of pain, and literally dozens of others (Gracely 1999; Gracely et al. 2003). Due to this heterogeneity, findings with a particular stimulus type (e.g., age differences in mechanical pain thresholds) may not be consistently observed using other stimulus modalities. Generally, across modalities, forms of psychophysical pain assessment can be categorized into three types: assessment of pain threshold, suprathreshold scaling, and psychophysical assessment of central pain processing. Studies of interrelationships between differing pain responses and differing stimulus modalities often, but not always (Edwards et al. 2003b), reveal at least moderate correlations across measures, leading to discussion of a "pain phe-notype" (Kim et al. 2004). For example, pain threshold and tolerance are moderately to strongly correlated across modalities of stimulation (Edwards and Fillingim 2001a; Granot et al. 2003b; Fillingim et al. 2004). In spite of these fairly robust inter-modality associations, however, differing pain as-sessment procedures will often produce variable results when groups of young and elderly subjects are compared, as described later in the chapter.

AGE DIFFERENCES IN PAIN THRESHOLD

Pain threshold is conceptually the simplest measure of pain sensitivity and pain processing. Pain threshold represents the lowest stimulus intensity (or duration) at which pain is felt; biologically, measures of pain threshold represent the acuity or sensitivity of pain's early-warning-system function (Gibson and Farrell 2004), an often-overlooked adaptive aspect of pain. In fact, while having an exceeding low threshold for pain places an individual at undue risk for experiencing frequent clinical pain (Edwards et al. 2005), which in turn would impair function and decrease quality of life, having an overly elevated pain threshold risks unacceptable delays in action taken to alleviate the effects of tissue-damaging stimuli.

As noted in a comprehensive recent review (Gibson and Farrell 2004), the extensive literature regarding aging and pain thresholds includes over 40 studies of noxious thermal, mechanical, and electrical stimuli. Collectively, the preponderance of evidence suggests increases in cutaneous pain thresh-old with advancing age; within the studies summarized in the review by Gibson and Farrell (2004), including our recent report (Edwards et al. 2003a), 55.0% of findings suggested a statistically significant increase in heat or electrical pain thresholds among older subjects. No studies that included elderly subjects have reported an overall age-related decrease in thermal or electrical pain thresholds. Indeed, even among published reports of negative findings, elderly participants tend to show elevated heat or electrical pain thresholds; it is simply the substantial within-group variability and small sample sizes that prevent the effect from achieving statistical significance. For example, our earlier examination (Edwards and Fillingim 2001a) of age differences in heat pain responses revealed 14% higher thermal pain thresh-olds among older adults ($P > 0.05$); though this is classified as a "negative" finding, the magnitude and direction of the effect is consistent with other "positive" studies. Collectively, the published findings to date are consistent with a small increase in cutaneous pain threshold in healthy older adults. Previous reviews emphasized the variability in study findings and the lack of definitive data (Harkins and Scott 1996), but as summarized recently, if there were a true absence of an aging effect one would expect a more even spread of findings between an age-related increase, a decrease, or no change in pain threshold (Gibson and Farrell 2004). The fact that a slight majority of the findings suggest age-related increases in threshold, taken together with the fact that no studies of elderly participants report an age-related decrease in cutaneous pain thresholds, argues against a conclusion that there is no consistent effect of age on pain thresholds.

AGE DIFFERENCES IN SUPRATHRESHOLD PAIN RESPONSES

Since pain thresholds are theoretically and empirically related to responses to suprathreshold noxious stimuli (e.g., individuals with lower thresholds generally have lower pain tolerances and rate more highly the painfulness of suprathreshold stimuli), it is natural to expect aging effects for suprathreshold pain responses to parallel the threshold findings. However, available data suggest, on balance, that the opposite may in fact be true: while older age is associated with reduced sensitivity to threshold level stimuli, sensitivity to suprathreshold stimuli may be enhanced among older adults (see Yehuda and Carasso 1997; Gagliese and Melzack 1997; Gibson and Helme 2001; Gibson and Farrell 2004). Pain tolerance is operationalized as the stimulus intensity or duration at which the subject terminates the stimulus, indicating an unwillingness to endure further pain; conceptually, it is a behavioral index of the motivational dimension of the pain experience. Generally, reports of associations between age and pain tolerance suggest that tolerance for cold pain (Walsh et al. 1989; Edwards et al. 2003a), for mechanical muscle pain (Woodrow et al. 1972; Edwards and Fillingim 2001a), and for exercise-induced ischemic muscle pain (Edwards and Fillingim 2001a) declines with increasing age, though tolerance for cutaneous contact heat has not been reported to vary in older relative to younger adults (Edwards and Fillingim 2001a; Edwards et al. 2003a). These findings appear to suggest an accelerating pain function among older adults (i.e., a steeper slope and narrower range to the curve relating stimulus intensity to pain). Several older studies of electrical pain (Harkins and Chapman 1976, 1977) and an investigation of suprathreshold scaling of noxious thermal stimuli (Harkins et al. 1986) have suggested that the effects of age on pain responses vary with the physical intensity of the noxious stimulus, with elderly subjects rating more intense stimuli as more painful than younger subjects and less intense stimuli as less painful (i.e., "under-rating" and "over-rating" at the lower and upper extremes of the intensity spectrum; Harkins et al. 1986). In our studies, we have noted similar findings for mechanical stimuli, with no apparent age differences near threshold, but more rapidly increasing ratings with increasing stimulus intensity among older, relative to younger, subjects (Edwards and Fillingim 2001a). Insights into the impact of aging on suprathreshold scaling of other stimulus modalities are not currently available. However, the available evidence indicates that the senescent pain-processing system retains and even enhances its acuity for conveying information concerning highly intense and potentially physically damaging stimuli. In functional terms, this evidence suggests a reduced range from pain threshold to pain tolerance, as well as an accelerating association between stimulus properties (intensity, duration) and the amount of pain experienced. Putative explanations for this potentially puzzling phenomenon may relate to the differential effects of aging on peripheral versus central pain-processing mechanisms (Edwards and Fillingim 2001a,b; Edwards et al. 2003a), such as a decrement in excitatory transmission in the periphery coupled with an opposing decrement in central pain-inhibitory processes.

VARIABLES INFLUENCING AGE-PAIN RELATIONSHIPS

The variability in findings across studies of aging-related differences in pain perception has engendered investigation into the factors that may account for some of the discrepancies. As noted above, stimulus intensity appears to serve as an important moderating variable, with older adults showing reduced sensitivity to less intense, threshold-level stimuli, but greater sensitivity to more intense suprathreshold stimuli. Several additional variables, described below, also seem to influence the likelihood of producing and detecting age-associated differences in pain responses. Overall, it is important to note that aging also does not produce uniform changes in the functioning of non-pain-related systems; for example, age-related alterations in the processing of auditory stimuli depend on stimulus frequency, with profound changes in some domains and negligible changes in others (Sakamoto et al. 1998). Similarly, even non-sensory domains of functioning demonstrate differential effects of aging. For example, some cognitive and intellectual abilities improve with age, some decline, and some remain relatively constant (Hedden and Gabrieli 2004; Henry et al. 2004). Thus, it would be unreasonable to expect that age-associated alterations in the perception and processing of pain would be perfectly consistent across differing stimulus properties. Rather, the study of variation in age effects as a function of variation in stimulus characteristics provides an additional opportunity to more fully elucidate changes in pain processing across the lifespan.

STIMULUS MODALITY

As noted above, laboratory pain induction procedures differ from one another along a variety of dimensions. Broadly speaking, age-related increases in pain thresholds are most likely to be observed for superficial cutaneous stimuli relative to noxious stimuli that affect deeper structures such as muscles and joints. Recent results from our laboratory indicated that healthy older subjects had significantly lower thresholds for ischemic muscle pain, and similar pressure pain thresholds over two muscle groups, while slight elevations in thermal pain sensitivity were recorded (Edwards and Fillingim 2001a). Even within the classification of "cutaneous" stimuli, differing results are obtained in summarizing studies that utilize contact or radiant heat compared to those that utilize electricity (Gibson and Farrell 2004). Approximately 87% of published studies applying radiant heat or thermal stimuli using a CO_2 laser find age-related increases in pain thresholds, while electrical pain thresholds seem to be relatively constant across the age spectrum. Given that electrical stimuli bypass receptors and directly stimulate nerve fibers (of all types), it is reasonable to hypothesize that altered receptor mechanisms may play a part in the observed aging effects for cutaneous thermal stimuli.

STIMULUS SITE

In general, physiological aging is proposed to take place in a distal-proximal fashion, with earlier effects evident in the periphery of the body. Moreover, the lower limbs appear to evidence more rapid age-related changes than the upper limbs. These findings probably stem from the fact that the longest peripheral nerve fibers, which span the lower body, are most prone to damage or degeneration with age. Several studies have compared younger to older participants on thermal pain responses at both upper- and lower-limb sites. These reports are unanimous in suggesting that age-related decreases in pain sensitivity are maximal in the leg relative to the arm (Lautenbacher and Strian 1991; Harkins et al. 1994; Yarnitsky et al. 1995; Edwards et al. 2003a). Interestingly, innervation of visceral tissue may also decline with disproportionate rapidity as a function of aging. While cutaneous pressure pain thresholds show variable relationships with age, the few existing studies of mechanical pain thresholds in the digestive tract and the esophagus have reported age-related increases in thresholds on the order of 50% (Lasch et al. 1997; Mertz et al. 1998). Similarly, while our group has previously demonstrated age-related decreases in thresholds for ischemic muscle pain (Edwards and Fillingim 2001a), other studies have suggested that ischemic pain thresholds in cardiac muscle may show substantial increases in elderly adults (Miller et al. 1990; Ambepitiya et al. 1994). Collectively, these findings indicate that age-related reductions in pain sensitivity are most likely to be observed in the periphery, especially in the legs, or in visceral tissue.

STIMULUS DURATION

At least one recent study directly suggests that age-related differences in pain thresholds vary as a function of stimulus duration. Helme and colleagues (2004) studied 100-fold variations in thermal and electrical stimulus duration in healthy older and younger subjects; they noted that the older group showed a substantially-increased threshold for thermal and electrical pain only if the duration of the stimulus was short (e.g., 1 vs. 100 seconds for heat stimuli). The authors suggest that this effect may explain much of the variability in aging effects on pain threshold. Indeed, an overview of the previous literature utilizing similarly sized contact heat thermodes does suggest that the majority of such studies that report no age differences in heat pain thresholds employ slower temperature rise times (e.g., generally under 1.0°C/s; e.g., Kenshalo 1986; Edwards and Fillingim 2001a), while "positive" studies often utilize steeper temperature ramps (e.g., above 4°C/s; e.g., Harkins et al. 1986; Lautenbacher and Strian 1991).

STIMULUS AREA

The magnitude of age-related changes in thermal pain thresholds is much greater for the very small skin areas stimulated by laser stimuli compared to the findings for contact heat thermodes, because the stimulation area of the latter may be orders of magnitude greater than in most laser paradigms (Gibson and Farrell 2004). This finding suggests that smaller stimulus areas magnify the effects of aging. However, while spatial summation of afferent information concerning noxious stimuli is an important consideration in determining pain thresholds (Stohler and Kowalski 1999; Lautenbacher et al. 2001; Polianskis et al. 2002), no published studies have yet rigorously evaluated the impact of age on the magnitude of pain-related spatial summation. It is interesting to speculate that since spatial summation is a central process dependent on endogenous pain-modulatory systems (Staud et al. 2004), enhanced summation in the elderly might be observed, given the findings of diminished central pain inhibition as a function of advancing age. However, such speculation must await empirical investigation.

RESPONSE MODALITY

While the characteristics of the stimulus are clearly important in shaping age-related differences in pain responses (i.e., either magnifying or obscuring such effects), the use of differing response modalities also appears to play an influential role. We have already noted that age-related findings differ for threshold-level responses vs. tolerance-level responses, although in this case, differences in response types are confounded by differences in stimulus duration. However, the assessment tool that is utilized to measure pain also appears to influence the magnitude and direction of aging effects. In studies that compare ratings of clinical or experimental pain stimuli in young and elderly adults, verbal and numerical pain rating scales often produce discrepant findings. For example, in situations in which older and younger groups did not differ in either numeric or visual analogue scale ratings of postsurgical pain intensity (Gagliese and Katz 2003), chronic pain intensity (Gagliese and Melzack 2003), or cold pressor pain intensity (Edwards et al. 2003a), older adults reported lower sensory and affective pain on the McGill Pain Questionnaire (MPQ). Similarly, while ratings of pain intensity and unpleasantness are highly correlated (Price et al. 1987), it has been suggested that aging may produce decrements in some sensory dimensions of pain while enhancing the affective processing of noxious stimuli (Yehuda and Carasso 1997; Gibson and Farrell 2004). However, several studies have reported similar age effects on pain ratings regardless of whether the rating scale assesses the intensity or unpleasantness of pain (Edwards and Fillingim 2001b), and therefore such propositions must remain speculative at present, in the absence of definitive data.

AGE DIFFERENCES IN ENDOGENOUS PAIN MODULATION

While most prior studies of relationships between aging and pain have focused on age-associated alterations in the transmission of afferent input, a more thorough understanding of aging effects should include characterization of efferent processes, such as spinal and supraspinally initiated influences on the central processing of pain. Information concerning noxious stimuli is actively modulated by multiple endogenous neural and hormonal systems (Fields and Basbaum 1999; Melzack 2001), and such central processing networks may be either antinociceptive or pronociceptive. On the basis of animal work, pain-inhibitory systems have been classified according to their opioid-dependence and neural vs. hormonal mechanisms of operation (Bodnar et al. 1988; Gagliese and Melzack 2000), with most studies documenting a general decline in the efficacy of neural opioid and non-opioid analgesic mechanisms in aged animals (Hamm and Knisely 1985; Hamm et al. 1986).

Several recent studies have suggested the presence of deficits in endogenous pain inhibition in older humans as well. Washington and colleagues (2000) recently examined the effects of repeated immersion of the hand in cold water on thermal and electrical pain thresholds in samples of young and elderly volunteers. Increases in thresholds in response to immersion of the hand were found to be significantly greater in young adults (~50% increase) when compared with older persons (~40% increase). A later study of cold-pain-induced endogenous analgesia offered similar results (Edwards et al. 2003a). In this investigation, diffuse noxious inhibitory controls (DNIC) were assessed in healthy younger and older adults. DNIC (Le Bars et al. 1979, 1981) refers to the phenomenon of one noxious stimulus inhibiting the perception of pain produced by application of a second noxious stimulus via widespread, supraspinally generated inhibition of spinal neurons. Study findings indicated that the nature of DNIC responses differ as a function of age. In fact, while heterotopic noxious stimulation (i.e., a cold pressor test) produced DNIC effects (i.e., a reduction in thermal pain ratings) among younger subjects, older participants actually showed increases in thermal pain ratings during concurrent stimulation with noxious cold, revealing a net facilitatory or additive effect of multiple noxious stimuli (Edwards et al. 2003a). Interestingly, additional studies of patients with osteoarthritis have suggested that chronic nociceptive input may impair the functioning of such pain-modulatory systems (Kosek and Ordeberg 2000a,b), hinting that older age may be associated with decrements in DNIC-like mechanisms as a consequence of a longer history of exposure to natural noxious stimuli.

Other studies have also noted that the reversal of centrally mediated sensitization is a more prolonged process in older adults, suggesting decrements in the effectiveness of endogenous inhibitory processes. For example, Zheng and colleagues (2000) reported that topical application of capsaicin produced a much longer-lasting secondary mechanical hyperalgesia among older subjects. In a study utilizing repeated cold pressor tasks (Edwards et al. 2003a), age differences were not apparent on the initial task, but by the fourth consecutive cold water immersion, older adults demonstrated a reduced tolerance relative to their younger counterparts, suggesting an age-associated deficit in habituation or adaptation. The consistency of such findings certainly appears to suggest age-associated reductions in the capacity of the central nervous system (CNS) to reverse pain-induced sensitization at spinal and supraspinal levels.

Still another form of endogenous analgesia appears to be dependent on the functioning of the cardiovascular system (Bruehl and Chung 2004), with elevations in blood pressure contributing to arousal-regulating homeostatic feedback loops in the presence of painful stimuli. Such interactions depend on opioid and noradrenergic mechanisms (Bruehl and Chung 2004; Edwards et al. 2004), systems that have both been described as showing age-related declines. To our knowledge, only one study has examined the influence of age on associations between pain and high blood pressure. We previously reported that while increased arterial blood pressure was generally associated with increased pain thresholds and tolerances, these relationships were somewhat weaker among older subjects, suggesting a potential age-related impairment of mechanisms linking enhanced cardiovascular activity and baroreceptor activation to endogenous analgesic mechanisms (Edwards and Fillingim 2001a).

It is also important to note that endogenous pain-facilitatory (as well as pain-inhibitory) mechanisms may be altered as a function of aging. In this regard, considerable attention has been directed toward contributions of second-order neurons in the dorsal horn to the initiation and maintenance of hyperalgesic states (Pedersen et al. 1998; Herrero et al. 2000; Melzack et al. 2001). The phenomenon of "wind-up" refers, in animal models, to plastic changes in the spinal cord in which repeated noxious stimuli result in a state of sensitization (Herrero et al. 2000). Temporal summation, the psychophysical analogue to wind-up in human studies, is a well-characterized phenomenon that consists of a C-fiber-dependent enhancement of central neuronal responses to unchanging afferent inputs applied with a frequency greater than 0.3 Hz (Price and McHaffie 1988; Staud et al. 2001; Price et al. 2002). Three studies have addressed age-related alterations in patterns of the temporal summation of noxious stimuli. First, for trains of moderately high-intensity thermal stimuli, older people, relative to younger, reported greater summation of thermal pain (i.e., larger increases in pain ratings across stimuli) on the upper extremities, but less summation of pain in the foot, although only this latter effect achieved statistical significance (Harkins 1994). Second, a later study from our laboratory found more pronounced temporal summation in the arm among older participants for mild to moderately intense thermal stimuli (47°C and 50°C) (Edwards and Fillingim 2001b). In addition to greater summation, older adults also showed reduced habituation (i.e., prolonged maintenance of the summation) compared to their younger counterparts. Finally, as summarized in a recent review (Gibson and Farrell 2004), the threshold for temporal summation is apparently lower in older compared to younger adults; repeated electrical stimuli applied to the ankle elicit reports of increasingly intense pain at frequencies as low as 0.2 Hz in older people, whereas frequencies of at least 0.3 Hz are required for younger subjects.

Collectively, findings from these studies suggest that when peripheral input is well preserved, the older CNS is more prone to upregulation of pain processing in the context of repeated noxious stimulation, which dovetails nicely with the previously reported findings of diminishing pain tolerance as a function of older age. Overall, this apparently enhanced sensitizability of the older CNS, in concert with the reduced efficacy of endogenous analgesic systems, is likely to result in more severe pain following prolonged noxious stimulation, making it more difficult for persons of advanced age to manage persistent clinical pain conditions.

CLINICAL RELEVANCE OF THE PSYCHOPHYSICAL ASSESSMENT OF PAIN PERCEPTION

Inter-individual variation in pain perception is substantial (Gracely 1999), with threshold, tolerance, and ratings in response to a variety of painful stimuli being approximately normally distributed in the general population. However, there has been little consensus on whether findings from psychophysical studies of pain are relevant to the clinical experience of pain (Edwards et al. 2005; Kim et al. 2004). Recently, however, a number of studies have highlighted the potential value of experimental pain assessment in predicting and understanding the experience of clinical pain. Several cross-sectional studies have examined associations between psychophysical pain responses and reports of daily pain symptoms among healthy adults. For example, healthy young adults reporting high numbers of recent pain episodes such as headache or backache showed significantly lower heat pain tolerances than those with less frequent clinical pain (Fillingim et al. 1999); similarly, heat pain tolerance was also negatively associated with the number of pain sites reported over the past month (Edwards and Fillingim 1999, 2001b). More recently, an index of the magnitude of DNIC, reflecting endogenous pain-inhibitory capacity, was shown to be significantly related to several indices of pain and physical function among younger and older adults, such that greater DNIC was associated with less pain and better physical functioning in day-to-day life (Edwards et al. 2003b). Similarly, even in groups of patients with chronic pain, findings from psychophysical assessments often correlate with clinical pain reports; for example, lower ischemic pain tolerance was associated with greater clinical pain severity in a heterogeneous group of chronic pain patients (Edwards et al. 2001) and among patients with temporomandibular joint disorders (Fillingim et al. 1996).

Several recent prospective studies have also examined preoperative experimental pain responses as predictors of postoperative pain. Among individuals undergoing limb amputation, pre-amputation pressure pain sensitivity correlated with post-amputation stump pain and phantom pain (Nikolajsen et al. 2000). In addition, preoperative thermal QST responses predicted postoperative pain scores in women undergoing cesarean section, explaining up to 54% of the variance in postsurgical pain (Granot et al. 2003a). Importantly, suprathreshold pain ratings were highly positively correlated with postoperative pain, while thermal pain thresholds were not. Other investigations have produced comparable results. Following anterior cruciate ligament repair, preoperative suprathreshold pain ratings, but not pain thresholds, were strongly correlated with joint pain ratings (Werner et al. 2004). Finally, preoperative cold pressor pain tolerance predicted postoperative pain after laparoscopic cholecystectomy, even though the investigators controlled for neuroticism (Bisgaard et al. 2001). In every case, greater sensitivity to experimental pain (i.e., lower tolerance, higher ratings) was associated with greater reported clinical pain severity. Taken together, these findings identify suprathreshold experimental pain responses (but not necessarily pain thresholds) as important predictors of acute pain following surgery; long-term prospective studies will be necessary to evaluate QST as a predictor of chronic pain. Thus, age-associated increases in sensitivity to intense noxious stimuli and age-related decrements in endogenous pain inhibition are likely to have important detrimental consequences for the experience of acute and chronic pain in day-to-day life. Indeed, the fact that more widespread, disabling pain is observed in elderly relative to young persons may well be due in part to just such age-related changes in central processing of information concerning noxious stimuli.

POTENTIAL MECHANISMS UNDERLYING AGE DIFFERENCES IN PAIN RESPONSES

PERIPHERAL NERVOUS SYSTEM

Animal and human studies have revealed potentially pain-relevant structural and functional changes in the aging peripheral nervous system. In particular, there is an age-related loss of both myelinated and unmyelinated fibers, with fiber loss being greater (i.e., up to 50% reduction in density in the oldest-old) for unmyelinated fiber types (Ochoa and Mair 1969a,b; Verdu et al. 2000). In addition to age-related changes in absolute numbers of fibers, the proportion of sensory fibers, both myelinated and unmyelinated, with anatomical abnormalities or signs of degeneration also shows a marked increase at the upper limits of the age distribution (Knox et al. 1989). Relatedly, there is also a clear decrement in nerve conduction velocity in elderly compared to young adults, most likely as a consequence of these pathological changes (Kakigi 1987; Verdu et al. 2000). Interestingly, a psychophysical study employing selective nerve blocks suggested a selective age-related impairment of myelinated fiber function during pain perception and an increasing reliance with advancing age on (unmyelinated) C-fiber input (Chakour et al. 1996). In addition to these considerations of peripheral nervous system changes, responses to cutaneous stimuli are also influenced by changes in senescent skin, including decreases in microcirculation and thinning of several dermal layers (Harkins and Scott 1996). Biochemical studies in the periphery have also documented reductions in the substance P content of aged human skin (Gibson and Farrell 2004), and rat studies have confirmed that both substance P and calcitonin gene-related peptide (CGRP), major transmitters utilized by primary afferent nociceptive fibers, exhibit substantial functional declines in aged animals (Bergman et al. 1996). Collectively, psychophysical, histological, and biochemical studies all hint at age-associated decrements in peripheral nerve fiber function; these changes are likely to be prime contributors to the small but potentially significant age-related increases in pain thresholds.

CENTRAL NERVOUS SYSTEM

Within the aging CNS, a broad array of changes takes place, many of which have implications for the processing of pain. Readers are referred to several recent, thorough reviews of the literature describing age-related alterations in CNS structure and function (Peters 2002a,b,c; Peters and Rosene 2003). Generally, primate studies reveal a small loss of absolute numbers of neurons, with this loss being most pronounced in the neocortex as opposed to midbrain and brainstem regions. In addition to neuronal losses from the neocortex, magnetic resonance imaging in both humans and monkeys shows that significant amounts of white matter are also lost. This effect appears as an increase in ventricle size and gyral atrophy on the order of 15–30%. Paralleling the losses of neurons are reductions in dendritic length and in the number of dendritic spines and synapses of existing neurons. For example, aged monkeys show roughly a 20% loss of synapses from the prefrontal cortex (Peters 2002b). Interestingly, two recent neuroimaging investigations have identified the prefrontal cortex as the locus of placebo analgesia (Lieberman et al. 2004; Wager et al. 2004), and this region probably also participates in other forms of cognitively induced endogenous analgesic responses, such as hypnotic analgesia or adaptive cognitive coping with pain. Thus, structural changes in brain volume and connectivity may have important functional implications for pain processing (e.g., reductions in the efficacy of endogenous analgesic systems).

Pathological changes in myelin and in cellular structures have also been noted with age (Peters 2002c). Splitting of myelin sheaths, in conjunction with an increase in the frequency of redundant myelin, suggest that while production of myelin continues with age, myelin's effectiveness as an insulator of nerve cells declines, potentially accounting for observed decreases in conduction velocities. With age, most cortical neurons also acquire increasing amounts of lipofuscin granules in their cytoplasm. Such lipofuscin accumulations serve as a biomarker for cellular aging and may interfere with normal cell functioning (Peters 2002a). In general, the inhibitory nonpyramidal cells seem to acquire more lipofuscin than the excitatory pyramidal neurons, which may manifest as a more rapid age-related decrement in pain-inhibitory relative to pain-excitatory processes.

At the neurotransmitter level, cholinergic, serotonergic, and noradrenergic pathways all begin to demonstrate functional decrements over the course of normal aging (Ko et al. 1997); each of these systems has been reported to participate in centrally mediated pain inhibition. For example, descending serotonergic projections are thought to partially mediate the analgesic effects of morphine and presumably of the endogenous opioids as well (Wigdor and Wilcox 1987). Substantial evidence derived from animal and human studies has indicated progressive decrements in absolute levels of serotonin within the CNS, in serotonergic function, and in serotonin receptor density (Morgan and May 1992). Diminished levels of CGRP, substance P, and somatostatin are also prevalent in individuals of advanced age (Hukkanen et al. 2002). Finally, CNS indices of endogenous opioids, including β-endorphins and enkephalins, also decline with advancing age (Gambert et al. 1980; Crisp et al. 1994), and exogenously administered opioids produce progressively decreasing analgesic effects in aged animals (Hoskins et al. 1986; Kramer and Bodnar 1986), suggesting functional decrements in opioidergic systems.

In summary, the aged CNS shows substantial and widespread changes in structure, neurochemistry, and function. Obviously, the vast majority of studies documenting these effects are not performed by pain researchers, and so there is a dearth of information documenting the functional pain-related consequences of such CNS alterations. Additional translational work will become increasingly important as researchers attempt to characterize the neural and cellular processes that underpin the observed age-related changes in the perception, processing, and experience of pain.

PSYCHOSOCIAL PROCESSES

While we know about dozens of psychosocial factors that influence the chronic pain experience (Turk and Okifuji 2002; Keefe et al. 2005), the association of these factors with pain thresholds or pain-modulatory processes is not clear. Moreover, only scant research attention has been dedicated to examining age-related changes specifically in pain-relevant psychological variables. However, several variables show promise as potential contributors to age-related differences in the experience of pain. First, recent work by Gibson and colleagues on the construct of stoicism has suggested that older people may demonstrate some reticence in labeling brief, mildly noxious stimuli as painful; for example, they documented an age-related increase in stoical attitudes toward pain (Yong et al. 2001). This increasingly cautious approach to the identification of pain has been proposed as a potential explanation for aging effects on pain threshold (Gibson and Farrell 2004). A conceptually related literature involves the use of sensory decision theory (SDT) methodology to assess "response bias," or the willingness to report pain at varying levels of stimulation. While SDT techniques and the conclusions they generate are rather controversial (Rollman 1977), SDT study findings dovetail with the stoicism findings described above, revealing a greater reluctance among older subjects to report low-intensity electrical stimuli as painful (Clark and Mehl 1971; Harkins and Chapman 1976, 1977).

There is also evidence for age-related differences in the strategies individuals use for coping with pain. For example, some research has indicated that older adults make less use of cognitive pain-coping strategies than their younger counterparts (Sorkin et al. 1990). In addition, especially in the context of less severe pain from chronic conditions, older adults' coping repertoire includes more maladaptive pain-management strategies (Watkins et al. 1999). However, within a sample of healthy adults, free from chronic pain, we have observed lower levels of catastrophizing, a primary maladaptive pain-related coping strategy (Sullivan et al. 2001), among older compared to younger subjects (Edwards and Fillingim 2000). Thus, it is likely that age effects on psychosocial variables may be sample-specific, with potentially opposite findings in community-based vs. clinic-based samples. Interestingly, in this same community-based sample of healthy adults (Edwards and Fillingim 2000), older participants reported higher levels of hypervigilance to somatic sensations; this construct has demonstrated important links to chronic pain (McDermid et al. 1996), and further investigations of senescent changes in somatic focus as it relates to the perception of pain seem warranted.

SUMMARY AND METHODOLOGICAL CRITIQUE
OF EXISTING STUDIES

In general, while prior studies of age-related changes in pain perception and pain processing have provided a good deal of valuable information, much obviously remains to be learned. Rather than attempt to replicate prior findings, future studies may benefit from attention to some of the methodological difficulties evidenced in previous work. First, inadequate statistical power is a nearly ubiquitous problem. For example, assuming that there is a small increase in pain thresholds in the elderly (i.e., corresponding to an effect size, Cohen's d, of 0.30), it would take a total of nearly 300 participants in order to reliably (i.e., 80% of the time) detect an existing difference in pain thresholds between a young group and an elderly group. It is the rare psychophysical study that achieves this sample size. Second, there is a clear need to include a wide range of ages or age groups in cross-sectional studies. As an example, our recent report of age-related differences in pain inhibition included two groups: younger adults, mostly in their early twenties, and older adults, mostly in their sixties (Edwards et al. 2003a). Hence, we were unable to provide information on endogenous pain-inhibitory processes in middle-aged adults or in the oldest-old. Third, longitudinal investigations are sorely needed, as these are the best means to study mediators of age effects. Cross-sectional analyses confound age effects with cohort effects and do not permit evaluation of individual differences in patterns of sensory changes with advancing age. Fourth, additional information related to the contribution of comorbidities would be quite valuable. Most psychophysical studies include groups that are highly selected for healthiness, whereas the vast majority of older adults have one or more medical conditions—such as hypertension or diabetes—that might affect the experience of pain. For example, while most investigations of electrical pain thresholds show no age differences in healthy volunteers, a larger study that included subjects with major medical conditions showed increased thresholds in older subjects (Tucker et al. 1989), suggesting that aging effects on pain are influenced by the presence or absence of major medical conditions. Fifth, future studies would do well to continue investigating efferent, as well as afferent, processes; many age-related changes are probably effected by changes in central processing that require further understanding.

Overall, the experience of pain is dependent on a complex neural processing system incorporating excitatory and inhibitory mechanisms that are affected by numerous attributes of the stimulus and the environment. Collectively, increasing age appears to have a small but significant effect on the threshold for pain, with thresholds increasing gradually as a function of older age. Such effects are maximized when stimuli are brief, when their spatial area is minimal, and when they are applied to the distal limbs or to visceral organs. This overall effect may represent a slight but damaging decrement in the "early warning" functions of pain (Gibson and Farrell 2004), decreasing the likelihood that adaptive action will be taken to obviate the effects of tissue-damaging stimuli. In addition, suprathreshold responses to pain appear to be amplified during senescence, potentially making prolonged or severe pain more disabling among the elderly. Older adults show progressive decrements in multiple endogenous analgesic systems, showing an increased propensity for sensitization of central pain-processing systems in the face of prolonged or repeated noxious stimulation. These effects are presumed to be at least partially mediated by maladaptive neurophysiological and biochemical changes in the aging central nervous system, changes which may also contribute to the more widespread, persistent clinical pain experienced by the elderly, as documented in numerous epidemiological studies (Verhaak et al. 1998; Gureje et al. 2001). In summary, changes in the perception of pain with advancing age are complex and incompletely understood, although they represent an increasing focus of research attention (Gagliese and Melzack 1997). What can be stated with certainty is that the prior conventional wisdom, that older age brings an increasing insensitivity to pain, is hardly defensible at this point. Indeed, the opposite position, that increasing age confers greater vulnerability to the deleterious impact of persistent pain, seems likely to become the newly dominant paradigm in the next generation of research on the interrelationship between pain and aging.

REFERENCES

Ambepitiya G, Roberts M, Ranjadayalan K, Tallis R. Silent exertional myocardial ischemia in the elderly: a quantitative analysis of anginal perceptual threshold and the influence of autonomic function. *J Am Geriatr Soc* 1994; 42:732–737.

Bergman E, Johnson H, Zhang X, Hokfelt T, Ulfhake B. Neuropeptides and neurotrophin receptor mRNAs in primary sensory neurons of aged rats. *J Comp Neurol* 1996; 375:303–319.

Bisgaard T, Klarskov B, Rosenberg J, Kehlet H. Characteristics and prediction of early pain after laparoscopic cholecystectomy. *Pain* 2001; 90:261–269.

Bodnar RJ, Romero MT, Kramer E. Organismic variables and pain inhibition: roles of gender and aging. *Brain Res Bull* 1988; 21:947–953.

Bruehl S, Chung OY. Interactions between the cardiovascular and pain regulatory systems: an updated review of mechanisms and possible alterations in chronic pain. *Neurosci Biobehav Rev* 2004; 28:395–414.

Chakour MC, Gibson SJ, Bradbeer M, Helme RD. The effect of age on A delta- and C-fibre thermal pain perception. *Pain* 1996; 64:143–152.

Clark WC, Mehl L. A sensory decision theory analysis of the effect age and sex on *d'*, various response criteria, and 50% pain threshold. *J Abnorm Psychol* 1971; 78:202–212.

Coghill RC, Eisenach J. Individual differences in pain sensitivity: implications for treatment decisions. *Anesthesiology* 2003; 98:1312–1314.

Crisp T, Stafinsky JL, Hoskins DL, et al. Effects of aging on spinal opioid-induced antinociception. *Neurobiol Aging* 1994; 15:169–174.

Edwards RR, Fillingim RB. Ethnic differences in thermal pain responses. *Psychosom Med* 1999; 61:346–354.

Edwards RR, Fillingim RB. Differential relationships between pain-coping strategies and responses to noxious stimuli in healthy older and younger adults. Poster presented at: Annual Meeting of the American Pain Society, November 2000, Atlanta.

Edwards RR, Fillingim RB. Age-associated differences in responses to noxious stimuli. *J Gerontol A Biol Sci Med Sci* 2001a; 56:M180–M185.

Edwards RR, Fillingim RB. Effects of age on temporal summation of thermal pain: clinical relevance in healthy older and younger adults. *J Pain* 2001b; 2:307–317.

Edwards RR, Doleys DM, Fillingim RB, Lowery D. Ethnic differences in pain tolerance: clinical implications in a chronic pain population. *Psychosom Med* 2001; 63:316–323.

Edwards RR, Fillingim RB, Ness TJ. Age-related differences in endogenous pain modulation: a comparison of diffuse noxious inhibitory controls in healthy older and younger adults. *Pain* 2003a; 101:155–165.

Edwards RR, Ness TJ, Weigent DA, Fillingim RB. Individual differences in diffuse noxious inhibitory controls (DNIC): association with clinical variables. *Pain* 2003b; 106:427–437.

Edwards RR, Ness TJ, Fillingim RB. Endogenous opioids, blood pressure, and diffuse noxious inhibitory controls: a preliminary study. *Percept Mot Skills* 2004; 99:679–687.

Edwards RR, Sarlani E, Wesselmann U, Fillingim RB. Quantitative assessment of experimental pain perception: multiple domains of clinical relevance. *Pain* 2005; 114:315–319.

Fields HL, Basbaum A. Central nervous system mechanisms of pain modulation. In: Wall P, Melzack R (Eds). *Textbook of Pain*. New York: Churchill Livingstone, 1999, pp 309–329.

Fillingim RB, Maixner W, Kincaid S, Sigurdsson A, Harris MB. Pain sensitivity in patients with temporomandibular disorders: relationship to clinical and psychosocial factors. *Clin J Pain* 1996; 12:260–269.

Fillingim RB, Edwards RR, Powell T. The relationship of sex and clinical pain to experimental pain responses. *Pain* 1999; 83:419–425.

Fillingim RB, Ness TJ, Glover TL, et al. Experimental pain models reveal no sex differences in pentazocine analgesia in humans. *Anesthesiology* 2004; 100:1263–1270.

Gagliese L, Katz J. Age differences in postoperative pain are scale dependent: a comparison of measures of pain intensity and quality in younger and older surgical patients. *Pain* 2003;103:11–20.

Gagliese L, Melzack R. Chronic pain in elderly people. *Pain* 1997; 70:3–14.

Gagliese L, Melzack R. Age differences in nociception and pain behaviours in the rat. *Neurosci Biobehav Rev* 2000; 24:843–854.

Gagliese L, Melzack R. Age-related differences in the qualities but not the intensity of chronic pain. *Pain* 2003;104:597–608.

Gambert SR, Garthwaite TL, Pontzer CH, Hagen TC. Age-related changes in central nervous system beta-endorphin and ACTH. *Neuroendocrinology* 1980; 31:252–255.

Gibson SJ, Farrell M. A review of age differences in the neurophysiology of nociception and the perceptual experience of pain. *Clin J Pain* 2004; 20:227–239.

Gibson SJ, Helme RD. Age-related differences in pain perception and report. *Clin Geriatr Med* 2001; 17:433–456.

Gracely R. Studies of pain in human subjects. In: Wall P, Melzack R (Eds). *Textbook of Pain*. New York: Churchill Livingstone, 1999, pp 385–407.

Gracely RH, Grant MA, Giesecke T. Evoked pain measures in fibromyalgia. *Best Pract Res Clin Rheumatol* 2003; 17:593–609.

Granot M, Lowenstein L, Yarnitsky D, Tamir A, Zimmer EZ. Postcesarean section pain prediction by preoperative experimental pain assessment. *Anesthesiology* 2003a; 98:1422–1426.

Granot M, Sprecher E, Yarnitsky D. Psychophysics of phasic and tonic heat pain stimuli by quantitative sensory testing in healthy subjects. *Eur J Pain* 2003b; 7:139–143.

Gureje O, Simon GE, Von Korff M. A cross-national study of the course of persistent pain in primary care. *Pain* 2001; 92:195–200.

Hamm RJ, Knisely JS. Environmentally induced analgesia: an age-related decline in an endogenous opioid system. *J Gerontol* 1985; 40:268–274.

Hamm RJ, Knisely JS, Watson A. Environmentally-induced analgesia: age-related differences in a hormonally-mediated, nonopioid system. *J Gerontol* 1986; 41:336–341.

Harkins SW, Chapman CR. Detection and decision factors in pain perception in young and elderly men. *Pain* 1976; 2:253–264.

Harkins SW, Chapman CR. The perception of induced dental pain in young and elderly women. *J Gerontol* 1977; 32:428–435.

Harkins SW, Scott RB. Pain and presbyalgos. In: Birren JE (Ed). *Encyclopedia of Gerontology: Age, Aging, and the Aged.* San Diego: Academic Press, 1996.

Harkins SW, Price DD, Martelli M. Effects of age on pain perception: thermonociception. *J Gerontol* 1986; 41:58–63.

Harkins SW, Davis MD, Bush FM, Kasberger J. Suppression of first pain and slow temporal summation of second pain in relation to age. *J Gerontol* 1994; M260–M265.

Hedden T, Gabrieli JD. Insights into the ageing mind: a view from cognitive neuroscience. *Nat Rev Neurosci* 2004; 5:87–96.

Helme RD, Gibson SJ. The epidemiology of pain in elderly people. *Clin Geriatr Med* 2001; 17:417–431.

Helme RD, Meliala A, Gibson SJ. Methodologic factors which contribute to variations in experimental pain threshold reported for older people. *Neurosci Lett* 2004; 36:1144–146.

Henry JD, MacLeod MS, Phillips LH, Crawford JR. A meta-analytic review of prospective memory and aging. *Psychol Aging* 2004; 19:27–39.

Herrero JF, Laird JM, Lopez-Garcia JA. Wind-up of spinal cord neurones and pain sensation: much ado about something? *Prog Neurobiol* 2000; 61:169–203.

Hoskins B, Burton CK, Ho IK. Differences in morphine-induced antinociception and locomotor activity in mature adult and aged mice. *Pharmacol Biochem Behav* 1986; 25:599–605.

Hukkanen M, Platts LA, Corbett SA, et al. Reciprocal age-related changes in GAP-43/B-50, substance P and calcitonin gene-related peptide (CGRP) expression in rat primary sensory neurones and their terminals in the dorsal horn of the spinal cord and subintima of the knee synovium. *Neurosci Res* 2002; 42:251–260.

Kakigi R. The effect of aging on somatosensory evoked potentials following stimulation of the posterior tibial nerve in man. *Electroencephalogr Clin Neurophysiol* 1987; 68:277–286.

Keefe FJ, Abernethy AP, Campbell L. Psychological approaches to understanding and treating disease-related pain. *Annu Rev Psychol* 2005; 29:601–630.

Kenshalo DR. Somaesthetic sensitivity in young and elderly humans. *J Gerontol* 1986; 41:732–742.

Kim H, Neubert JK, Rowan JS, et al. Comparison of experimental and acute clinical pain responses in humans as pain phenotypes. *J Pain* 2004; 5:377–384.

Knox CA, Kokmen E, Dyck PJ. Morphometric alteration of rat myelinated fibers with aging. *J Neuropathol Exp Neurol* 1989; 48:119–139.

Ko ML, King MA, Gordon TL, Crisp T. The effects of aging on spinal neurochemistry in the rat. *Brain Res Bull* 1997; 42:95–98.

Kosek E, Ordeberg G. Abnormalities of somatosensory perception in patients with painful osteoarthritis normalize following successful treatment. *Eur J Pain* 2000a; 4:229–238.

Kosek E, Ordeberg G. Lack of pressure pain modulation by heterotopic noxious conditioning stimulation in patients with painful osteoarthritis before, but not following, surgical pain relief. *Pain* 2000b; 88:69–78.

Kramer E, Bodnar RJ. Age-related decrements in morphine analgesia: a parametric analysis. *Neurobiol Aging* 1986; 7:185–191.

Lasch H, Castell DO, Castell JA. Evidence for diminished visceral pain with aging: studies using graded intraesophageal balloon distension. *Am J Physiol* 1997; 272:G1–3.

Lautenbacher S, Strian F. Similarities in age differences in heat pain perception and thermal sensitivity. *Funct Neurol* 1991; 6:129–135.

Lautenbacher S, Nielsen J, Andersen T, Arendt-Nielsen L. Spatial summation of heat pain in males and females. *Somatosens Mot Res* 2001; 18:101–105.

Le Bars D, Dickenson AH, Besson JM. Diffuse noxious inhibitory controls (DNIC). I. Effects on dorsal horn convergent neurones in the rat. *Pain* 1979; 6:283–304.

Le Bars D, Chitour D, Clot AM. The encoding of thermal stimuli by diffuse noxious inhibitory controls (DNIC). *Brain Res* 1981; 230:394–399.

Lieberman MD, Jarcho JM, Berman S, et al. The neural correlates of placebo effects: a disruption account. *Neuroimage* 2004; 22:447–455.

Macfarlane GJ, McBeth J, Silman AJ. Widespread body pain and mortality: prospective population based study. *BMJ* 2001; 323:662–665.

McDermid AJ, Rollman GB, McCain GA. Generalized hypervigilance in fibromyalgia: evidence of perceptual amplification. *Pain* 1996; 66:133–144.

Melzack R. Pain and the neuromatrix in the brain. *J Dent Educ* 2001; 65:1378–1382.

Melzack R, Coderre TJ, Katz J, Vaccarino AL. Central neuroplasticity and pathological pain. *Ann NY Acad Sci* 2001; 933:157–174.

Mertz H, Fullerton S, Naliboff B, Mayer EA. Symptoms and visceral perception in severe functional and organic dyspepsia. *Gut* 1998; 42:814–822.

Miller PF, Sheps DS, Bragdon EE, et al. Aging and pain perception in ischemic heart disease. *Am Heart J* 1990; 120:22–30.

Mogil JS, Yu L, Basbaum AI. Pain genes? natural variation and transgenic mutants. *Annu Rev Neurosci* 2000; 23:777–811.

Morgan D, May PC. Age-related changes in synaptic neurochemistry. In: Schneider E, Rowe JW (Eds). *Handbook of the Biology of Aging*. New York: Academic Press, 1992, pp 219–254.

Nikolajsen L, Ilkjaer S, Jensen TS. Relationship between mechanical sensitivity and postamputation pain: a prospective study. *Eur J Pain* 2000; 4:327–334.

Ochoa J, Mair WG. The normal sural nerve in man. I. Ultrastructure and numbers of fibres and cells. *Acta Neuropathol (Berl)* 1969a; 13:197–216.

Ochoa J, Mair WG. The normal sural nerve in man. II. Changes in the axons and Schwann cells due to ageing. *Acta Neuropathol (Berl)* 1969b; 13:217–239.

Pedersen JL, Andersen OK, Arendt-Nielsen L, Kehlet H. Hyperalgesia and temporal summation of pain after heat injury in man. *Pain* 1998; 74:189–197.

Peters A. Structural changes in the normally aging cerebral cortex of primates. *Prog Brain Res* 2002a; 136:455–465.

Peters A. Structural changes that occur during normal aging of primate cerebral hemispheres. *Neurosci Biobehav Rev* 2002b; 26:733–741.

Peters A. The effects of normal aging on myelin and nerve fibers: a review. *J Neurocytol* 2002c; 31:581–593.

Peters A, Rosene DL. In aging, is it gray or white? *J Comp Neurol* 2003; 462:139–143.

Polianskis R, Graven-Nielsen T, Arendt-Nielsen L. Spatial and temporal aspects of deep tissue pain assessed by cuff algometry. *Pain* 2002; 100:19–26.

Price DD, McHaffie JG. Effects of heterotopic conditioning stimuli on first and second pain: a psychophysical evaluation in humans. *Pain* 1988; 34:245–252.

Price DD, Harkins SW, Baker C. Sensory affective relationships among different types of clinical and experimental pain. *Pain* 1987; 28:297–307.

Price DD, Staud R, Robinson ME, et al. Enhanced temporal summation of second pain and its central modulation in fibromyalgia patients. *Pain* 2002; 99:49–59.

Rollman G. Signal detection theory measurement of pain: a review and critique. *Pain* 1977; 3:187–211.

Sakamoto M, Sugasawa M, Kaga K, Kamio T. Average thresholds in the 8 to 20 kHz range as a function of age. *Scand Audiol* 1998; 27:189–192.

Sorkin BA, Rudy TE, Hanlon RB, Turk DC, Stieg RL. Chronic pain in old and young patients: differences appear less important than similarities. *J Gerontol* 1990; 45:P64–P68.

Staud R, Vierck CJ, Cannon RL, Mauderli AP, Price DD. Abnormal sensitization and temporal summation of second pain (wind-up) in patients with fibromyalgia syndrome. *Pain* 2001; 91:165–175.

Staud R, Vierck CJ, Robinson ME, Price DD. Spatial summation of heat pain within and across dermatomes in fibromyalgia patients and pain-free subjects. *Pain* 2004; 111:342–350.

Stohler CS, Kowalski CJ. Spatial and temporal summation of sensory and affective dimensions of deep somatic pain. *Pain* 1999; 79:165–173.

Sullivan MJ, Thorn B, Haythornthwaite JA, et al. Theoretical perspectives on the relation between catastrophizing and pain. *Clin J Pain* 2001; 17:52–64.

Tucker MA, Andrew MF, Ogle SJ, Davison JG. Age-associated change in pain threshold measured by transcutaneous neuronal electrical stimulation. *Age Ageing* 1989; 18:241–246.

Turk DC. Clinical effectiveness and cost-effectiveness of treatments for patients with chronic pain. *Clin J Pain* 2002; 18:355–365.

Turk DC, Okifuji A. Psychological factors in chronic pain: evolution and revolution. *J Consult Clin Psychol* 2002; 70:678–690.

Verdu E, Ceballos D, Vilches JJ, Navarro X. Influence of aging on peripheral nerve function and regeneration. *J Peripher Nerv Syst* 2000; 5:191–208.

Verhaak PF, Kerssens JJ, Dekker J, Sorbi MJ, Bensing JM. Prevalence of chronic benign pain disorder among adults: a review of the literature. *Pain* 1998; 77231–239.

Wager TD, Rilling JK, Smith EE, et al. Placebo-induced changes in fMRI in the anticipation and experience of pain. *Science* 2004; 303:1162–1167.

Walsh NE, Schoenfeld L, Ramamurthy S, Hoffman J. Normative model for cold pressor test. *Am J Phys Med Rehab* 1989; 68:6–11.

Washington LL, Gibson SJ, Helme RD. Age-related differences in the endogenous analgesic response to repeated cold water immersion in human volunteers. *Pain* 2000; 89:89–96.

Watkins KW, Shifren K, Park DC, Morrell RW. Age, pain, and coping with rheumatoid arthritis. *Pain* 1999; 82:217–228.

Werner MU, Duun P, Kehlet H. Prediction of postoperative pain by preoperative nociceptive responses to heat stimulation. *Anesthesiology* 2004; 100:115–119.

Wigdor S, Wilcox GL. Central and systemic morphine-induced antinociception in mice: contribution of descending serotonergic and noradrenergic pathways. *J Pharmacol Exp Ther* 1987; 242:90–95.

Woodrow KM, Friedman GD, Siegelaub AB, Collen MF. Pain tolerance: differences according to age, sex and race. *Psychosom Med* 1972; 34:548–556.

Woolf CJ, Max MB. Mechanism-based pain diagnosis: issues for analgesic drug development. *Anesthesiology* 2001; 95:241–249.

Yarnitsky D, Sprecher E, Zaslansky R, Hemli JA. Heat pain thresholds: normative data and repeatability. *Pain* 1995; 60:329–332.

Yehuda S, Carasso R. A brief history of pain perception and pain tolerance in aging. In: Mostofsky D, Lomranz J (Eds). *Handbook of Pain and Aging*. New York: Plenum Press, 1997.

Yong HH, Gibson SJ, Horne DJ, Helme RD. Development of a pain attitudes questionnaire to assess stoicism and cautiousness for possible age differences. *J Gerontol B Psychol Sci Soc Sci* 2001; 56:279–284.

Zheng Z, Gibson SJ, Khalil Z, Helme RD, McMeeken JM. Age-related differences in the time course of capsaicin-induced hyperalgesia. *Pain* 2000; 85:51–58.

Correspondence to: Robert R. Edwards, PhD, Department of Psychiatry and Behavioral Sciences, Johns Hopkins University School of Medicine, 600 N Wolfe St., Meyer 1-108, Baltimore, MD 21287, USA. Tel: 410-955-4871; Fax: 410-614-3366; email: redwar10@jhmi.edu.

Pain in Older Persons, Progress in Pain
Research and Management, Vol. 35, edited
by Stephen J. Gibson and Debra K. Weiner,
IASP Press, Seattle, © 2005.

4

Age Differences in Clinical Pain States

Gisèle Pickering

*Clinical Pharmacology Center, University Hospital, Medical Faculty,
Clermont-Ferrand, France*

AGE DIFFERENCES IN CLINICAL PAIN STATES

Living organisms are fortunate in having an early warning system that springs immediately into action after nociceptive stimulation, enabling them to protect themselves from further damage. With aging this dynamic system may become less effective. Age may blunt the protective and warning mechanisms of pain, which are an integral part of survival. All sensory signals become fainter and slower with aging, not only those concerning pain but also other enteroceptive systems such as those governing hydration and thirst, hemodynamic adaptation and physical exercise, and reaction time and vigilance (Pickering et al. 1997).

The "pain system" consists of a set of controls and balances between facilitatory and inhibitory pathways. Disruption of this equilibrium may lead to chronic pain, and aging appears to be associated with a loss of "buffering" capacity, in which compensatory mechanisms become overwhelmed by pain. A variety of other intervening factors such as past pain experience, cognitive impairment, social isolation, altered body image, and depression add to the complexity of the pattern of clinical pain presentation in the elderly. Over the past few decades, growing evidence has emerged to show that aging has a profound impact on the presentation of illness, especially pain. Epidemiological studies (Gagliese and Melzack 1997; Pickering et al. 2001; Gibson and Farrell 2004), reinforced by experimental findings (Pickering et al. 2002; Helme et al. 2004) and preclinical studies (Gagliese and Melzack 2000; Jourdan et al. 2002), have improved our knowledge of the evolution of pain in this heterogeneous population. Indeed, from the healthy community-dwelling individual to the frail "oldest old" person in a nursing home, older adults have a broad range in health status, characterized by heterogeneity even among those of the same age. Individuals age at remarkably different rates, and deficits of all kinds associated with advanced age will determine the differences between biological and chronological ages, determining each individual's experience of pain. With the increasing number of people over 65 years old in industrialized countries, clinicians will treat more older patients than in the past and will have to anticipate absent, atypical, or exacerbated presentations of acute or chronic pain.

AGE AND ACUTE PAIN

Acute pain, whether visceral or somatic in origin, is short lasting and usually manifests in ways that can be easily described and observed. A large part of the literature on age differences has focused on acute visceral pain, which often occurs suddenly and may be distressing and even life-threatening. Conditions associated with visceral pain such as myocardial infarction, renal disease, gallstones, and pleuritic pain involve vital functions and play a large part in the morbidity and the mortality of older persons. Although pain is a cardinal feature in patients with pathologies of visceral origin, atypical presentations are prevalent in older persons for a number of abdominal, cardiac, and pulmonary conditions. Another complexity of the process of visceral pain initiation and transmission compared to somatic pain is that it is often poorly localized, it is often referred to other locations, and it is not always linked to tissue injury (Raja et al. 1999), which makes its diagnosis even more difficult in the elderly.

ABDOMINAL PAIN

The main causes accounting for acute abdominal pain in older adults (Espinoza et al. 2004) are biliopancreatic diseases, intestinal obstruction, complicated hernia, peptic and duodenal ulcer disease and perforation, appendicitis, and peritonitis. Concerning abdominal pathologies, atypical pain presentation is an almost universal clinical observation. As laboratory screening tests for evaluation of abdominal pain in the elderly do not differentiate nonsurgical conditions from those requiring surgery, physicians who evaluate older patients with acute abdominal pain must be aware that their clinical impression is of greater importance than laboratory tests in the decision to request special studies or surgical consultation (Parker et al. 1996).

Cholecystitis. Cholecystitis is the most common cause of acute abdominal pain (31%) in the geriatric population, mainly because the incidence of gallstones increases with age. The typical epigastric or right upper quadrant abdominal pain in adults is absent in about 85% of adults of advanced age. Even diffuse abdominal pain may be absent in about 5% of elderly patients. Radiation pain in the back or in the flank, a classic symptom of cholecystitis in younger populations, is experienced by only 61% of elderly patients (Parker et al. 1997). Given that no single clinical finding or laboratory test carries sufficient weight to establish or exclude cholecystitis without further investigation, deficient presentation often retards appropriate diagnosis (Trowbridge et al. 2003).

Ulcer disease. Absence of abdominal pain is confirmed in approximately 30% of older patients with peptic ulcer disease compared to only 7–19% in younger adults (Clinch et al. 1984; Hilton et al. 2001). Upper gastrointestinal bleeding that accompanies the ulcer is commonly painless in older patients; pain is present in less than 15% of elderly patients and tends to be milder than in younger adults (Scapa et al. 1989). However, failure to systematically report consumption of steroids and NSAIDs for other conditions could play a distorting role in the relative lack of pain. The absence of pain as a major symptom in older patients means that they often present late and are admitted with acute complications including perforation (50%) or bleeding (30%), with the result that diagnosis is delayed and mortality is high (Watson et al. 1985).

Achalasia. Aging also significantly alters the intensity and frequency of presentation of esophageal or chest pain associated with achalasia (constriction of the lower part of the esophagus) (Clouse et al. 1991; Eckardt et al. 1999).

Appendicitis and peritonitis. The classical symptoms of periumbilical pain, nausea, vomiting, and lower right quadrant pain observed in 90% of adults are not usually present in the aged; only 22% of elderly patients with appendicitis or peritonitis present with diffuse abdominal pain (Albano et al. 1975). Unlike younger patients, the aged have concomitant underlying diseases (Bender 1989) and tend to present later in the course of their disease, after a prolonged period (several hours) of moderate pain associated with an underlying perforated appendix (Lee et al. 2000). Patients older than 70 years are more likely to manifest appendicitis associated with perforation (Gurleyick and Gurleyick 2003) or intra-abdominal abscess (Franz et al. 1995). Peritonitis and other intra-abdominal infections (Cooper et al. 1994) are especially relevant in the elderly, and even in advanced peritonitis, abdominal pain is observed in only 55% of cases (Wroblewski and Mikulowski 1991).

Pancreatitis. Although acute pancreatitis in the aged is often of gallstone etiology, recognition of pancreatitis is more difficult because of unclear etiology in 30–40% of older patients (Browder et al. 1993) and because of the atypical clinical presentation (Gullo et al. 1994). Typically, the patient will complain of strong pain in the upper abdomen, radiating to the back. The clinical presentation in older persons differs from this typical picture because abdominal pain is absent in 90% of cases, leading to misdiagnosis; in fact, diagnosis is often first made at autopsy (Wilson and Imrie 1988; Lankisch et al. 1991).

CARDIAC PAIN

Recent large sample studies, including mostly patients over 65 years, have reported atypical pain presentation in 33% of cases of acute myocardial infarction and in 50% of cases of confirmed unstable angina pectoris (Lusiani et al. 1994; Jouriles 1998; Canto et al. 2000, 2002; Dorsch et al. 2001). Although atypical presentation in younger people is not uncommon (14.2% in those <65 versus 40.6% in those 65–74 years old), age has been found to be an independent predictor of atypical pain presentation of angina pectoris, with older patients being 1.09 times more likely to present with atypical pain of unstable angina pectoris with every decade of life (Canto et al. 2002). During the 30-year follow-up of the Framingham study (Kannel and Abbott 1984), 25% of cases of acute myocardial infarction were apparent only after examination of the electrocardiogram (ECG) results. Half of these patients had no symptoms, and the other half had atypical symptoms; ECGs are, however, often nondiagnostic and do not demonstrate ST elevation or Q waves (Mehta et al. 2001). Instead of the typical crushing substernal chest pain, the most frequent symptoms associated with atypical presentation in the elderly are pain in the arm (11.5%), epigastrium (8.1%), shoulder (7.4%), or neck (5.9%), as well as dyspnea and syncope. Intensity of pain tends to be lower by around 15–20% in the aged person. Another point is that even with pain, older patients often withstand moderate pain longer, as for example in exertional myocardial ischemia, and tend to delay more than 6 hours in seeking medical assistance after onset of pain, leading to worsened diagnosis and increased mortality (Tresch 1996).

PULMONARY DISEASE

Atypical presentations of pulmonary pathologies are also more likely in older adults: in pneumonia and acute pneumothorax (Liston et al. 1994), the classical symptom of acute onset pleuritic chest pain is often absent (74% versus 45% in younger persons). In pulmonary embolism characterized by shortness of breath and pleuritic chest pain, pain may also be absent or attenuated in 74% of elderly patients and in 47–61% of younger adults

(Ramos et al. 2000; Ceccarelli et al. 2003; Timmons et al. 2003; Punukollu et al. 2005).

SOMATIC PAIN

Musculoskeletal acute pain.   Studies on the age differences in clinical states of acute somatic pain are scarce. Acute pain arising from deep structures and that arising from superficial structures probably represent different types of pain (Bonica 1990). Acute pain intensity associated with cutaneous structures and with muscle, joint, and tendon strain probably changes minimally with advancing age, although acute situations occur against a background of age-associated degenerative musculoskeletal conditions such as osteoarthritis. The prevalence of most fractures does, however, increase with age, since between 60 and 90 years of age the apparent incidence of vertebral fracture rises 20-fold in women; women of this age group have a 50-fold increase in risk of hip fracture compared to women under 60 (Kanis and McCloskey 1992). Nonetheless, the intensity of acute pain in the young-old (65–74 years), middle-old (75–84 years) and old-old (85+ years) is not reported to change with age.

Acute oral pain.   Most studies on toothache and pain in the jaw, face, and oral mucosa show that older age groups are less likely to report pain and discomfort than younger age groups (Locker et al. 1987; Pau et al. 2003). Also, younger people anticipate much more potential pain and experience higher pain intensity than older persons (Watkins et al. 2002).

IMPLICATIONS OF ALTERED VISCERAL AND SOMATIC PAIN WITH ADVANCING AGE

The main consequence of painless disease presentation in the aged person is that when the warning and protective functions of pain as a defense mechanism, as first described by Descartes in the 17th century, are lost or impaired, most pathologies that can be diagnosed early if pain is present will usually be diagnosed at a later stage. As a result, the risk of increased complications is greater. Consequences of absent visceral pain are numerous and include delayed diagnosis, misdiagnosis, and a higher mortality rate. For example, hemorrhage and perforation are the physical symptoms of peptic ulcer disease in the emergency department, especially in the older population. Cardiac failure, cardiogenic shock, and an increased incidence of new coronary events will follow ischemic problems. Patients without pain will be less likely to receive management or treatment strategies of proven prognostic value, and beneficial strategies will often be overlooked. Even though thrombolytic therapy and revascularization procedures reduce hospital mortality in both younger and older patients (50% and 48%, respectively), treatment will be delayed (Rich 1996, 1998). Such treatments are reportedly given less often to adults of advanced age than to younger patients (17% and 32%, respectively).

Absent or atypical pain is part of a set of factors including age, delayed report of illness, physiological changes, comorbidities, and polypharmacy that increase mortality in the older population. A comparison of older and younger patients (n = 2582) presenting with chest pain showed that older patients with ischemic chest pain delayed more than 6 hours in seeking medical assistance after onset of pain, even though more than 50% had a history of documented coronary artery disease (Tresch 1996). Physiological changes and comorbidities that accompany aging may predispose patients with a frequent history of congestive heart failure, left ventricular impairment (Dorsch et al. 2001), or diabetes to an increased risk of mortality. Older patients are often maintained on a fragile homeostasis and have difficulty coping with any additional stress (Vreeburg et al. 1997). Added to this problem is the increased risk of drug interactions and adverse drug events in the older patient (Pickering 2004).

AGE AND CANCER PAIN

Over half of cancer patients are aged 60 years or older (Balducci 2003). An international survey of cancer pain characteristics and syndromes showed that a large majority of patients of all ages (92.5%) experienced one or more pains caused directly by the cancer, while in 20.8% of patients pain was caused by cancer therapies. Although syndromes and inferred pathophysiologies are very heterogeneous, somatic pain (71.6%), visceral pain (34.7%), and neuropathic pain (39.7%) are the most frequent (Caraceni et al. 1999). Various studies have explored the relationship between age and intensity of cancer-related pain for all primary cancer sites (with lung, breast, colorectal, and prostate sites being the most common) (McMillan 1989; Brescia et al. 1992; Walsh et al. 2000), for a specific pathology (colorectal carcinoma; Curless et al. 1994), or for metastatic cancer (Caraceni et al. 1999). In these studies, higher pain intensity was associated with patients younger than 60–65 years. Younger patients are 1.2 to 4 times more likely to report pain than older patients (Curless et al. 1994; Caraceni et al. 1999; Walsh et al. 2000) and 1.5 times more likely to report pain rated higher than 7 on a 0–10-point visual analogue scale (Caraceni et al. 1999). Age therefore affects the prevalence and severity of pain symptoms (with a 0–15% decrease in intensity of pain with age; Walsh et al. 2000) and is an independent predictor of cancer pain intensity.

AGE AND POSTOPERATIVE PAIN

Several studies show that older people have the highest rate of surgical procedures (Gagliese et al. 1999) and report lower postsurgical pain intensity than younger patients (Bellville et al. 1971; Oberle et al. 1990). There is a reduction in pain intensity of approximately 10–20% per decade after 60 years (Thomas et al. 1998). However, some studies have found no correlation between age and pain (Giuffre et al. 1991; Duggleby and Lander 1994; Gagliese et al. 2000). These differences may be due to methodological differences between studies and across age groups, and may be dependent on the type of pain scale used (Gagliese and Katz 2003). It has been suggested that verbal descriptors are more appropriate than visual analogue scales in measuring pain in older persons (see Chapter 6); the fact that older patients report lower pain levels with verbal descriptors may signify age differences in the quality, but not in the intensity, of pain (Gagliese and Melzack 2003).

A distinction should be made between pain assessment in the early versus the late postsurgical periods. In the early period, pain is associated with cardiac, renal, or respiratory dysfunction (Cousins 1994) and with delirium (Duggleby and Lander 1994). The residual analgesic effect of drugs, especially anesthetics administered in the pre-and perioperative periods, may constitute a bias in pain evaluation and pain report. Also, aging is accompanied by changes in the pharmacokinetic and pharmacodynamic properties of drugs, and analgesics are fully influenced by these modifications (see Chapter 10). Although many studies have reported lower opioid doses in older adults, few have controlled for pain intensity or pain relief in the postoperative period. A recent study (Sauaia et al. 2005) reported that 62% of older patients experience severe postoperative pain, with 30% reporting a level of 10 on the visual analogue scale. Despite high levels of pain, 87% of older patients were satisfied with their treatment. This paradoxical relationship between pain report and satisfaction stresses the problem of underreport or perhaps stoicism in older segments of the population (Yong et al. 2003). In longer-term postsurgical pain, functional impairment and chronic pain may develop or increase in persons of advanced age (Katz 1997). One of the most common forms of surgery in the elderly is hip fracture repair. Persistent hip pain is a frequent symptom associated with skeletal muscle weakness of the fractured leg. It is also associated with symptoms of depression, particularly in frail older adults (Herrick et al. 2004), who may have limited capacities in accommodating any stress (Woodhouse et al. 1988).

AGE AND CHRONIC PAIN

Chronic pain affects 50% to 80% of older persons, as they are more likely to suffer from musculoskeletal pain (arthritis and bone, joint, and back disorders) (Verhaak et al. 1998). Well over half the older adults in the United States report chronic joint symptoms (Leveille 2004), and low back pain (LBP) is among the most disabling pain conditions (Weiner et al. 2004; Weiner and Ernst 2004). Elderly persons may suffer also from neuropathic pain such as trigeminal and postherpetic neuralgia, poststroke central or thalamic pain, post-amputation phantom limb pain, or diabetic neuropathic pain. Literature on chronic pain in the aged has largely focused on prevalence. Several studies report that the prevalence of persistent pain increases with advancing age (Crook et al. 1984; Verhaak et al. 1998; Helme and Gibson 2001). Older age might even be a predictor of both the onset of a persistent pain condition and the failure to recover from it (Gureje et al. 2001). Other authors have recorded that the prevalence of pain complaints peaks around middle age and decreases thereafter, not only in terms of overall pain complaints (Andersson et al. 1993; Gagliese and Melzack 1999) but also regarding specific pathologies (Cook et al. 1989; Lipton et al. 1993; Wright et al. 1995). In addition, the prevalence of pain that interferes with everyday life increases incrementally with age (Thomas et al. 2004), probably because osteoarthritis dominates the pain pattern in older adults (March and Bagga 2004) and because comorbidity amplifies the level of restriction. An age-related decrease in the prevalence of pain in sites other than the joints (Sternbach 1986; Gagliese and Melzack 1997) or the lower limb region has also been reported. Hence, epidemiological findings are not entirely consistent as to whether the prevalence of pain is higher in older age groups than in younger age groups; this topic is further discussed in Chapter 1.

Studies that have focused on changes in intensity and unpleasantness of chronic pain in young and old patients have also led to differing conclusions. Some have suggested that intensity and unpleasantness are similar in patients of quite different ages attending a chronic pain management center (Puder 1988; Harkins et al. 1994). Other studies have reported age differences, with an increase in pain intensity (Brattberg et al. 1996) and more people complaining of "much" and "very much" pain with increasing age: 15% (in those aged 75–79 years), 18% (80–84 years), 22% (85–89 years), and 28% (90 years and older) (Jakobsson et al. 2003).

MUSCULOSKELETAL DISEASE AND ARTHRITIS

Musculoskeletal disease and arthritis are extraordinarily frequent among geriatric patients; it is suggested that the pattern of pain has multiple localizations and differs in body regions as a function of advancing age (Thomas et al. 2004). People over 60 years of age are 1.5 times more likely to suffer from hip/knee or foot pain compared to adults under 60 years old (Picavet and Schouten 2003). Hip and knee pain symptoms are complex in older people, and most older patients (52%) have more than one hip or knee affected (Dawson et al. 2004). Knee pain is severe in 19–44% of patients, and those over 75 years old are 2.2 times more likely to report pain than those between 65 and 75 (Jinks et al. 2002; Picavet and Schouten 2003). Sex differences in pain severity have been described. More women report severe pain than men in five locations (the hip, knee, hand, shoulder, and elbow); pain complaints tend to decrease in women with advancing age, so that 40.3% of women aged 77 report mild or severe pain compared to 36.7% of women aged 98. On the other hand, more men report severe pain at age 98 (35.6%) than at age 77 (24.6%).

Foot pain, while uncommon in younger persons, may play a key role in disability in older persons. Severe foot pain (7–10 on a scale of 0–10) of at least one month's duration has been reported in 14% of women and is more common in persons aged 65 to 75 (especially if they are obese or have hand or knee osteoarthritis) (Leveille et al. 1998) than in persons aged 75 and older.

Chronic back pain prevalence is not accurately known, but it ranges from 7% to 49% in persons older than 65 years and is one of the most important factors affecting the health status of older persons. Persistent back pain lasting for 3 months has been reported in 55% of those over 65 years old, while back pain lasting for 6 months has been described in 49% (Andersson et al. 1993). The pain was described as continuous in 34% and as intermittent in 66% of the sample. Gender differences have been reported in the severity of back pain with age: severe pain increases in men with age (9.8% of 77–79-year-olds had pain compared to 13.6% of those 85 years old or more), while women have a higher prevalence as they age, but no change in pain intensity (Brattberg et al. 1996).

Frequency of pain associated with osteoarthritis and chronic back pain is daily in 44.4% of patients, and persons around 65 with poor self-rated health are 3.2 times more likely to report pain at least several times a week than those with good self-rated health, compared to an increased likelihood of pain report of 1.6 in a younger group (Mantyselka et al. 2003).

Although the underlying pathophysiology may differ for neck and shoulder pain, the resulting muscle involvement is often similar, and elderly patients do not always differentiate between the two pain sites. The frequency for moderate and severe intensity of neck pain amounts to 7.7% in 70–79-year-old individuals, while it is reported to affect approximately 4.6% in the working population (Côté et al. 1998). Moderate and severe shoulder pain affects 12.7% of persons in their seventies (Vogt et al. 2003), especially women (Brattberg et al. 1996). Interestingly, elderly patients with severe or extreme neck pain are about 15 times more likely to report moderate or worse shoulder pain, and vice versa (Vogt et al. 2003).

Overall, it appears that the prevalence of musculoskeletal pain symptoms shows a large age-related increase and is uniformly more common in women regardless of site. This age-related increase in the frequency of pain in the knee, hip, foot, back, neck, and shoulder is thought to reflect the increasing prevalence of osteoarthritis in older segments of the community. Less information is available on age differences in pain severity, although it appears that severe pain may be more common in the young old (65–74 years) than in persons of very advanced age.

ABDOMINAL AND CHEST PAIN

Abdominal and chest pain is not subject to significant age differences in intensity within the elderly population (Brattberg et al. 1996), although there may be a slight decrease in the rate of chronic painless pancreatitis (Kamisawa et al. 2004).

HEADACHE

Headache is the eighth-most prevalent chronic pain condition, with a prevalence of 12.5% (Bingefors and Isacson 2004). It is characterized by major gender differences, with women being more likely to report more severe pain. The prevalence of migraine and cluster headache declines with age, while the prevalence of secondary headache disorders (temporal arteritis, mass lesions, and drug-induced headache) remains unchanged. Symptomatology also varies with age, but intensity of pain has not been demonstrated to change with age.

CHRONIC OROFACIAL PAIN

Chronic orofacial pain (temporomandibular, facial, and dental pain, oral sores, and burning mouth syndrome) is a substantial health problem in the older segments of the population. Between 55 and 75 years of age, pain does not differ in intensity, but the oldest old patients (85 or older) report a higher number of disability days (Chung et al. 2004). Compared to persons less than 65 years old, elderly persons complain less of temporomandibular pain related to jaw movement (16% versus 9%) (Agerberg and Carlsson 1972) or of facial pain, but more of burning mouth syndrome (Lipton et al. 1993).

NEUROPATHIC PAIN

Disease states such as herpes zoster are more prevalent in senescent individuals. Age is a risk factor for the incidence of herpes zoster in individuals aged 50–60 years, and the older patient is at much greater risk for postherpetic neuralgia (PHN). Long-standing pain of clinical importance after herpes zoster may be severe, is often disabling, and persists for at least a year in 50% of herpes zoster patients over 70 (Jung et al. 2004). After a first episode of herpes zoster, the probability of having severe PHN decreases with time (7% at 3 months, 3% at 12 months), while only 2% of patients under 60 years present with mild pain 3 months after infection. Antiviral therapy given rapidly at the onset of the skin rash can markedly reduce the percentage of patients who develop PHN (Jung et al. 2004) and may be a useful preventive measure for patients over 60 years old, although further data on risk factors for neuralgia are needed (Helgason et al. 2000).

Other types of neuropathy, including trigeminal neuralgia, post-thoracotomy pain, entrapment neuropathy (carpal tunnel syndrome), and diabetic neuropathy, are often associated with age-related comorbidities, and older adults are heterogeneous in their degree of development of chronic pain and in their response to persistent pain (Weiner et al. 2001).

Consequences of chronic pain are numerous, including sleep disturbance (Foley et al. 2004), impaired ambulation, loss of independence related to impaired physical function (Weiner et al. 2004), increased health care costs, decreased socialization (Peat et al. 2004), and adverse events from multiple drug prescriptions. Unrelieved pain detracts from the quality of life and psychological well-being of the elderly.

REASONS FOR AGE DIFFERENCES IN CLINICAL PAIN STATES

NEUROPHYSIOLOGICAL CHANGES WITH ADVANCING AGE

An age-related dysfunction in the components along the pain pathways including peripheral afferent fibers, spinal, supraspinal, and cerebral locations has been advanced as a reason for age differences in pain (Gibson and Helme 2001; Gibson and Farrell 2004; Moore and Clinch 2004). Anatomical, physiological, and biochemical studies (see review in Gibson and Farrell 2004) have reported a loss of both myelinated and unmyelinated nerve fibers with age, as well as reduced peripheral levels of calcitonin gene-related peptide (CGRP) and substance P, and experimental studies have suggested differential age-related impairment in Aδ- versus C-fiber-mediated pain perception, with a consequent impairment in Aδ-fiber function (Chakour et al. 1996). Cardiac and other visceral organs are innervated by silent sympathetic afferents, which are activated by myocardial ischemia. Mechanically insensitive sympathetic afferents may function as cardiac nociceptors (Pan and Chen 2002). The latter may, however, be less functional in the elderly, in whom age-related cardiovascular autonomic dysfunction has been reported (Jones et al. 2003; Laitinen et al. 2004).

A number of neurophysiological changes have been observed with age at the level of the dorsal horn of the spinal cord and in supraspinal locations, a situation that could explain altered pain transmission. These changes include decreased levels of CGRP and substance P, lower levels of serotonin in the medulla, spinal cord, and brain, altered serotonin metabolism, and increased serotonin turnover (Marazitti et al. 1989; Yonezewa et al. 1989; Gozlan et al. 1990). There is also a decline in the expression and in the density of *N*-methyl-D-aspartate (NMDA) receptors in central nervous system structures (Piggott et al. 1992). At supraspinal locations, neurochemical studies have shown a decline with age in the synthesis, transport, uptake, and binding of neurotransmitters involved in pain processing, such as γ-aminobutyric acid (GABA), dopamine, norepinephrine, acetylcholine, glutamate, and opioid receptors (Spokes 1979; Amenta et al. 1991; Barili et al. 1998). Nociceptive processing occurs in a number of regions including the prefrontal cortex, somatosensory cortex, hippocampus, anterior cingulate gyrus, insula, and thalamus, some of which are also devoted to cognition, emotion, and memory. Collectively, such age-related changes might be expected to modulate pain integration. Finally, evidence points to a role of the baroreflex system in modulating nociception: transmission of noxious stimuli at the spinal level may be attenuated secondary to descending inhibitory influences that are projected from brainstem sites involved in cardiovascular regulation, and this process may depend on baroreceptor activation or on a central "drive." Hypertension-related hypoalgesia may have clinically relevant consequences, especially in silent myocardial ischemia and unrecognized myocardial infarction (Ghione 1996). Conversely, after intense levels of stimulation, for example in neuropathic pain, the reduced efficacy of the endogenous pain-inhibitory system will result in more severe pain.

PSYCHOSOCIAL FACTORS AND ADVANCING AGE

Psychosocial factors may also modify the pain experience of older individuals. Depressive symptoms, clinical depression, and anxiety, often linked to isolation or widowhood, are known to be associated with chronic pain (Fishbain et al. 1997; Bradbeer et al. 2003, Strine et al. 2004).

Chronic, persistent, or recurrent pain may have a greater impact on physical and psychosocial functioning in the elderly (Gibson et al. 1994). Also, old age is associated with greater expectations of chronic pain and greater interference with daily activities (Gibson et al. 1994; Harkins 1996; Kendig et al. 2000). Persistent nonmalignant pain may often be neglected when older adults do not complain because they consider chronic pain to be a characteristic of normal aging. Chronic pain is related to self-rated health and is an indicator of morbidity (Mantyselka et al. 2003). Neglect of persistent pain is even further amplified in the frail elderly (Pickering 2004) when cognitive impairment makes it difficult to localize acute pain. Cognitive impairment in neurodegenerative disorders (e.g., Alzheimer's disease) is associated with less pain report, lower consumption of analgesics, and a reduced area of cerebral activation (Benedetti et al. 2004; Scherder et al. 2005), stressing the importance of central processing in pain experience. However, little is known so far about the link between pain and mild cognitive decline. In addition, previous pain-associated physical and psychological experiences may leave scars and prejudices, thereby accounting for altered meaning of pain symptoms with increasing experience and with increased age (Arntz and Claassens 2004).

Comorbidities may also represent another important age-associated factor that modulates pain and often leads to increased intake of a variety of medications. Drug side effects and drug interactions may often result, further confounding the expression of pain.

CONCLUSION

The evidence of studies on age differences in clinical pain presentation suggests a dichotomy between acute and chronic pain states in elderly persons. Repeated demonstrations of atypical, less frequent, and even absent pain symptoms in acute and life-threatening pathologies suggest the need for common sense, excellent observational skills, and patience on the part of the medical team in order to reach the correct diagnosis. Similarly, a consensus view from several studies would suggest that cancer pain and postoperative pain may be less frequent and less intense in persons of advanced age.

Conversely, the frequency of chronic pain is much greater in older segments of the population, particularly in the joints, presumably reflecting the well-recognized age-related increase in the prevalence of osteoarthritis. However, further work is needed to establish clear patterns of age differences in the severity and quality of pain symptoms in chronic musculoskeletal disorders. The heterogeneity and complexity of chronic pain mandate the use of adequate pain assessment tools to estimate correctly the impact of pain on patient well-being. Evaluation of risk factors for developing chronic pain will also help clinicians to adapt adequate pharmacological or nonpharmacological preventive strategies in order to ameliorate unbearable and distressing pain. Several directions can be suggested for future research—improvement of pain assessment tools, development of neurochemical techniques, and imaging research studies. These efforts must be directed toward older persons and especially the oldest age cohorts, to make possible a comprehensive assessment of their cognitive, psychosocial, and health states.

REFERENCES

Agerberg G, Carlsson GE. Functional disorders of the masticatory system. I. Distribution of symptoms according to age and sex as judged from investigation by questionnaire. *Acta Odontol Scand* 1972; 30(6):597–613.

Albano WA, Zielinski CM, Organ CH. Is appendicitis in the aged really different? *Geriatrics* 1975; 30(1 Sz):81–88.

Amenta F, Zaccheo D, Collier WL. Neurotransmitters, neuroreceptors and aging. *Mech Ageing Dev* 1991; 61(3):249–273.

Andersson HI, Ejilertsson G, Leden I, Rosenberg C. Chronic pain in a geographically defined population: studies of differences in age, gender, social class and pain localization. *Clin J Pain* 1993; 9:174–182.

Arntz A, Claassens L. The meaning of pain influences its experienced intensity. *Pain* 2004; 109(1–2):20–25.

Balducci L. Management of cancer pain in geriatric patients. *J Support Oncol* 2003; 1(3):175–191.

Barili P, De Carolis G, Zaccheo D, Amenta F. Sensitivity to ageing of the limbic dopaminergic system: a review. *Mech Ageing Dev* 1998; 106(1–2):57–92.

Bellville JW, Forrest WH Jr, Miller E, Brown BW Jr. Influence of age on pain relief from analgesics. A study of postoperative patients. *JAMA* 1971; 217:1835–1841.

Bender JS. Approach to the acute abdomen. *Med Clin North Am* 1989; 73(6):1413–1422.

Benedetti F, Arduino C, Vighetti S, et al. Pain reactivity in Alzheimer patients with different degrees of cognitive impairment and brain electrical activity deterioration. *Pain* 2004; 111(1–2):22–29.

Bingefors K, Isacson D. Epidemiology, co-morbidity, and impact on health-related quality of life of self-reported headache and musculoskeletal pain—a gender perspective. *Eur J Pain* 2004; 8(5):435–450.

Bonica JJ. *The Management of Pain,* 2nd ed. Philadelphia: Lea & Febiger, 1990.

Bradbeer M, Helme RD, Yong HH, Kendig HL, Gibson SJ. Widowhood and other demographic associations of pain in independent older people. *Clin J Pain* 2003; 19:247–254.

Brattberg G, Parker MG, Thorslund M. The prevalence of pain among the oldest old in Sweden. *Pain* 1996; 67(1):29–34.

Brescia FJ, Portenoy RK, Ryan M, Krasnoff L, Gray G. Pain, opioid use, and survival in hospitalized patients with advanced cancer. *J Clin Oncol* 1992; 10(1):149–155.

Browder W, Patterson MD, Thompson JL, Walters DN. Acute pancreatitis of unknown etiology in the elderly. *Ann Surg* 1993; 217(5):469–474.

Canto JG, Shlipak MG, Rogers WJ, et al. Prevalence, clinical characteristics, and mortality among patients with myocardial infarction presenting without chest pain. *JAMA* 2000; 283(24):3223–3229.

Canto JG, Fincher C, Kiefe CI, Allison JJ, et al. Atypical presentations among Medicare beneficiaries with unstable angina pectoris. *Am J Cardiol* 2002; 90(3):248–253.

Caraceni A, Portenoy RK. An international survey of cancer pain characteristics and syndromes. IASP Task Force on Cancer Pain. International Association for the Study of Pain. *Pain* 1999; 82(3):263–274.

Ceccarelli E, Masotti L, Barabesi L, Forconi S, Cappelli R. Pulmonary embolism in very old patients. *Aging Clin Exp Res* 2003;15(2):117–122.

Chakour MC, Gibson SJ, Bradbeer M, et al. The effect of age on A-Delta and C fiber thermal pain perception. *Pain* 1996; 64:143–152.

Chung JW, Kim JH, Kim HD, et al. Chronic orofacial pain among Korean elders: prevalence, and impact using the graded chronic pain scale. *Pain* 2004; 112(1–2):164–170.

Clinch D, Banerjee AK, Ostick G. Absence of abdominal pain in elderly patients with peptic ulcer. *Age Ageing* 1984; 13(2):120–123.

Clouse RE, Abramson BK, Todorczuk JR. Achalasia in the elderly. Effects of aging on clinical presentation and outcome. *Dig Dis Sci* 1991; 36(2):225–228.

Cook NR, Evans DA, Funkenstein HH, et al. Correlates of headache in a population cohort of elderly. *Arch Neurol* 1989; 46:1338–1344.

Cooper GS, Shlaes DM, Salata RA. Intraabdominal infection: differences in presentation and outcome between younger patients and the elderly. *Clin Infect Dis* 1994; 19(1):146–148.

Côté P, Cassidy JD, Carroll L. The Saskatchewan Health and Back Pain Survey. The prevalence of neck pain and related disability in Saskatchewan adults. *Spine* 1998; 1:23(15):1689–1698.

Cousins M. Acute and postoperative pain. In: Wall PD, Melzack R (Eds). *Textbook of Pain.* Edinburgh: Churchill Livingstone, 1994, pp 284–305.

Crook J, Rideout E, Browne G. The prevalence of pain complaints in a general population. *Pain* 1984; 18:299–314.

Curless R, French J, Williams GV, James OF. Comparison of gastrointestinal symptoms in colorectal carcinoma patients and community controls with respect to age. *Gut* 1994; 35(9):1267–1270.

Dawson J, Linsell L, Zondervan K, et al. Epidemiology of hip and knee pain and its impact on overall health status in older adults. *Rheumatology* 2004; 43:497–504.

Dorsch MF, Lawrance RA, Sapsford RJ, et al. EMMACE Study Group. Poor prognosis of patients presenting with symptomatic myocardial infarction but without chest pain. *Heart* 2001; 86(5):494–498.

Duggleby W, Lander J. Cognitive status and postoperative pain in older adults. *J Pain Symptom Manage* 1994; 9:19–27.

Eckardt VF, Stauf B, Bernhard G. Chest pain in achalasia: patient characteristics and clinical course. *Gastroenterology* 1999; 116(6):1300–1304.

Espinoza R, Balbontin P, Feuerhake S, Pinera C. Acute abdomen in the elderly. *Rev Med Chil* 2004; 132(12):1505–1512.

Fishbain DA, Cutler R, Rosomoff HL, Rosomoff RS. Chronic pain-associated depression: antecedent or consequence of chronic pain? A review. *Clin J Pain* 1997; 13(2):116–137.

Foley D, Ancoli-Israel S, Britz P, Walsh J. Sleep disturbances and chronic disease in older adults: results of the 2003 National Sleep Foundation Sleep in America Survey. *J Psychosom Res* 2004; 56(5):497–502.

Franz MG, Norman J, Fabri PJ. Increased morbidity of appendicitis with advancing age. *Am Surg* 1995; 61(1):40–44.

Gagliese L, Katz J. Age differences in postoperative pain are scale dependent: a comparison of measures of pain intensity and quality in younger and older surgical patients. *Pain* 2003; 103(1–2):11–20.

Gagliese L, Melzack R. Chronic pain in elderly people. *Pain* 1997; 70(1):3–14.

Gagliese L, Melzack R. Age differences in the response to the formalin test in rats. *Neurobiol Aging* 1999; 20(6):699–707.

Gagliese L, Melzack R. Age differences in nociception and pain behaviours in the rat. *Neurosci Biobehav Rev* 2000; 24(8):843–854.

Gagliese L, Melzack R. Age-related differences in the qualities but not the intensity of chronic pain. *Pain* 2003; 104(3):597–608.

Gagliese L, Katz J, Melzack R. Pain in the elderly. In: Wall PD, Melzack R (Eds). *Textbook of Pain.* New York: Churchill Livingstone, 1999, pp 991–1006.

Gagliese L, Jackson M, Ritvo P, Wowk A, Katz J. Age is not an impediment to effective use of patient controlled analgesia by surgical patients. *Anesthesiology* 2000; 93:601–610.

Ghione S. Hypertension-associated hypalgesia. Evidence in experimental animals and humans, pathophysiological mechanisms, and potential clinical consequences. *Hypertension* 1996; 28(3):494–504.

Gibson SJ, Farrell M. A review of age differences in the neurophysiology of nociception and the perceptual experience of pain. *Clin J Pain* 2004; 20(4):227–239.

Gibson SJ, Helme RD. Age-related differences in pain perception and report. *Clin Geriatr Med* 2001; 17(3):433–456.

Gibson SJ, Katz B, Corran TM, Farrell MJ, Helme RD. Pain in older persons. *Disabil Rehabil* 1994; 16(3):127–139.

Giuffre M, Asci J, Arnstein P, Wilkinson C. Postoperative joint replacement pain: description and opioid requirements. *J Post Anesth Nurs* 1991; 6:239–245.

Gozlan H, Daval G, Verge D, et al. Aging associated changes in serotoninergic and dopaminergic pre- and postsynaptic neurochemical markers in the rat brain. *Neurobiol Aging* 1990; 11:437–449, 2002

Gullo L, Sipahi HM, Pezzilli R. Pancreatitis in the elderly. *J Clin Gastroenterol* 1994; 19(1):64–68.

Gureje O, Simon GE, Von Korff M. A cross-national study of the course of persistent pain in primary care. *Pain* 2001; 92(1–2):195–200.

Gurleyik G, Gurleyik E. Age-related clinical features in older patients with acute appendicitis. *Eur J Emerg Med* 2003; 10(3):200–203.

Harkins SW. Geriatric pain. Pain perceptions in the old. *Clin Geriatr Med* 1996; 12(3):435–459.

Harkins SW, Price DD, Bush FM, Small RE. Geriatric pain. In: Wall PD, Melzack R (Eds). *Textbook of Pain.* Edinburgh: Churchill Livingstone, 1994, pp 769–782.

Helgason S, Petursson G, Gudmundsson S, Sigurdsson JA. Prevalence of postherpetic neuralgia after a first episode of herpes zoster: prospective study with long term follow up. *BMJ* 2000; 321(7264):794–796.

Helme RD, Gibson SJ. The epidemiology of pain in elderly people. *Clin Geriatr Med* 2001; 17(3):417–431.

Helme RD, Meliala A, Gibson SJ. Methodologic factors which contribute to variations in experimental pain threshold reported for older people. *Neurosci Lett* 2004; 6,361(1–3):144–146.

Herrick C, Steger-May K, Sinacore DR, et al. Persistent pain in frail older adults after hip fracture repair. *J Am Geriatr Soc* 2004; 52(12):2062–2068.

Hilton D, Iman N, Burke G, et al. Absence of abdominal pain in older persons with endoscopic ulcers: a prospective study. *Am J Gastroenterol* 2001; 96:380–384.

Jinks C, Jordan K, Croft P. Measuring the population impact of knee pain and disability with the Western Ontario and McMaster Universities Osteoarthritis Index (WOMAC). *Pain* 2002; 100(1–2):55–64.

Jones PP, Christou DD, Jordan J, Seals DR. Baroreflex buffering is reduced with age in healthy men. *Circulation* 2003; 107(13):1770–1774.

Jourdan D, Pickering G, Marchand F, et al. Impact of ageing on the antinociceptive effect of reference analgesics in the Lou/c rat. *Br J Pharmacol* 2002; 137(6):813–820.

Jouriles NJ. Atypical chest pain. *Emerg Med Clin North Am* 1998; 16(4):717–740.

Jung BF, Johnson RW, Griffin DR, Dworkin RH. Risk factors for postherpetic neuralgia in patients with herpes zoster. *Neurology* 2004; 62(9):1545–1551.

Kamisawa T, Yoshiike M, Egawa N, et al. Chronic pancreatitis in the elderly in Japan. *Pancreatology* 2004; 4(3–4):223–227.

Kanis JA, McCloskey EV. Epidemiology of vertebral osteoporosis. *Bone* 1992; 13:S1–10.

Kannel WB, Abbott RD. Incidence and prognosis of unrecognized myocardial infarction. An update on the Framingham study. *N Engl J Med* 1984; 311(18):1144–1147.

Katz J. Pain begets pain: predictors of long-term phantom limb pain and post-thoracotomy pain. *Pain Forum* 1997; 6:140–144.

Kendig H, Browning CJ, Young AE. Impacts of illness and disability on the well-being of older people. *Disabil Rehabil* 2000; 22:15–22.

Laitinen T, Niskanen L, Geelen G, Lansimies E, Hartikainen J. Age dependency of cardiovascular autonomic responses to head-up tilt in healthy subjects. *J Appl Physiol* 2004; 96(6):2333–2340.

Lankisch PG, Schirren CA, Kunze E. Undetected fatal acute pancreatitis: why is the disease so frequently overlooked? *Am J Gastroenterol* 1991; 86(3):322–326.

Lee JF, Leow CK, Lau WY. Appendicitis in the elderly. *Aust N Z J Surg* 2000; 70(8):593–596.

Leveille SG. Musculoskeletal aging. *Curr Opin Rheumatol* 2004; 16(2):114–118.

Leveille SG, Guralnick JM, Ferrucci L, et al. Foot pain and disability in older women. *Am J Epidemiol* 1998; 148:657–665.

Lipton RB, Pfeffer D, Newman LC, Solomon S. Headaches in the elderly. *J Pain Symptom Manage* 1993; 8:87–97.

Liston R, McLoughlin R, Clinch D. Acute pneumothorax: a comparison of elderly with younger patients. *Age Ageing* 1994; 23(5):393–395.

Locker D, Grushka M. Prevalence of oral and facial pain and discomfort: preliminary results of a mail survey. *Commun Dent Oral Epidemiol* 1987; 15(3):169–172.

Lusiani L, Perrone A, Pesavento R, Conte G. Prevalence, clinical features, and acute course of atypical myocardial infarction. *Angiology* 1994; 45(1):49–55.

McMillan SC. The relationship between age and intensity of cancer-related symptoms. *Oncol Nurs Forum* 1989; 16(2):237–241.

Mantyselka PT, Turunen JH, Ahonen RS, Kumpusalo EA. Chronic pain and poor self-rated health. *JAMA* 2003; 290(18):2435–2442.

Marazitti D, Falcone MF, Rotondo A, et al. Age-related differences in human platelet serotonin uptake. *Naunyn-Schmiedebergs Arch Pharmacol* 1989; 340:593–594.

March LM, Bagga H. Epidemiology of osteoarthritis in Australia. *Med J Aust* 2004; 180(5 Suppl):S6–10.

Mehta RH, Rathore SS, Radford MJ, et al. Acute myocardial infarction in the elderly: differences by age. *J Am Coll Cardiol* 2001; 38(3):736–741.

Moore AR, Clinch D. Underlying mechanisms of impaired visceral pain perception in older people. *J Am Geriatr Soc* 2004; 52(1):132–136.

Oberle K, Paul P, Wry J. Pain, anxiety and analgesics: a comparative study of elderly and younger surgical patients. *Can J Ageing* 1990; 9:13.

Pan HL, Chen SR. Myocardial ischemia recruits mechanically insensitive cardiac sympathetic afferents in cats. *J Neurophysiol* 2002; 87(2):660–668.

Parker JS, Vukov LF, Wollan PC. Abdominal pain in the elderly: use of temperature and laboratory testing to screen for surgical disease. *Fam Med* 1996; 28(3):193–197.

Parker LJ, Vukov LF, Wollan PC. Emergency department evaluation of geriatric patients with acute cholecystitis. *Acad Emerg Med* 1997; 4(1):51–55.

Pau AK, Croucher R, Marcenes W. Prevalence estimates and associated factors for dental pain: a review. *Oral Health Prev Dent* 2003; 1(3):209–220.

Peat G, Thomas E, Handy J, Croft P. Social networks and pain interference with daily activities in middle and old age. *Pain* 2004; 112(3):397–405.

Picavet HS, Schouten JS. Musculoskeletal pain in the Netherlands: prevalences, consequences and risk groups, the DMC(3)-study. *Pain* 2003; 102(1–2):167–178.

Pickering G. Frail elderly, nutritional status and drugs. *Arch Gerontol Geriat* 2004; 38:174–180.

Pickering GP, Fellmann N, Morio B, et al. Effects of endurance training on the cardiovascular system and water compartments in elderly subjects. *J Appl Physiol* 1997; 83(4):1300–1306.

Pickering G, Deteix A, Eschalier A, Dubray C. Impact of pain on recreational activities of nursing home residents. *Aging* 2001; 13(1):44–48.

Pickering G, Jourdan D, Eschalier A, Dubray C. Impact of age, gender and cognitive functioning on pain perception. *Gerontology* 2002; 48(2):112–118.

Piggott MA, Perry EK, Perry RH, Court JA. [³H]MK-801 binding to the NMDA receptor complex, and its modulation in human frontal cortex during development and aging. *Brain Res* 1992; 588:277–286.

Puder RS. Age analysis of cognitive-behavioral group therapy for chronic pain outpatients. *Psychol Aging* 1988; 3(2):204–207.

Punukollu H, Khan IA, Punukollu G, et al. Acute pulmonary embolism in elderly: clinical characteristics and outcome. *Int J Cardiol* 2005; 99(2):213–216.

Raja SN, Meyer RA, Ringkamp M, et al. Peripheral neural mechanisms of nociception. In: Melzack R, Walls PD (Eds). *Textbook of Pain,* 4th ed. London: Churchill Livingstone, 1999, pp 11–45.

Ramos A, Murillas J, Mascias C, Carretero B, Portero JL. Influence of age on clinical presentation of acute pulmonary embolism. *Arch Gerontol Geriatr* 2000; 30(3):189–198.

Rich MW. Therapy for acute myocardial infarction. *Clin Geriatr Med* 1996; 12:141–168.

Rich MW. Management of the older patient with acute myocardial infarction: difference in clinical presentations between older and younger patients. *J Am Geriatr Soc* 1998; 46:1302–1307.

Sauaia A, Min SJ, Leber C, et al. Postoperative pain management in elderly patients: correlation between adherence to treatment guidelines and patient satisfaction. *J Am Geriatr Soc* 2005; 53(2):274–282.

Scapa E, Horowitz M, Waron M, Eshchar J. Duodenal ulcer in the elderly. *J Clin Gastroenterol* 1989; 11(5):502–506.

Scherder E, Oosterman J, Swaab D, et al. Recent developments in pain in dementia. *BMJ* 2005; 330(7489):461–464.

Spokes EG. An analysis of factors influencing measurements of dopamine, noradrenaline, glutamate decarboxylase and choline acetylase in human post-mortem brain tissue. *Brain* 1979; 102(2):333–346.

Sternbach RA. Survey of pain in the United States: the Nuprin Pain Report. *Clin J Pain* 1986; 2:49–53.

Strine TW, Chapman DP, Kobau R, Balluz L, Mokdad AH. Depression, anxiety, and physical impairments and quality of life in the U.S. non-institutionalized population. *Psychiatr Serv* 2004; 55(12):1408–1413.

Thomas T, Robinson C, Champion D, McKell M, Pell M. Prediction and assessment of the severity of post-operative pain and of satisfaction with management. *Pain* 1998; 75(2–3):177–185.

Thomas E, Peat G, Harris L, Wilkie R, Croft PR. The prevalence of pain and pain interference in a general population of older adults: cross-sectional findings from the North Staffordshire Osteoarthritis Project (NorStOP). *Pain* 2004;110(1–2):361–368.

Timmons S, Kingston M, Hussain M, Kelly H, Liston R. Pulmonary embolism: differences in presentation between older and younger patients. *Age Ageing* 2003; 32(6):601–605.

Tresch DD. Signs and symptoms of heart failure in elderly patients. *Am J Geriatr Cardiol* 1996; 5(1):27–33.

Trowbridge RL, Rutkowski NK, Shojania KG. Does this patient have acute cholecystitis? *JAMA* 2003; 289(1):80–86.

Verhaak PF, Kerssens JJ, Dekker J, Sorbi MJ, Bensing JM. Prevalence of chronic benign pain disorder among adults: a review of the literature. *Pain* 1998; 77(3):231–239.

Vogt MT, Simonsick EM, Harris TB, et al. Neck and shoulder pain in 70- to 79-year old men and women: findings from the Health, Aging and Body Composition Study. *Spine J* 2003; 3:435–441.

Vreeburg EM, Snel P, De Bruijne JW, et al. Acute upper gastrointestinal bleeding in the Amsterdam area. Incidence, diagnosis and clinical outcome. *Am J Gastroenterol* 1997; 92:236–243.

Walsh D, Donnelly S, Rybicki L. The symptoms of advanced cancer: relationship to age, gender, and performance status in 1,000 patients. *Support Care Cancer* 2000; 8(3):175–179.

Watson RJ, Hooper TL, Ingram G. Duodenal ulcer disease in the elderly: a retrospective study. *Age Ageing* 1985; 14(4):225–229.

Watkins CA, Logan HL, Kirchner HL. Anticipated and experienced pain associated with endodontic therapy. *J Am Dent Assoc* 2002; 133(1):45–54.

Weiner DK, Ernst E. Complementary and alternative approaches to the treatment of persistent musculoskeletal pain. *Clin J Pain* 2004; 20(4):244–255.

Weiner DK, Rudy TE, Gaur S. Are all older adults with persistent pain created equal? Preliminary evidence for a multiaxial taxonomy. *Pain Res Manage* 2001; 6(3):133–141.

Weiner DK, Rudy TE, Kim YS, Golla S. Do medical factors predict disability in older adults with persistent low back pain? *Pain* 2004; 112(1–2):214–220.

Wilson C, Imrie CW. Deaths from acute pancreatitis: why do we miss the diagnosis so frequently? *Int J Pancreatol* 1988; 3(4):273–281.

Woodhouse KW, Wynne H, Baillie S, James OF, Rawlins MD. Who are the frail elderly? *Q J Med* 1988; 68(255):505–506.

Wright D, Barrow S, Fisher AD, et al. Influence of physical, psychological and behavioural factors on consultations for back pain. *Br J Rheumatol* 1995; 34:156–161.

Wroblewski M, Mikulowski P. Peritonitis in geriatric inpatients. *Age Ageing* 1991; 20(2):90–94.

Yonezewa Y, Kondo H, Nomaguchi TA. Age-related changes in serotonin content and its release in rat platelets. *Mech Ageing Dev* 1989; 47:65–75.

Yong HH, Bell R, Workman B, Gibson SJ. Psychometric properties of the Pain Attitudes Questionnaire (revised) in adult patients with chronic pain. *Pain* 2003; 104:673–681.

Correspondence to: Gisèle Pickering, MD, PhD, DPharm, Centre de Pharmacologie Clinique, Bâtiment 3C, Centre Hospitalier Universitaire, 63009 Clermont-Ferrand, France. Tel: 33-04-7317-8416; email: gisele.pickering@u-clermont1.fr.

Pain in Older Persons, Progress in Pain
Research and Management, Vol. 35, edited
by Stephen J. Gibson and Debra K. Weiner,
IASP Press, Seattle, © 2005.

5

Age Differences in Psychosocial Aspects of Pain

Stephen J. Gibson

*National Ageing Research Institute, Parkville, Victoria; Department of
Medicine, University of Melbourne, Melbourne, Victoria; Caulfield Pain
Management and Research Centre, Caulfield, Victoria, Australia*

Pain is recognized as being a complex, multidimensional, personal experience with sensory-discriminative, affective-motivational, and cognitive-interpretive dimensions. Modern conceptualizations of pain emphasize a biopsychosocial perspective in which biological, psychological, and social factors all play a relevant role (Turk and Flor 1999). As a result, psychosocial factors are thought to be of great importance in two major ways—first, in shaping the experience of pain and the consequent levels of emotional and functional impact of any chronic pain problem, and second, in terms of the psychosocial dysfunction that occurs as part of the clinical presentation of chronic pain states. Indeed, the psychological and social impacts of chronic pain are now routinely assessed as part of most multidisciplinary pain management programs and comprise an integral component of the clinical status of chronic pain patients. The longer the pain persists, the greater the probability that the person will become depressed, socially withdrawn, irritable, and somatically preoccupied. Anger, frustration, and increased anxiety also frequently result as the person tries and fails with a variety of medical and non-medical therapies (Gibson et al. 1994). However, the relationship between psychosocial factors and pain is truly bidirectional. The social context in which noxious information is processed, the meanings attributed to pain symptoms, and more generic psychological attributes, such as beliefs, attitudes, personality, and mood all play a major role in shaping the clinical pain experience.

The list of relevant psychosocial factors is quite extensive and continues to grow with advances in the field. Some of the most common and important influences include attitudes, appraisals, beliefs, coping strategy use, mood state, personality traits, cognitive functioning, symptom meaning, and motivation as well as the role of family and social support networks, cultural norms, vocational responsibilities, and religious and economic circumstances. Many of these psychosocial influences are known to change as a function of advancing age; however, to date, there has been relatively little systematic empirical research into pain-related age differences in the psychosocial domain. This chapter provides a selective review of the major empirical studies, focusing on age differences in the psychosocial impacts of chronic pain and the mediational relationship between psychosocial influences, the perceptual experience of pain, and consequent levels of suffering.

IMPACT OF PAIN ON PSYCHOLOGICAL AND SOCIAL FUNCTIONING

Chronic pain has a pervasive impact upon the lives of those affected. A great deal of literature is devoted to pain interference and the complex interrelationships between pain and psychosocial dysfunction. Epidemiological research and studies of patients attending multidisciplinary pain management programs highlight the ubiquity of mood disturbance, poor sleep hygiene, impaired social and family functioning, and reduced quality of life. For instance, depression is thought to affect 40–80% of patients with chronic pain, and more than 50% of patients report sleep disturbance as an important clinical issue. Despite considerable heuristic interest in this topic, including numerous studies in older adult populations, relatively little research has examined age differences in psychosocial impacts of chronic pain. It is desirable to characterize age differences in pain interference because it helps to better inform age-appropriate treatment approaches and, perhaps of greater importance, can improve our understanding of the basic phenomenology and clinical characteristics of chronic pain in older adults. The following discussion focuses on some of the most pertinent aspects of psychosocial pain impacts, including psychopathology and mood disturbance, cognitive function, social integration, and family and marital relationships.

DEPRESSION, ANXIETY, AND PSYCHOPATHOLOGY

Using both cross-sectional (Stacey and Gatz 1991) and longitudinal designs (Costa et al. 1987), the general literature on age-related changes in mood suggests a peak prevalence of depressive symptoms, anxiety, and disturbance in other mood states in late middle-age and then a decline into advanced age. When compared to younger adults, community-dwelling adults of advanced age report fewer symptoms of depression (Blazer et al. 1991;

Gillis et al. 1995), anxiety (Spielberger 1983; Gibson 1997), anger (Kaye et al. 1988; Gibson 1997), and general mood disturbance (Chiriboga 1977; Schulz 1985; Costa 1987; Stacey and Gatz 1991). The likelihood of a clinical diagnosis of major depression, generalized anxiety disorders, or other affective disorders has also been reported to decline in older adults (Henderson et al. 1998; Jorm 2000). On the basis of this literature, one might expect to find lower levels of depressive symptoms and affective distress in older patients with chronic pain. However, the results with chronic pain patients are quite mixed and seem to depend upon the type of affective distress and psychopathology as well as the size of the population being monitored. In general, studies with a small sample are less likely to show significant age differences, which may reflect the reduced statistical power to detect a true age difference. With regard to the type of psychopathology, the majority of studies show no age-related difference in levels of self-rated depression (Middaugh et al. 1988; Sorkin et al. 1990; Herr et al. 1993; Corran et al. 1994; Turk et al. 1995; Gagliese and Melzack 1997a; Cossins et al. 1999) or in the rate of clinical diagnosis of a major depressive illness (Herr et al. 1993; Corran et al. 1994; Benbow et al. 1996; Wijeratne et al. 2001). Consistent with studies in young and middle-aged chronic pain samples, the prevalence of depressive disorders is reported at approximately 40% in all age cohorts that include adults across the entire lifespan (Herr et al. 1993; Corran et al. 1994; Turk et al. 1995; Wijeratne et al. 2001). In terms of the self-reported levels of depressive symptoms, there is a 5–15% lower mean score when psychometric measures of depression are used (Middaugh et al. 1988; Turk et al. 1995; Gagliese and Melzack 1997a; Gibson 1997; Cossins et al. 1999). Of interest, the only two studies to find a significant age-related reduction in self-rated depression had a sample size of 340 and 820 patients, respectively, and reported a mean decrease in symptom scores of 18% (Corran et al. 1997) and 23% (Riley et al. 2000), respectively.

Anxiety symptoms may be prominent in patients with chronic pain for several reasons. The often-unknown cause of continuing pain may lead to concern, and the uncertainty over how long pain will last and the stress of living with chronic pain can often elicit anxiety. Certain anxiety disorders, such as post-traumatic stress disorder, may share a common cause with chronic pain (e.g., a motor vehicle accident). Finally, similar to depression, anxiety disorders are thought to share common neurophysiological and neurochemical substrates with chronic pain, thereby contributing to a high comorbid presence of both conditions (Gallagher and Verma 2004). Older chronic pain patients appear to report fewer symptoms of anxiety than their younger counterparts, with a 25% lower mean score on the Spielberger Anxiety Inventory (Corran et al. 1994; Cossins et al. 1999) in older adults compared with younger adults and a 20% lower score on the Symptom Checklist-90 and other psychometric measures (Middaugh et al. 1988; McCracken et al. 1993; Riley et al. 2000). Consistent with these findings, in chronic pain patients of advanced age there is also evidence of a lower percentage of patients with a psychiatric diagnosis (defined according to the *Diagnostic and Statistical Manual of Mental Disorders*) of generalized anxiety disorder, phobic disorders, and personality traits of the anxious type, such as neuroticism (Benbow et al. 1996; Wijeratne et al. 2001). These findings are likely to be of clinical significance given the magnitude of age-related change and suggest that age may modify the well-established relationship between pain and anxiety.

Other psychiatric disorders associated with chronic pain include somatization disorder, substance abuse, conversion disorder, hypochondriasis, factitious disorder, and what used to be called psychogenic pain (DSM-III; American Psychiatric Association 1980), then somatoform pain (DSM-IIIR; American Psychiatric Association 1987), and is now referred to as pain disorder with associated psychological factors (DSM-IV; American Psychiatric Association 2000). There are very few reports of somatoform disorders and other psychiatric diagnoses in chronic pain patients across the lifespan. In young adult populations, up to 23% of chronic pain patients have substance abuse problems (Hoffman et al. 1995), and there is a relatively high concurrence between chronic pain and post-traumatic stress disorder, which affected about 10% of patients attending a multidisciplinary pain clinic (Benedikt and Kolb 1986). The reported prevalence of somatoform pain disorder was found to be 17% in a large representative sample of the general population (Grabe et al. 2003), and more recent work suggests that about 75% of chronic pain patients may meet the criteria for at least one DSM-defined diagnosis at some point in their lives (Polatin et al. 1993; Kouyanov et al. 1998). With regard to older adults, Helme et al. (1996) reported that 8.7% of patients attending a geriatric pain clinic were diagnosed with somatoform pain disorder. Age differences in the rate of hypochondriasis (12.3% in adults less than 65 years old versus 8.1% in those aged 65 or older), secondary gain (19% versus 6.2%) and hysteria (3.8% versus 1.3%) were reported in a large pain clinic population of 3,000 patients (Benbow et al. 1996). Younger chronic pain patients are more likely to be preoccupied with somatic discomfort and to display impulsive personality traits, but not somatoform disorder (Wijeratne et al. 2001). It remains unclear, therefore, whether there is a differential age related-risk for somatoform disorders in chronic pain populations.

In explaining age differences in pain-related mood disturbance and psychopathology, one can consider several potential reasons. It has been suggested that older adults are less emotionally labile, have greater emotional control, and do not exhibit the same emotional highs and lows common to younger adults (Stacey and Gatz 1991). Evidence also indicates that older adults may not be as willing to report emotional problems and prefer to portray themselves in a good light by only endorsing socially desirable traits (Chiriboga 1977; Gibson 1997). Both of these changes could result either from developmental processes—a so-called psychological immunization due to repeated exposure to adverse events (Jorm 2000)—or from a cohort effect in which emotional stoicism is a more valued attribute. Physiological changes in arousal and autonomic responsivity (see Chapter 2; see Gibson and Farrell 2004 for a review) may also play some role in decreased emotional expression among adults of very advanced age. Regardless of the exact reasons for the modest age-related reduction in certain types of mood disturbance and psychopathology, it is important to recognize the profound and wide-ranging psychological effects of chronic pain in older persons. Compared to age-appropriate norms, older adults with chronic pain still exhibit significant elevations in mood disturbance (Gibson 1997) and are 4–5 times more likely to be diagnosed with a major depressive disorder (Ohayon and Schatzberg 2003). Thus, despite the observed age differences in the pain-mood nexus, pain-related psychological/psychiatric distress is still a major issue for older adults.

COGNITIVE AND NEUROPSYCHOLOGICAL FUNCTIONING

Aging is associated with a well-documented decline in cognitive functioning (Craik et al. 1995). Major changes in short-term episodic memory (events that have occurred in the recent past) and encoding, a reduced rate of information processing, and deficits in certain aspects of language and novel problem-solving capacity have frequently been reported. These deficits in concentration, learning, and remembering new information can be quite large even with normal healthy aging and may begin quite early (fifth or sixth decade of life) and accumulate across the lifespan (Salthouse 2004). However, not all cognitive abilities decline with age; semantic memory (knowledge about the world), or what has been called crystallized intelligence, remains largely intact and may even increase over the entire adult lifespan (Salthouse 2004).

Recent times have seen considerable heuristic interest in characterizing the neuropsychological impairments associated with acute and chronic pain problems. Statistically significant deficits in attention, immediate and delayed recall of verbal and nonverbal material, abstract thinking, problem solving, mental flexibility, and executive functioning have been noted (Eccleston 1994, 1995; Eccleston et al. 1997; Iezzi et al. 1999). Both pain and its related problems (depression, sleep disturbance, and opioid use) are thought to contribute to the observed neuropsychological impairments (Iezzi et al. 1999; Nicholson et al. 2001; Ersek et al. 2004); studies have even started to explore the precise central nervous system mechanisms responsible for these effects (Buffington et al. 2005). Unfortunately, almost all of these studies have been undertaken in middle-aged or young adult populations, and information is scarce on neuropsychological impairments in older persons with chronic pain.

A very recent study has shown that older adults with chronic low back pain demonstrate impaired performance on several measures of neuropsychological function as compared with pain-free individuals, and that the severity of pain is strongly associated with degree of cognitive impairment (Weiner et al. 2005). Duggleby and Lander (1994) assessed 60 older adults (aged 50–80 years) undergoing total hip replacement surgery to investigate the impact of postoperative pain on cognitive functioning. One-third of patients showed a drop in mental status (as indexed by the Mini Mental State Examination), which was reported to be due to pain, rather than to analgesic intake. Delirium (an acute confusional state) is a common occurrence in older adults following surgery and is usually attributed to the effects of anesthesia. However, postoperative pain, rather than the duration of surgery or the dose or type of anesthetic used, was found to be related to the magnitude of neuropsychological impairment in adults aged over 60 years (Heyer et al. 2000). In a large case series, about 10% of older patients (mean age 67 years) developed delirium within the postoperative period. After the investigators controlled for other known risk factors including age, alcohol intake, premorbid cognitive status, and type of surgery, persons with higher pain scores were more likely to suffer from delirium within the first three postoperative days (Lynch et al. 1998). Moreover, Morrison et al. (2003) showed that higher doses of parenteral morphine administered following hip fracture surgery significantly decreased the risk of delirium, suggesting that improved pain control is an important factor in preserving cognitive functioning. These results support the need for good postoperative pain control in older adults and emphasize the important interrelationships between unrelieved pain and cognitive function. Finally, in the only published study to make an age-based comparison of neuropsychological impairment and pain, Brown et al. (2002) examined the relationships between pain and cognitive performance in 121 patients with rheumatoid arthritis (aged 34–84 years). Pain was associated with worse performance on measures of reasoning ability, working and episodic memory, as well as speed of information processing, although depression mediated the entire relationship between pain and cognitive performance. Advanced age had an independent negative impact on cognitive performance, but it did not alter the relationship between cognitive function and having pain and/or depression. These findings suggest that the negative impacts of pain on neuropsychological functioning are quite similar across the lifespan. Overall, it appears that pain and its related problems can have a major impact on neuropsychological performance, particularly in the areas of attention and memory. The limited available data show that age does not influence this effect, although further specific tests of age differences in the magnitude of pain-related cognitive impairments are needed in order to confirm this view.

SOCIAL INTEGRATION AND FAMILY RELATIONSHIPS

Existing literature supports a strong bidirectional relationship between chronic pain and sociocultural context, including social roles, family functioning, and social integration. It is argued that social factors play a major role in the etiology and maintenance of chronic pain through social modeling, reinforcement of illness behavior, and conditioning of a "sick role" (Payne and Norfleet 1986). Conversely, chronic pain can have an adverse effect on the family, on social functioning, and on vocational roles. For instance, a qualitative study of 18 young adult patients with chronic pain and their partners and family revealed high levels of social isolation, tension in social and vocational roles, marital conflict, and loss of contact with friends and relatives (Snelling 1994). Almost 50% of migraine sufferers noted a moderate or greater impact on family home life and social leisure activities as well as a greater number of missed days of family/leisure activities than of work-related activities (MacGregor et al. 2004). In working adults, the range of limitations is typically quite broad, including parenting roles, housework, leisure activities, and spiritual engagement, quite apart from the vocational disruption (Strunin and Boden 2004). Given the age-related changes in family and social circumstances over the lifespan, one can reasonably ask whether similar effects occur in older populations.

Using a random community-dwelling sample of 205 older adults, Roy and colleagues (1996) found that chronic pain was without apparent effect on participation in organized social activities (such as social trips), visiting family or friends, and more physical recreational activities including lawn bowling, walking, aerobics, and swimming. Moreover, with the exception of physical recreational activities, there was no difference between "younger" old adults (65–70 years) and the so-called "old" old (80–89 years) in the impact of pain. Over 30% of the younger group reported interference with physical recreation compared to only 2% of adults aged 80 years or older. However, the extent of pain's impact on social functioning may depend upon the type of sample; for instance, older adults attending a pain clinic reported significant impact of pain on church attendance and visiting friends, but more frequent social interaction with family when compared to age-matched controls (Roy et al. 1996). In a study of cancer patients across a broad age range (27–91 years), pain and depression were strongly related to the level of self-rated adequacy of social support, satisfaction with family functioning, and the size of the social support network (Hann et al. 2002). There were no significant age differences in the strength of this relationship, although a larger social network, which helped prevent depression in younger persons, was not necessarily protective of depressed mood in older adults. Finally, a study of young (20–39 years), middle-aged (40–59 years), and older (60–85 years) patients with fibromyalgia revealed no age differences in the relationship between psychosocial factors and symptomatology (pain, sleep disturbance, and tender point count), despite significant age differences in most of the clinical variables measured (Cronan et al. 2002). Based on this limited evidence, it is clear that pain has serious adverse effects on most aspects of social functioning, including family and vocational roles, personal intimacy, social leisure activities, and spiritual engagement. Older age does not appear to moderate the social impacts of pain, nor the perceived satisfaction and importance of social support structures.

PSYCHOSOCIAL MEDIATORS OF PAIN

Beliefs, attitudes, and appraisals of chronic pain symptoms, coping strategy use, and social environment are major targets of cognitive-behavioral treatment programs because they are known to play important roles in shaping the pain experience and the consequent levels of emotional distress and physical disability. A number of recent studies have started to examine age differences in the psychosocial mediators of pain, and there is now growing evidence of some important differences over the adult lifespan.

APPRAISALS AND MEANING OF PAIN SYMPTOMS

Studies have demonstrated that patients with chronic pain are eight times more likely to rate their health status as being poor (Mantyselka et al. 2003). However, it appears that pain may have a bigger impact on self-rated health in younger rather than older adults (Benyamini et al. 2003; Kerns et al. 2003; Mantyselka et al. 2003). In particular, mild pain symptoms have a strong influence on self-rated health in younger adults, especially when health is perceived as poor (Mangione et al. 1993; Kaplan and Baron-Epel

2003). In marked contrast, older adults do not place a high value on pain when making judgments about perceived health (Pinquart 2001; Benyamini et al. 2003). The one exception to this apparent age-related change in the relationship between the presence of pain symptoms and self-rated health occurs when pain is judged as bothersome or severe (Leventhal and Prohaska 1986; Reyes-Gibby et al. 2002). In a representative community-dwelling sample of over 5,000 older adults, logistic regression analysis revealed that those who reported bothersome pain were more than twice as likely as pain-free controls to perceive their health to be poor, even after the authors controlled for differences in clinical health status (Reyes-Gibby et al. 2002).

There are several possible reasons to explain the age-associated decrease in the relationship between pain symptoms and self-rated health. With older age, individuals may redefine the criteria for making judgements about good health, such that a lack of illness or pain may have lower importance. There may be a greater acceptance of pain as a normal companion of old age; Helme and Allen (1992) have reported that almost 80% of older adults agree with the statement: "You have to expect more pain as you get older." Others have confirmed this view that pain is more accepted by older persons (Hofland 1992; Liddell and Locker 1997; Weiner and Rudy 2002), although there have been some exceptions showing no correlation between age and scores on the pain acceptance questionnaire (McCracken 1998). Another possible explanation may relate to the misattribution of pain symptoms to the normal aging process. Older persons are very aware of the increased prevalence of disease and pain in their peer group and are more likely to attribute mild aches and joint pain to aging rather than interpreting them as a warning sign of disease (Leventhal and Prohaska 1986; Prohaska et al. 1987; Stoller 1993). Indeed, 15% of older adults with cancer or arthritis do not regard pain as a sign of illness or disease (Ruzicka 1998). When compared to younger adults, older persons complain of less back pain than might be expected on the basis of physical pathology (Mechanic and Angel 1987), and they may have less concern about pain as a cause of disability (Gibson 2003). In contrast, using a composite pain beliefs questionnaire with items on expectation (pain is to be expected as a person ages), how bothersome pain is (people my age are bothered by pain) and attribution of pain symptoms (pain is part of the aging process), Gagliese and Melzack (1997b) reported no age-related differences between young (18–35 years), middle-aged (36–64 years), and older adults (65–86 years). They also noted a lack of age difference in the psychological (depression makes pain worse) and organic (pain results from tissue damage) subscales of this questionnaire.

The study of age differences in symptom attribution has important implications for our understanding of pain in older adults. Pain has obvious biological significance as a warning signal of disease or tissue injury. If older adults do attribute mild pain symptoms to the normal aging process rather than to disease, then the fundamental meaning of pain is altered. Pain is likely to be less threatening, there is a reduced likelihood of making a report of pain, and pain will provide less motivation to seek appropriate treatment or to modify those behaviors associated with increased pain. In summary, although there is a lack of universal agreement, the weight of current evidence does support some age-related changes in pain acceptance, expectation, and the misattribution of pain symptoms. These changes may alter the cognitive import and fundamental meaning of mild pain symptoms in adults of advanced age.

OTHER TYPES OF PAIN ATTITUDES AND BELIEFS

The range of questionnaires designed to monitor various attitudinal and cognitive beliefs that are thought to be of relevance to chronic pain has grown immensely over the past two decades. Moreover, many of these beliefs and attitudes have started to attract increased attention from researchers interested in the study of age differences. Using a newly developed questionnaire of pain attitudes, pain-free older adults living in the community displayed a greater degree of stoicism and reluctance to label a sensation as painful (Yong et al. 2001). Follow-up studies in a sample with chronic pain (aged 20–97 years) confirmed an age-related increase in stoic attitudes ("Get on with life despite pain," "It's no good complaining") and cautiousness in making a judgement about pain (Yong et al. 2003). These findings are consistent with earlier work using signal detection theory techniques to demonstrate a more stringent response criterion for the report of low-intensity pain and a reduced willingness to label a sensation as painful by adults of advanced age (Clark and Mehl 1971; Harkins and Chapman 1976, 1977). Thus, the increased stoicism with increased age may lead to the underreporting of pain by older adults and may partly explain the observed age-related reduction in psychosocial impact described above.

Beliefs about control over pain have proven to be one of the more enduring cognitive constructs in the pain literature. An examination of the degree to which individuals believe that pain severity is controlled by factors of chance, by the actions of others (e.g., their doctor), or by their own behavior revealed a higher chance locus of control in adults over 80 years of age (Gibson and Helme 2000). This contrasts with younger chronic pain patients, who endorse their own actions as the most important determinant of pain severity. A chance locus of control was shown to be associated with increased pain, mood disturbance, and disability and with more frequent use of maladaptive coping strategies. Moreover, an internal locus was found to predict reduced levels of self-rated depression in this older cohort (Gibson and Helme 2000). This finding might suggest that older adults, with a typically higher chance locus than their younger counterparts, would have poorer psychosocial adjustment to pain. However, in addition to the orientation or locus of control as discussed above, beliefs about control also involve the degree of control and the extent of self-efficacy in being able to deal with chronic pain. The ability to decrease pain, control pain severity, and increase one's self-rated efficacy in using appropriate coping strategies to help manage pain do not appear to change as a function of age. Indeed, there is unanimous agreement across multiple studies, using several different instruments, to show a lack of age differences in self-rated control over pain (Harkins et al. 1984; Keefe and Williams 1990; Keefe et al. 1991; Strong et al. 1992; Kotler-Cope and Gerber 1993; Corran et al. 1994; Gagliese et al. 2000) or even an increased level of self-efficacy in older adults (Chong et al. 2001; Gibson 2003; LaChapelle and Hadjistavropoulos 2005). These findings highlight a relative stability in perceived self-competence across the lifespan regardless of the preferred orientation of control (i.e., chance locus versus internal locus). Further research is needed to disentangle the strength and direction of the relationship between psychosocial impact and the locus and degree of control in adults of varying age.

Other reports have demonstrated age differences in most of the beliefs assessed by the Cognitive Risks Profile (Cook et al. 1999). Older adults (aged 60–90 years) were reported to exhibit a lower cognitive risk of helplessness, less absence of emotional support, and lower self-blame, but increased desire for a medical cure and a denial of pain-related mood disturbance. Similar age differences have been reported using the Survey of Pain Attitudes, with older chronic pain patients endorsing a higher conviction in finding a medical cure and greater belief that pain causes disability (Gibson 2003). The extent of age differences in a quite diverse collection of pain beliefs further illustrates the pervasive nature of change in the cognitive interpretation and meaning of pain. This altered cognitive interpretation is likely to influence pain self-report, the desire to seek treatment, and the perceived impact of pain on mood, function, and quality of life.

COPING STRATEGIES

Several different conceptual models of coping with chronic pain have been examined with respect to age differences. These models include problem-focused versus emotion-focused coping (Lazarus and Folkman 1984), active versus passive coping (Brown and Nicassio 1987), and adaptive versus maladaptive cognitive coping efforts (Rosenstiel and Keefe 1983). A recent study using Lazarus and Folkman's transactional model of coping noted a significant age-related reduction in the use of most problem-focused coping strategies (avoidance, confrontive coping, seeking social support, and targeted problem solving) as well as some emotion-focused strategies (self-controlling, accepting responsibility, and positive reappraisal) (LaChapelle and Hadjistavropoulos 2005). Others have also reported an age-related reduction in the use of active coping methods including handling or confronting pain (Ramirez-Maestre et al. 2004; Soares et al. 2004) or cognitive coping strategies including relaxation, distraction, and problem solving (Sorkin et al. 1990), all of which might be considered as further examples of problem-focused coping methods. In the context of chronic pain, problem-focused coping has been shown to be more adaptive than emotion-focused efforts, and so it has been suggested that pain treatment programs for older adults should concentrate on the enhancement of adaptive strategies as a priority (LaChapelle and Hadjistavropoulos 2005). This advice contrasts with the current emphasis on the reduction of maladaptive coping strategies as commonly taught in pain management programs for younger adults with chronic pain.

Several studies have examined age differences in the use of adaptive and maladaptive cognitive coping strategies as measured by the coping strategies questionnaire (Rosenstiel and Keefe 1983); the results have been somewhat mixed. Studies by Keefe and colleagues (Keefe and Williams 1990; Keefe et al. 1991) show no age differences in the frequency of use of adaptive techniques (e.g., coping self-statements) or maladaptive strategies (e.g., catastrophizing), although there was a strong trend for older adults to use more praying and hoping to cope with pain. In a large sample of pain clinic patients ($N = 350$, aged 18–92 years), a significant age difference in the use of praying and hoping and ignoring pain sensations emerged in those aged over 60 years (Corran et al. 1994). Mosley et al. (1993) also found an age-related increase in praying and hoping and both studies reported no age difference in catastrophizing or other maladaptive strategies. In contrast, a study on young-adult (aged 34–50), middle-aged (51–65), and older adult (66–85) patients with rheumatoid arthritis found clear age differences when coping with pain of mild intensity (Watkins et al. 1999). Middle-aged and older patients reported a more frequent use of catastrophizing, praying, and hoping, but less use of self-coping statements, when compared to younger adults. However, when pain was severe, the tendency to use these type of coping strategies was similar in all age groups (Watkins et al. 1999). Thus, it would appear that even in the same patient group, any age differences observed in coping strategy use might depend on the intensity of the pain problem. Further work is needed to reconcile the disparate findings of age differences in the various subscales from the coping strategies questionnaire, although a reasonably consistent observation is that older adults with chronic pain have an increased use of praying and hoping. This increased reliance on prayer by older adults is more likely to be due to a sociocultural cohort effect than to a maturational-developmental change (Corran et al. 1994).

To date, only one study has examined possible age-related differences in the relationship between coping strategy use and the self-rated levels of pain, mood disturbance, and disability (Corran et al. 1994). Consistent with earlier studies in young adult populations (see Jensen et al. 1991 for a review), the use of catastrophizing was found to be a maladaptive coping strategy and was the strongest predictor of negative adjustment to chronic pain (Corran et al. 1994). Catastrophizing was found to account for between 20% and 30% of the variance in self-rated depression, anxiety, and disability. However, it was in the use of other coping strategies that age differences started to emerge. In older patients with chronic pain, making self-coping statements was a significant predictor of positive psychosocial adjustment, and diverting one's attention was related to increased pain and disability. In younger adults, ignoring pain was the major positive strategy, with reinterpreting pain sensations and diverting attention being maladaptive. These coping strategies were all of secondary importance to catastrophizing, accounting for less than 10% of the variance in pain, depression, anxiety, and disability scores. As a result, the observed age differences probably represent a subtle shift in the choice and effectiveness of coping methods rather than some major age-related shift in the mediational relationship between coping methods and chronic pain.

SOCIAL INFLUENCES

There has been a substantial amount of research examining how social, vocational, and family relationships can influence chronic pain (Payne and Norfleet 1986; Turk et al. 1987). However, relatively few studies have focused on older segments of the population. The family is often regarded as the primary agent in the socialization of health care attitudes, behaviors, and compliance with treatment, and it provides the major socioenvironmental context for chronic pain patients. The role of the family in the etiology and maintenance of chronic pain problems has been investigated in terms of early learning theory and social modeling; family systems theory, in which codependence and over-closeness result in the perpetuation of an illness role; and operant conditioning models, whereby family members provide a major source of positive and negative reinforcement for the development and maintenance of pain behaviors. In particular, spouses or other primary caregivers who are overly solicitous, nurturing, and protective, or else overly critical and punishing, are thought to have a negative influence, corresponding to higher self-rated levels of pain and disability in patients with chronic pain due to the reinforcement of overt expressions of distress and suffering and a lack of reinforcement of healthy behaviors (Romano et al. 1995). In contrast, appropriate social support from family and friends may buffer the negative consequences of chronic pain by improving the ability to cope (Kerns et al. 2002; Evers et al. 2003). The older person with chronic pain often lives alone, is widowed, and has a smaller social support network (Roy et al. 1996; Corran et al. 1997). As a result, expressions of pain may be particularly relevant for older persons because they are likely to elicit caretaking behavior by family and friends and perhaps provide a source of social contact that would otherwise be unavailable (Fordyce 1978; Kwentus et al. 1985). However, the frequency of social contact has been shown to be similar in older adults with and without chronic pain (Roy and Thomas 1987), and older adults are apparently less likely to manifest signs of pain and illness behavior to family and friends (Riley et al. 2000). Moreover, in a recent longitudinal study of mostly older adults with rheumatoid arthritis (mean age 62 years), initially low levels of social support were shown to significantly predict increased pain and functional disability at 5-year follow-up (Evers et al. 2003). The authors concluded that by increasing the access to social resources one can moderate the less favorable outcomes in older patients with rheumatoid arthritis and actually reduce expressions of pain and suffering.

Within the context of family dynamics and social support, one of the most salient threats to older persons is the loss of a lifetime partner. The loneliness and bereavement associated with the death of a spouse represent the major psychosocial stressor in those of advanced age and often lead to depression, long-standing grief, and even death (Lichtenstein et al. 1998; Pitt 1998). In 1,000 community-dwelling adults aged over 65 years, approximately one-third were widowed and one-third were living alone (Bradbeer et al. 2003). Those living alone had 1.5 times the risk of suffering from moderate to severe pain at worst, whereas those recently widowed were 3.4 times more likely to report strong to severe current pain (Bradbeer et al. 2003). Furthermore, being widowed was shown to be a more important predictor of self-rated pain intensity than any other measured sociodemographic variable, including age, gender, living alone, education level, number of children, work participation, and socioeconomic status. A path analysis revealed that the mood disturbance associated with recent spousal bereavement mediated the entire relationship between being widowed and the increased likelihood of more severe pain (Bradbeer et al. 2003). Others have noted that bereavement may aggravate pain (Prigerson et al. 1995; Turk et al. 1995). In older populations, loss of a spousal partner may represent the single most important social determinant of self rated pain, disability, and suffering.

Other social influences that are thought to be of importance in the maintenance and etiology of chronic pain in younger adult populations include vocational factors, involvement in compensation and litigation, cultural background, and ethnicity. One study of injured workers with chronic low back pain demonstrated significant age differences in the duration of pain-related disability and the likelihood of returning to work (Mayer et al. 2001). Those more than 55 years old (mean age 59) were 5.7 times more likely to return to the same job, if they did return to work, whereas those aged less than 25 years found a new employer or a different job within the same occupational setting. The authors make the point that the current social security system provides the older worker with opportunities for financial support without the need for continuing work—an option that often is not available to younger workers (Mayer et al. 2001). This situation might suggest a differential socioeconomically sanctioned maintenance of chronic pain and disability in older workers, although other factors—reduced employment opportunity, less transferable skills, and longer duration of disability—may also play a role in explaining the worse rates of return to work. A better knowledge of socioeconomic factors across the lifespan is required for a more comprehensive understanding of age differences in the experience of pain. To date, no other studies have systematically examined socioeconomic and vocational factors across the adult lifespan as they relate to pain, and this area should be considered a priority for future research.

CONCLUDING REMARKS

There is widespread acknowledgment of the integral role of psychological and social factors in shaping the experience of pain and as a constituent of the multidimensional clinical pain experience. The process of growing older is often considered as a predictable biological process that begins from the moment of conception. However, this process always occurs within a sociocultural context, and the cognitive, affective, and social transitions associated with advancing age are equally important in defining the stage of life for any individual. As a result, there are major areas of contextual overlap between the aging process and the clinical experience of pain, yet relatively little research has focused on this topic. The limited available evidence does show some clear age differences in many types of pain beliefs, coping mechanisms, attributions of pain symptoms, attitudes, and acceptance of pain. These changes in beliefs and in the misattribution of pain symptoms to the normal aging process are likely to alter the fundamental meaning of pain, diminish the importance of mild aches and pains as a warning sign of injury and disease, and consequently reduce the likelihood of seeking appropriate treatment. In contrast, lower levels of social support, and particularly the loss of a lifetime partner and bereavement, may exacerbate the pain and suffering experienced by older adults. Despite the obvious age differences in many of the psychosocial mediators of pain, the impact of chronic pain on psychosocial adjustment shows a relatively modest change as a function of age. There is some evidence of an age-related reduction in depression, anxiety, and certain types of psychopathology, but relatively little age difference in the effect of pain on cognitive functioning and social integration. At present, it is not entirely clear why the pervasive age-related change in psychosocial mediators does not parallel a similar magnitude of change in the psychosocial impacts of chronic pain. Such questions must await further research, and there is a clear need for greater awareness of age differences in the psychosocial domain, if we are ever to develop a more comprehensive understanding of the clinical pain experience in adults of advanced age.

REFERENCES

American Psychiatric Association. *Diagnostic and Statistical Manual of Mental Disorders,* 3rd ed. Washington, DC: American Psychiatric Association, 1980.

American Psychiatric Association. *Diagnostic and Statistical Manual of Mental Disorders,* 3rd ed., revised. Washington, DC: American Psychiatric Association, 1987.

American Psychiatric Association. *Diagnostic and Statistical Manual of Mental Disorders,* 4th ed. Washington, DC: American Psychiatric Association, 2000.

Benbow S, Cossins L, Bowsher D. A comparison of young and elderly patients attending a regional pain centre. *Pain Clinic* 1996; 8:323–332.

Benedikt RA, Kolb LC. Preliminary findings on chronic pain and PTSD. *Am J Psychiatry* 1986; 143:908–910.

Benyamini Y, Leventhal EA, Leventhal H. Elderly people's ratings of the importance of health-related factors to their self-assessments of health. *Soc Sci Med* 2003; 56:1661–1667.

Blazer D, Burchett B, Service C, George L. The association of age and depression among the elderly: an epidemiologic exploration. *J Gerontol* 1991; 46:M210–M215.

Bradbeer M, Helme RD, Yong HH, Kendig HL, Gibson SJ. Widowhood and other demographic associations of pain in independent older people. *Clin J Pain* 2003; 19:247–254.

Brown GK, Nicassio PM. Development of a questionnaire for the assessment of active and passive coping strategies in chronic pain patients. *Pain* 1987; 31:53–64.

Brown SC, Glass JM, Park DC. The relationship of pain and depression to cognitive function in rheumatoid arthritis patients. *Pain* 2002; 96:279–284.

Buffington AL, Hanlon CA, McKeown MJ. Acute and persistent pain modulation of attention-related anterior cingulate fMRI activations. *Pain* 2005; 113:172–184.

Chiriboga D. Perceptions of well being. In: Lowenthal MF, Thurnher D, Chiriboga D (Eds). *Four Stages of Life: A Comparative Study of Women and Men Facing Transitions.* San Francisco: Josey Bass, 1977, pp 109–132.

Chong GS, Cogan D, Randolph P, Racz G. Chronic pain and self-efficacy: the effects of age, sex, and chronicity. *Pain Practice* 2001; 1:338–343.

Clark WC, Mehl L. Thermal pain: a sensory decision theory analysis of the effect of age and sex on *d'*, various response criteria, and 50 per cent pain threshold. *J Abnorm Psychol* 1971; 78:202–212.

Cook AJ, DeGood DE, Chastain DC. Age differences in pain beliefs. *Abstracts: 9th World Congress on Pain.* Seattle: IASP Press, 1999, pp 557–558.

Corran TM, Gibson SJ, Farrell MJ, Helme RD. Comparison of chronic pain experience between young and elderly patients. In: Gebhart GF, Hammond DL, Jensen TS (Eds). *Proceedings of the 7th World Congress on Pain,* Progress in Pain Research and Management, Vol. 2. Seattle: IASP Press, 1994, pp 895–906.

Corran TM, Farrell MJ, Helme RD, Gibson SJ. The classification of patients with chronic pain: age as a contributing factor. *Clin J Pain* 1997; 13:207–214.

Costa PT, Zonderman AB, McCrae RR, et al. Longitudinal analyses of psychological well being in a national sample. *J Gerontol* 1987; 42:50–55.

Cossins L, Benbow S, Wiles JR. A comparison of outcome in young and elderly patients attending a pain clinic. *Abstracts: 9th World Congress on Pain.* Seattle: IASP Press, 1999, p 90.

Craik FIM, Anderson ND, Kerr SA, Li KZH. Memory changes in normal ageing. In: Baddeley AD, Wilson BA, Watts FN (Eds). *Handbook of Memory Disorders.* New York: John Wiley & Sons, 1995, pp 23–34.

Cronan TA, Serber ER, Walen HR, Jaffe M. The influence of age on fibromyalgia symptoms. *J Aging Health* 2002; 14:370–384.

Duggleby W, Lander J. Cognitive status and postoperative pain: older adults. *J Pain Symptom Manage* 1994; 9:19–27.

Eccleston C. Chronic pain and attention: a cognitive approach. *Br J Clin Psychol* 1994; 33:535–547.

Eccleston C. Chronic pain and distraction: an experimental investigation into the role of sustained and shifting attention in the processing of chronic pain. *Behav Res Ther* 1995; 33:391–405.

Eccleston C, Crombez G, Aldrich S, Stannard C. Attention and somatic awareness in chronic pain. *Pain* 1997; 72:209–215.

Ersek M, Cherrier MM, Overman SS, Irving GA. The cognitive effects of opioids. *Pain Manage Nurs* 2004; 5:75–93.

Evers AWM, Kraaimaat FW, Geenen R, Jacobs JWG, Bijlsma WJ. Pain coping and social support as predictors of long term functional disability and pain in early rheumatoid arthritis. *Behav Res Ther* 2003; 41:1295–1310.

Fordyce WE. Evaluating and managing chronic pain. *Geriatrics* 1978; 33:59–62.

Gagliese L, Melzack R. Age differences in the quality of chronic pain: a preliminary study. *Pain Res Manag* 1997a; 2:157–162.

Gagliese L, Melzack R. Lack of evidence for age differences in pain beliefs. *Pain Res Manag* 1997b; 2:19–28.

Gagliese L, Jackson M, Ritvo P, Wowk A, Katz J. Age is not an impediment to effective use of patient-controlled analgesia by surgical patients. *Anesthesiology* 2000; 93:601–610.

Gallagher RM, Verma S. Mood and anxiety disorders in chronic pain. In: Dworkin RH, Breitbart W (Eds). *Psychosocial Aspects of Pain: A Handbook for Health Care Providers,* Progress in Pain Research and Management, Vol. 27. Seattle: IASP Press, 2004, pp 139–178.

Gibson SJ. The measurement of mood states in older adults. *J Gerontol* 1997; 52:P167–P174.

Gibson SJ. Pain and ageing: a comparison of the pain experience over the adult life span. In: Dostrovsky JO, Carr DB, Koltzenburg M (Eds). *Proceedings of the 10th World Congress on Pain,* Progress in Pain Research and Management, Vol. 24. Seattle: IASP Press, 2003, pp 767–790.

Gibson SJ, Farrell M. A review of age differences in the neurophysiology of nociception and the perceptual experience of pain. *Clin J Pain* 2004; 20:227–239.

Gibson SJ, Helme RD. Cognitive factors and the experience of pain and suffering in older persons. *Pain* 2000; 85:375–383.

Gibson SJ, Katz B, Corran TM, Farrell MJ, Helme RD. Pain in older persons. *Disabil Rehabil* 1994; 16:127–139.

Gillis MM, Haaga DAF, Ford GT. Normative values for the Beck Depression Inventory, Fear Questionnaire, Penn State Worry Questionnaire and Social Phobia and Anxiety Inventory. *Psychol Assess* 1995; 7:450–455.

Grabe HJ, Meyer C, Hapke U, et al. Somatoform pain disorder in the general population. *Psychother Psychosom* 2003; 72:88–94.

Hann D, Baker F, Denniston M, et al. The influence of social support on depressive symptoms in cancer patients: age and gender differences. *J Psychosom Res* 2002; 52:279–283.

Harkins SW, Chapman CR. Detection and decision factors in pain perception in young and elderly men. *Pain* 1976; 2:253–264.

Harkins SW, Chapman CR. The perception of induced dental pain in young and elderly women. *J Gerontol* 1977; 32:428–435.

Harkins SW, Kwentus J, Price DD. Pain in the elderly. *Adv Pain Res Ther* 1984; 7:103–112.

Helme RD, Allen F. *Use of Medications in a Community Based Elderly Population: Report to the Australian Council on the Aging.* Melbourne: NARI Press, 1992, pp 1–86.

Helme RD, Katz B, Gibson SJ, et al. Multidisciplinary pain clinics for older people. Do they have a role? *Clin Geriatr Med* 1996; 12:563–582.

Henderson AS, Jorm AF, Korten AE, Buck RD. Symptoms of depression and anxiety during adult life: evidence for a decline in prevalence with age. *Psychol Med* 1998; 28:1321–1328.

Herr KA, Mobily PR, Smith C. Depression and the experience of chronic back pain: a study of related variables and age differences. *Clin J Pain* 1993; 9:104–114.

Heyer EJ, Sharma R, Winfree CJ, et al. Severe pain confounds neuropsychological test performance. *J Clin Exp Neuropsychol* 2000; 22:633–639.

Hoffman NG, Olofsson O, Salon B, Wickstrom L. Prevalence of abuse and dependency in chronic pain patients. *Int J Addiction* 1995; 30:919–927.

Hofland SL. Elder beliefs: blocks to pain management. *Geriatr Nurs* 1992; 18:19–24.

Iezzi T, Archibald Y, Barnett P, Klinck A, Duckworth M. Neurocognitive performance and emotional status in chronic pain patients. *J Behav Med* 1999; 22:205–216.

Jensen MP, Turner JA, Romano JM, Karoly P. Coping with chronic pain: a critical review of the literature. *Pain* 1991; 47:249–283.

Jorm AF. Does old age reduce the risk of anxiety and depression? A review of epidemiological studies across the adult life span. *Psychol Med* 2000; 30:11–22.

Kaplan G, Baron-Epel O. What lies behind the subjective evaluation of health status? *Soc Sci Med* 2003; 56:1669–1676.

Kaye JM, Lawton MP, Gitlin LN, et al. Older people's performance on the Profile of Mood States (POMS). *Clin Gerontol* 1988; 7:35–56.

Keefe FJ, Williams DA. A comparison of coping strategies in chronic pain patients in different age groups. *J Gerontol* 1990; 45:P161–165.

Keefe FJ, Caldwell DS, Martinez S, et al. Analyzing pain in rheumatoid arthritis patients. Pain coping strategies in patients who have had knee replacement surgery. *Pain* 1991; 46:153–160.

Kerns RD, Otis JD, Wise E. Treating families of chronic pain patients: application of a cognitive-behavioral transactional model. In: Gatchel RJ, Turk DC (Eds). *Psychological Approaches to Pain Management.* New York: Guilford Press, 2002, pp 145–153.

Kerns RD, Otis J, Rosenberg R, Reid MC. Veterans' reports of pain and associations with ratings of health, health-risk behaviors, affective distress, and use of the healthcare system. *J Rehabil Res Dev* 2003; 40:371–379.

Kotler-Cope S, Gerber KE. Is age related to response to treatment for chronic pain? In: *Abstracts: 7th World Congress on Pain.* Seattle: IASP Press, 1993, p 100.

Kouyanov K, Pitcher C, Rabe-Hesketh SD, Wessley S. A comparative study of iatrogenesis, medication abuse and psychiatric comorbidity in chronic pain patients with and without medically explained symptoms. *Pain* 1998; 76:417–426.

Kwentus JA, Harkins SW, Lignon N, Silverman JJ. Current concepts of geriatric pain and its treatment. *Geriatrics* 1985; 40:48–54, 57.

LaChapelle DL, Hadjistavropoulos T. Age-related differences among adults coping with pain: evaluation of a developmental life-context model. *Can J Behav Sci* 2005; 37:123–137.

Leventhal EA, Prohaska TR. Age, symptom interpretation, and behavior. *J Am Geriatr Soc* 1986; 34:185–191.

Lichtenstein P, Gatz M, Berg S. A twin study of mortality after spousal bereavement. *Psychol Med* 1998; 28:635–643.

Liddell A, Locker D. Gender and age differences in attitudes to dental pain and dental control. *Community Dent Oral Epidemiol* 1997; 25:314–318.

Lynch EP, Lazor MA, Gellis JE, et al. The impact of postoperative pain on the development of postoperative delirium. *Anesth Analg* 1998; 86:781–785.

MacGregor EA, Brandes J, Eikermann A, Giammarco R. Impact of migraine on patients and their families: the Migraine and Zolmitriptan Evaluation (MAZE) survey—Phase III. *Curr Med Res Opin* 2004; 20:1143–1150.

McCracken LM. Learning to live with the pain: acceptance of pain predicts adjustment in persons with chronic pain. *Pain* 1998; 74:21–27.

McCracken LM, Gross RT. The pain anxiety symptoms scale: validation of a measure 017 anxiety associated with pain. In: *Abstracts: 7th World Congress on Pain.* Seattle: IASP Press, 1993, pp 583–584.

Mangione CM, Marcantonio ER, Goldman L, et al. Influences of age on measurement of health status in patients undergoing elective surgery. *J Am Geriatr Soc* 1993; 41:377–383.

Mantyselka PT, Turunen JH, Ahonen RS, Kumpusalo EA. Chronic pain and poor self-rated health. *JAMA* 2003; 290:2435–2442.

Mayer T, Gatchel RJ, Evans T. Effect of age on outcomes of tertiary rehabilitation for chronic disabling spinal disorders. *Spine* 2001; 26:1378–1384.

Mechanic D, Angel RJ. Some factors associated with the report and evaluation of back pain. *J Health Soc Behav* 1987; 28:131–139.

Middaugh SJ, Levin RB, Kee WG, Barchiesi FD, Roberts JM, Chronic pain: its treatment in geriatric and younger patients. *Arch Phys Med Rehabil* 1988; 69:1021–1026.

Morrison RS, Magaziner J, Gilbert M, et al. Relationship between pain and opioid analgesics on the development of delirium following hip fracture. *J Gerontol* 2003; 58:M76–M81.

Mosley TH, McCracken JJ, Gross RT, Penzien DB, Plaud JJ. Age, pain, and impairment: results from two clinical samples. In: *Abstracts: 7th World Congress on Pain.* Seattle: IASP Press, 1993, p 99.

Nicholson K, Martelli MF, Zasler ND. Does pain confound interpretation of neuropsychological test results? *NeuroRehabilitation* 2001; 16:225–230.

Ohayon MM, Schatzberg AF. Using chronic pain to predict depressive morbidity in a general population. *Arch Gen Psychiatry* 2003; 60:39–47.

Payne B, Norfleet MA. Chronic pain and the family: a review. *Pain* 1986; 26:1–22.

Pinquart M. Correlates of subjective health in older adults: a meta-analysis. *Psychol Aging* 2001; 16:414–426.

Pitt B. Loss in late life. *BMJ* 1998; 316:1452–1454.

Polatin P, Kinney R, Gatchel R, Lillo E, Mayer T. Psychiatric illness and chronic low back pain. *Spine* 1993; 18:66–71.

Prigerson HG, Maciejewski PK, Reynolds CF III, et al. Inventory of Complicated Grief: a scale to measure maladaptive symptoms of loss. *Psychiatry Res* 1995; 59:65–79.

Prohaska TR, Keller ML, Leventhal EA, Leventhal H. Impact of symptoms and aging attribution on emotions and coping. *Health Psychol* 1987; 6:495–514.

Ramirez-Maestre C, Martinez AEL, Zarazaga RE. Personality characteristics as differential variables of the pain experience. *J Behav Med* 2004; 27:147–165.

Reyes-Gibby CC, Aday L, Cleeland C. Impact of pain on self-rated health in the community-dwelling older adults. *Pain* 2002; 95:75–82.

Riley JL, Wade JB, Robinson ME, Price DD. The stage of pain processing across the adult lifespan. *J Pain* 2000; 1:162–170.

Romano JM, Turner JA, Jensen MP, et al. Chronic pain patient-spouse behavioral interactions predict patient disability. *Pain* 1995; 63:353–360.

Rosenstiel AK, Keefe FJ. The use of coping strategies in chronic low back pain patients: relationship to patient characteristics and current adjustment. *Pain* 1983; 17:33–44.

Roy RR, Thomas M. Elderly persons with and without pain: a comparative study (part 1). *Clin J Pain* 1987; 3:102–106.

Roy RR, Thomas M, Cook A. Social context of elderly chronic pain patients. In: Ferrell BR, Ferrell BA (Eds). *Pain in the Elderly*. Seattle: IASP Press, 1996, pp 111–117.

Ruzicka SA. Pain beliefs. What do elders believe? *J Holist Nurs* 1998; 16:369–382.

Salthouse TA. What and when of cognitive aging. *Curr Dir Psychol Sci* 2004; 13:140–144.

Schulz R. Emotion and affect. In: Birren JE, Schaie KW (Eds). *Handbook of the Psychology of Aging*. New York: Van Nostrand Reinhold, 1985, pp 106–123.

Soares JJ, Sundin O, Grossi G. The stress of musculoskeletal pain: a comparison between primary care patients in various ages. *J Psychosom Res* 2004; 56:297–305.

Sorkin BA, Rudy TE, Hanlon RB, Turk DC, Steig RL. Chronic pain in old and young patients: differences appear less important than similarities. *J Gerontol* 1990; 45:P64–68.

Snelling J. The effect of chronic pain on the family unit. *J Adv Nurs* 1994; 19:543–551.

Spielberger CD. *Manual for the State-Trait Anxiety Inventory*. Palo Alto: Consulting Psychologists Press, 1983.

Stacey CA, Gatz M. Cross-sectional age differences and longitudinal change on the Bradburn Affect Balance Scale. *J Gerontol* 1991; 46:P76–P78.

Stoller EP. Interpretations of symptoms by older people. *J Aging Health* 1993; 5:58–81.

Strong J, Ashton R, Chant D. The measurement of attitudes towards and beliefs about pain. *Pain* 1992; 48:227–236.

Strunin L, Boden LI. Family consequences of chronic back pain. *Soc Sci Med* 2004; 58:1385–1393.

Turk DC, Flor H. Chronic pain: a biobehavioral perspective. In: Gatchel RJ, Turk DC (Eds). *Psychosocial Factors in Pain: Critical Perspectives*. New York: Guilford Press, 1999, pp 18–74.

Turk DC, Flor H, Rudy TE. Pain and families. I. Etiology, maintenance, and psychosocial impact. *Pain* 1987; 30:3–27.

Turk DC, Okifuji A, Scharff L. Chronic pain and depression: role of perceived impact and perceived control in different age cohorts. *Pain* 1995; 61:93–101.

Weiner DK, Rudy TE. Attitudinal barriers to effective treatment of persistent pain in nursing home residents. *J Am Geriatr Soc* 2002; 50:2035–2040.

Watkins KW, Shifren K, Park DC, Morrell RW. Age, pain and coping with rheumatoid arthritis. *Pain* 1999; 82:217–228.

Weiner DK, Rudy TE, Morrow L, Slaboda J. Cognitive function in older adults with chronic low back pain: impairment is evident. *Abstracts: 11th World Congress on Pain*. Seattle: IASP Press, 2005, p 192.

Wijeratne C, Shome S, Hickie I, Koschera A. An age-based comparison of chronic pain clinic patients. *Int J Geriatr Psychiatry* 2001; 16:477–483.

Yong HH, Gibson SJ, Horne DJ, Helme RD. Development of a pain attitudes questionnaire to assess stoicism and cautiousness for possible age differences. *J Gerontol* 2001; 56:P279–P284.

Yong HH, Bell R, Workman B, Gibson SJ. Psychometric properties of the Pain Attitudes Questionnaire (revised) in adult patients with chronic pain. *Pain* 2003; 104:673–681.

Correspondence to: Prof. Stephen Gibson, PhD, National Ageing Research Institute, P.O. Box 31, Parkville, VIC 3052, Australia. Email: s.gibson@nari.unimelb.edu.au.

Part III

Pain Assessment in the Older Adult

Pain in Older Persons, Progress in Pain
Research and Management, Vol. 35, edited
by Stephen J. Gibson and Debra K. Weiner,
IASP Press, Seattle, © 2005.

6

Pain Assessment in the Older Adult with Verbal Communication Skills

Keela A. Herr

Adult and Gerontological Nursing, College of Nursing,
The University of Iowa, Iowa City, Iowa, USA

Appropriate assessment is vital for the successful identification and treatment of pain in all patients. However, the assessment of pain, particularly persistent pain, in older adults can be extremely challenging given the multiple comorbidities and issues that complicate pain presentation, as well as the impact of pain on the elder's quality of life and related outcomes. A comprehensive geriatric-focused assessment is necessary in order to recognize and effectively treat pain and associated pain-related problems such as depression, functional impairment, and social isolation. This chapter focuses on strategies for pain assessment in elders with verbal and cognitive ability to self-report. Chapter 7 complements this chapter by addressing assessment strategies in older adults with cognitive impairment, focusing on those unable to self-report.

AN APPROACH TO COMPREHENSIVE ASSESSMENT

Successful identification of the underlying physical pathologies is important in both acute and persistent pain states, but a comprehensive assessment must also include evaluation of physical function (e.g., impairment in performance of basic/instrumental/advanced activities of daily living, mobility, sleep, and appetite), psychosocial function (e.g., mood, interpersonal interactions, and fear of pain-related activity), and cognitive function (e.g., acute or subacute confusion and the patient's beliefs about pain) (Weiner 1999). The functional consequences of pain can affect the pain experience and impair the patient's ability to engage in and adhere to treatment recommendations, and thus must be identified in the comprehensive assessment.

Although monitoring pain intensity is the major outcome for acute pain treatment, effectiveness of persistent pain interventions must also be monitored in relation to changes in function (physical, psychological, and cognitive). Patients with persistent pain often respond more dramatically with respect to function than pain intensity (Flor et al. 1992), and functional outcomes are often key for older persons (Theiler et al. 2002; Ersek et al. 2003; Weiner et al. 2003). An improvement in quality of life for the older patient (reflected in optimum function in all domains) is an important indicator of the efficacy of pain management regimens and should be a goal of all health care providers when designing a pain management program.

OBTAINING SELF-REPORT

Self-report has been accepted as the most reliable source of information on the patient's pain and is considered the gold standard in most populations (American Geriatrics Society 2002; American Pain Society 2003). Although some obstacles may affect patients' ability to report their pain, discussion about pain is necessary with all older patients, and self-report should always be sought as a first step in any assessment (American Geriatrics Society 2002). Older adults are quite capable of providing self-report of pain. A structured pain interview that includes simple questions related to presence and absence of pain or discomfort, pain intensity, frequency, location, and impact on daily activities is a feasible approach to pain assessment, even in the cognitively impaired (Ferrell et al. 1990; Parmelee 1996; Weiner et al. 1999).

Given that cognitive, sensory, and motor deficits are common in older persons, it is important to determine the presence of any deficits and evaluate the patient's ability to complete the pain interview and to use available pain scales. The older adult should be provided clear, simple instructions on the use of the pain scales each time they are administered to assure understanding. In addition, sensory assistive devices (e.g., hearing aids) should be checked to make sure that they are working properly, and adjustments should be made to accommodate patients' sensory deficits, such as by providing written and oral instruction, using enlarged type and bold figures, and ensuring adequate lighting (Ferrell 1995; Herr and Garand 2001).

Although cognitive decline may require adaptations in assessment procedure and tool selection, reliable pain assessment can be obtained from individuals who are mildly or moderately cognitively impaired (Stein and Ferrell 1996; Feldt et al. 1998; Weiner et al. 1999; Krulewitch et al. 2000; Kaasalainen and Crook 2003; Taylor and Herr 2003; Herr et al. 2004; Pautex et al. 2005). Some authors have recently shown that even some older adults with severe dementia can report pain and use a simple pain scale (Krulewitch et al. 2000; Pautex et al. 2005). Research suggests that report of pain is more reliable when asking about present pain as compared to pain over time, such as average pain or pain last week (Parmelee 1996; Porter et al. 1996; Stein and Ferrell 1996; Feldt et al. 1998; Weiner et al. 1998a; Taylor and Herr 2003). It is also important to allow sufficient time for the older adult to process and respond to the assessment task (Ferrell et al. 1995; Weiner et al. 1998a). The health care provider should attempt to obtain self-report from all older adults, including the patient with dementia, before relying on surrogate reporters, due to potential discrepancies between caregiver and patient on report of pain severity (Horgas and Dunn 2001).

HISTORY AND PHYSICAL EXAMINATION

One of the most important first steps in obtaining the comprehensive assessment is a thorough history and physical examination to establish a diagnosis of underlying disease when possible. Initial questioning to elicit information and descriptions of current pain is followed by a more in-depth history and physical examination. As many older adults have multiple pain complaints, it is necessary to evaluate each as a distinct problem, because treatments may differ depending on the type, location, and etiology of the pain.

Present pain complaint. One cannot assume that older patients will automatically report pain. Many older adults will not report pain for a variety of reasons, including the belief that pain is expected and must be endured, not wanting to be a bother, expecting that the health care provider will know if pain is present, fear of the meaning of pain, fear of diagnostic tests and hospitalization, and fear of loss of independence (Herr and Garand 2001). Probing questioning must often be initiated by the health care provider. It is not uncommon for older adults to deny pain but admit to other sensations such as aching, hurting, soreness, or some other descriptor (Miller et al. 1996; Feldt et al. 1998; Bergh et al. 2000; Closs and Briggs 2002). Simple questions can be used to elicit information about pain presence, such as "Do you have any pain or discomfort today? What about aching or soreness?" (Weiner et al. 1999; Closs and Briggs 2002). Identifying and documenting the patient's preferred description of pain and using this terminology for subsequent reassessments can be useful in facilitating communication across health care providers (Miller et al. 1996).

A complete and systematic evaluation of the pain complaint by the health care provider is critical to ensure that a patient's pain complaint is fully understood. A thorough assessment of pain characteristics includes a detailed description of the pain's onset, pattern (including duration and frequency), intensity, quality, location, and any factors that exacerbate or alleviate the pain (Stein 1996; Luggen 1998; American Geriatrics Society 2002). Table I provides an example of a brief interview that will elicit information regarding the older adult's pain complaint. Specific tools for assessing pain intensity and other pain characteristics are discussed below.

Older persons, including those with dementia, can reliably identify the location of their pain by pointing to it or using a pain map or diagram (Weiner et al. 1998b; Wynne et al. 2000). With pain maps the extent of pain can be quantified and the pattern of pain used to guide therapy. It is important to identify the location of all the areas that hurt and prioritize those that are most bothersome. Pain drawings can be an effective way to communicate the older patient's pain problem and location to critical support staff in the nursing home. For example, a pain map placed on the wall at the head of the patient's bed could serve to remind the certified nursing assistant about body areas that are painful so that cautions can be taken when moving the patient during personal care or transfers.

Past history and physical examination. The history should explore conditions and illnesses that are more prevalent in older persons and can contribute to acute or persistent pain problems. Musculoskeletal pain is one

Table I

Assessment of brief pain impact for verbal patients

1. How strong is your pain (right now, worst/average over past week)?

2. How many days over the past week have you been unable to do what you would like to do because of your pain?

3. Over the past week, how often has pain interfered with your ability to take care of yourself, for example with bathing, eating, dressing, and going to the toilet?

4. Over the past week, how often has pain interfered with your ability to take care of your home-related chores such as going grocery shopping, preparing meals, paying bills, and driving?

5. How often do you participate in pleasurable activities such as hobbies, socializing with friends, and travel? Over the past week, how often has pain interfered with these activities?

6. How often do you do some type of exercise? Over the past week, how often has pain interfered with your ability to exercise?

7. Does pain interfere with your ability to think clearly?

8. Does pain interfere with your appetite? Have you lost weight?

9. Does pain interfere with your sleep? How often over the past week?

10. Has pain interfered with your energy, mood, personality, or relationships with other people?

11. Over the past week, how often have you taken pain medications?

12. How would you rate your health at the present time?

Source: Reprinted with permission from Weiner and Herr (2002).

of the most frequent causes of pain and thus should be given priority in the search for potential pain etiologies (Mobily et al. 1994; American Geriatrics Society 2002; Weiner and Herr 2002). A number of pain conditions affect multiple sites and are challenging to recognize and treat. Acute exacerbations of persistent pain may occur, and it is important to differentiate acute from persistent pain problems in order to tailor the treatment plan appropriately.

The primary purpose of the physical examination is to confirm any suspicions suggested by the history. Given that the most frequent types of pain in older adults are musculoskeletal and neurological, physical examination should focus on these two systems, although review of all systems is appropriate. It is not uncommon for coexisting conditions to exacerbate pain from other etiologies. An important consideration in the search for pain pathology is that an underlying cause of pain cannot always be identified. In this case, the practitioner is obligated to treat the pain as a disease (Brookoff 2000). It is also good pain practice to treat severe pain before an etiology is located—suffering of moderate to severe pain during ongoing evaluation and testing is unacceptable. Detailed discussion of history and physical examination approaches for older adults with specific pain conditions is provided in Part V of this volume.

Comorbidity evaluation and prior pain experience. The consequences of pain can have a major impact on the experience of pain and its treatment. Depression, sleep disturbance, anxiety, and fear are not uncommon in patients with persistent pain, and assessment for the existence of these comorbidities is essential in order to tailor the treatment plan effectively (Weiner and Hanlon 2001).

Functional assessment. Functional outcomes are a priority in assessment and treatment of pain in older persons. A strong relationship between pain and function in older adults has been documented (Mobily et al. 1994; Weiner et al. 1996; Lichtenstein et al. 1998; Won et al. 1999; Clifford et al. 2003; Cipher and Clifford 2004). Monitoring and maintaining optimum function in all areas is of utmost importance in assuring the best possible quality of life for older adults. Three key domains of function to be addressed in comprehensive assessment, including physical function, psychosocial function, and cognitive function, are noted in Table II, and further discussion of these domains is provided in several other chapters of this volume.

PAIN ASSESSMENT INSTRUMENTS

The purpose of pain assessment instruments is to measure severity of symptoms, determine the impact of pain on the person's quality of life, and

Table II
Assessing functional response to treatment of persistent
pain in older adults: suggested outcome measures

Functional Domain	Parameters	Comments
Physical	Basic and instrumental activities of daily living	Look at the degree of assistance needed.
	Mobility/activity level	Decreased activity, such as diminished participation in advanced activities of daily living in the community dweller, or decreased ability to participate in morning care in the nursing home resident may indicate pain.
	Sleep	Ask about pain awakening from sleep, difficulty falling asleep because of pain, and time spent in bed during the day.
	Appetite	Many persistent pain patients experience appetite suppression from pain. Follow caloric intake and weight.
	Pain intensity	May not be as responsive to treatment as functional capacity. In nursing home residents, use pain thermometer, behavioral indicators of pain, and rate of p.r.n. analgesic ingestion. In community dwellers, verbal scales are better than numeric.
Psychosocial	Mood	Anxiety and depression may coexist, and may worsen in patients with pain.
	Interpersonal interactions/ behavior	Reclusiveness and irritability or agitation may occur. In nursing home residents, the tone of interactions with staff, family, and other residents may be helpful.
Cognitive	Mental status	Consider pain as causative in the patient who experiences a decline in mental status or delirium. The mini-mental state exam may not be sensitive enough to detect subtle changes.
	Beliefs and attributions	Address fears and beliefs regarding pain. Has the patient changed his/her orientation from a "fix me" mentality to a "teach me" mentality?

Source: Adapted from Weiner and Hanlon (2001), with permission. Adapted version reprinted in Weiner and Herr (2002, p. 20).

serve as a benchmark for comparison of pathological conditions over time and the effectiveness of treatment interventions (Herr and Garand 2001). A number of pain assessment instruments exist for evaluating the presence and magnitude of pain for use with older adults (see Herr and Garand 2001 for review). These tools can be unidimensional, focusing on a single dimension of pain, usually pain intensity, or multidimensional, with multiple items that capture a variety of domains related to the pain problem. Documentation of pain assessments, whether a pain intensity score or a more comprehensive measure of pain impact, is an essential part of the medical record to permit monitoring of pain treatment effectiveness and facilitate communication across providers and settings (O'Connor 2003).

Decisions regarding which assessment tool to use in older adults focuses on reliability, validity, and utility of measures established in this population. Studies are accumulating that systematically examine the reliability and validity of common pain assessment tools when used with older adults. Face validity, concurrent validity, construct validity, and interrater reliability have been established for a number of useful instruments for assessing pain in older adults. Data on instrument stability is limited to those used for persistent pain problems, given the changing nature of acute pain. Table III provides an overview of selected pain instruments discussed in this chapter.

SELF-REPORT INSTRUMENTS

Pain intensity scales. Pain intensity scales are widely accepted as an assessment approach because they are easy to administer, require limited training of staff, and have demonstrated valid and reliable properties across populations. Pain intensity scales can be used to evaluate current pain or average, worst, or least pain in the past week or month.

For older adults who are cognitively intact, and even those with mild to moderate cognitive impairment, various scales are available to quantify pain intensity, including verbal descriptor scales (VDS), pain thermometers, numerical rating scales (NRS), and faces pain scales, which have acceptable validity when used among older adults (Herr and Garand 2001). A large proportion of older persons will not exhibit cognitive impairment and will have adapted to sensory losses with hearing aids and corrective lenses. Very few adaptations may be required when measuring pain with standard scales in these patients. There is considerable variability among individual patients as to preference for tool format, suggesting that several options should be available for selection.

The NRS, commonly used with a 0–10- or 0–20-point scale with wording such as "no pain" at one extreme and "worst pain possible" at the other, is a reliable and valid pain intensity scale and is often preferred when used by older adults (Weiner et al. 1998a; Bergh et al. 2000; Manz et al. 2000; Chibnall and Tait 2001; Taylor and Herr 2003; Herr et al. 2004). However, a substantial portion of older adults (both with and without cognitive impairment) have difficulty responding to this scale, particularly if administered verbally (Weiner et al. 1999; Wynne et al. 2000; Kaasalainen and Crook

Table III
Selected tools for pain assessment in older adults

Instrument	Pain Dimensions Measured	Psychometrics Established with Older Adults by Setting	Comments
Numeric Rating Scales Available in a variety of scale ranges, including 0–5, 0–10, and 0–20 scales	Intensity	Acute care Subacute care Pain clinic Long-term care Assisted-living facility Community-dwelling	Preferred by many older adults. Verbal version may be difficult for older persons with cognitive impairment. Requires abstract thought. Vertical version more suitable for older adults. Equal distance between pain categories useful for research. Sensitive to change in pain.
Verbal Descriptor Scales Available in a variety of scale types: Five-point Verbal Rating Scale (Closs 2004) Pain Thermometer (Herr and Mobily 1993) Present Pain Inventory (Melzack 1975) Graphic Rating Scale (Bergh et al. 2000)	Intensity	Acute Subacute care Pain clinic Long-term care Assisted-living facility Community-dwelling	Most preferred by older adults. Low failure rate even in cognitively impaired. Requires abstract thought. Unequal intervals between descriptive anchors. Limited number of response categories. Thermometer adaptation may assist with understanding of tool.
Pictorial Pain Scales Two main scales tested with older adults: Faces Pain Scale (Bieri et al. 1990) Wong-Baker FACES pain rating scale (Wong and Baker 1988, 1995)	Intensity	Acute care Subacute care Pain clinic Long-term care Assisted-living facility Community-dwelling	Preferred by many older adults. Most preferred by African-American older adults. Does not require language. Requires abstract thinking and has been found difficult to use for older adults with cognitive impairment. Questionable intervals between response categories. Limited number of response categories.
Visual Analogue Scales	Intensity	Acute care Pain clinic Long-term care Community-dwelling	Not preferred by many older adults. Higher failure rate. Requires use of paper and pencil or mechanical device. Requires greater abstract thought. Continuous variable enhances use for research. Highly sensitive to change in pain. Extra step in scoring adds source of error.
Other Instruments Short-Form McGill Pain Questionnaire (Melzack 1987)	Intensity Quality	Community-dwelling Pain clinics Acute care	Shorter than MPQ, so less burden. Not recommended for illiterate and cognitively impaired. May not discriminate between pain types.

Tool	Domains	Setting	Comments
Neuropathic Pain Scale (Galer and Jensen 1997)	Quality	Chronic pain in clinical trials (low back pain; osteoarthritis; postherpetic neuralgia; diabetic neuropathy)	Individual items may be more helpful than a change in total pain score. Distinguishes pain qualities of neuropathic and non-neuropathic pain. Sensitive to treatment changes. Useful for research.
Neuropathic Pain Questionaire (Krause and Backonja 2003)	Intensity Quality	Chronic pain clinic (mixed neuropathic/nociceptive pain patients)	Ability to differentiate neuropathic from nociceptive pain. Requires complex calculations to score. Not validated against treatment changes. Useful for clinical and research purposes.
Leeds Assessment of Neuropathic Symptoms and Signs Pain Scale (Bennett 2001)	Intensity Quality Location	Chronic pain clinic Community-dwelling (postal survey)	General assessment to differentiate neuropathic from nociceptive pain. Short, simple tool. Useful for clinical and research purposes.
Functional Pain Scale (Gloth 2001)	Intensity Function	Community-dwelling	Limited by indicators included in the tool. Short and easy to use.
Pain Disability Index (Tait et al. 1990)	Pain-related disability	Community-dwelling (chronic pain)	Short and easy to use. Useful for clinical and research purposes.
Brief Pain Inventory (Cleeland and Ryan 1994)	Intensity Interference	Multiple settings (cancer; chronic pain conditions; acute postsurgical pain); also older adults	Well-validated. Available in over 30 languages. Useful for clinical and research purposes.
Geriatric Pain Measure (Ferrell et al. 2000)	Intensity Interference Disengagement Pain with activity	Ambulatory geriatric clinic	Multidimensional. Limited evaluation data. Sensitivity to change unknown.
Multidimensional Pain Inventory (Kerns et al. 1985)	Pain intensity Interference Significant other support General activity	Multiple settings Chronic pain	Multidimensional. Well-established. Cross-culturally validated. Identifies adaptation styles and response to treatment. Length may affect its usefulness for clinical purposes.

2003). Vertical presentation of the NRS may be easier for persons with alterations in abstract thinking and is often preferred by older adults (Herr and Mobily 1993; Herr et al. 2004; see Fig. 1). Versions of the NRS using a smaller number orientation (0–5) may be less demanding and more effective in those with cognitive impairment; however, testing of this configuration is limited (Morrison et al. 1998). For research purposes, the 0–20 NRS is certainly advantageous given its increased response options and increased sensitivity to change in pain state.

The VDS (e.g., "no pain," "mild pain," "moderate pain," "severe pain," "extreme pain," and " the most intense pain imaginable") has demonstrated good reliability and validity, including increased sensitivity to change, and has a very low failure rate. It has been identified as the preferred instrument by many older adults and has overall strong psychometrics and utility (Herr and Mobily 1993; Bergh et al. 2000; Wynne et al. 2000; Herr et al. 2004). The VDS has been used successfully with cognitively impaired older adults (Feldt 2000; Kaasalainen and Crook 2003; Taylor and Herr 2003). A common VDS, the McGill Present Pain Inventory (Melzack 1975), has demonstrated good psychometric properties and feasibility in older adults (Gagliese and Melzack 1997; Manz et al. 2000; Gagliese and Katz 2003; Pautex et al. 2005). The Pain Thermometer, originally developed by Roland and Morris (1983), is a variation of the VDS that is preferred for patients with moderate to severe cognitive deficits or for patients who have difficulty with abstract thinking and verbal communication (Herr and Mobily 1993; Weiner et al. 1998a; Taylor and Herr 2003). A pain thermometer that has been evaluated for use with both cognitively intact and cognitively impaired older adults is illustrated in Fig. 1.

A third alternative format for assessing pain intensity is the use of a series of progressively distressed facial expressions that represent the severity or intensity of current pain. Several variations, initially developed for children, are available. The Faces Pain Scale (Bieri et al. 1990; Fig. 1) has been shown to be a reliable and valid alternative to assess pain intensity in cognitively intact and mild-to-moderately impaired older adults and is the preferred tool in studies focusing on African Americans (Herr et al. 1998, 2004; Stuppy 1998; Taylor and Herr 2002, 2003). However, a considerable proportion of patients, particularly those with moderate dementia, have more difficulty reliably using this tool (Scherder and Bouma 2000; Kaasalainen and Crook 2003). Because this scale does not require reading, writing, or expressive ability, it may be particularly useful in patients who are illiterate, dyslexic, or non-English speaking, although testing in these individuals is not currently available.

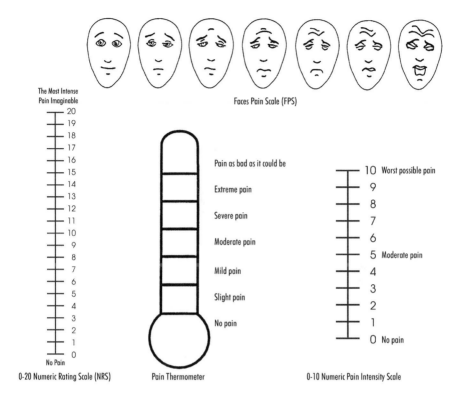

Fig. 1. Selected pain intensity scales—a vertical 0–10 and 0–20 point numeric rating scale (NRS), the Pain Thermometer, and the Faces Pain Scale (FPS). Source: The 0–20-point NRS and pain thermometer are used with permission from Keela Herr. The FPS is reprinted from Bieri et al. (1990), with permission from the International Association for the Study of Pain.

The key for clinical practice at this time is to find an assessment tool that the patient can easily use, to consistently use the same tool with each assessment, and to document the older adult's report of pain in an accessible location. The 0–10-point NRS is a good first choice for pain intensity measurement in many older adults because of its well-established psychometric properties, its increased ability to discriminate levels of pain, and its common use in clinical practice for other populations. If this scale is the standard in the setting in which the older adult is seen, attempting to use it is an appropriate first step. However, if the NRS is not an institutional standard, the VDS should be considered as the scale of choice for pain intensity assessment in older adults. If there is concern about the understanding and use of the NRS, other options should be tried to elicit self-report of pain intensity. For those with mild to moderate cognitive impairment, the pain

thermometer or another verbal descriptor scale is recommended, followed
by the Faces Pain Scale (Ferrell et al. 1995; Weiner et al. 1998b; Herr and
Garand 2001). Other tool variations are available with varying levels of
psychometric validation with older adults, but those discussed here have
received the most attention in recent years.

MULTIDIMENSIONAL PAIN ASSESSMENT TOOLS

Pain and disability scales. As noted above, pain intensity is only one
indicator of pain that can be used for assessing and reassessing pain. Multidimensional tools provide more comprehensive assessment information on
additional characteristics of the pain complaint (e.g., quality, location) and
on the impact of pain on selected domains of function. The Short-Form
McGill Pain Questionnaire (McGill-SF) (Melzack 1987) includes 15 pain
quality words scored on a Likert severity scale, plus the Present Pain Inventory and a visual analogue scale. This tool addresses two key aspects of the
primary pain complaint: intensity and quality. Testing in older persons suggests that it is reliable and valid for this population (Helme et al. 1996; Gagliese
and Melzack 1997; Luggen 1998; Gagliese and Katz 2003; Grafton et al. 2005).

Given the increased prevalence of neuropathic pain in older adults, newly
developed scales that focus on discriminating neuropathic from nociceptive
pain may be useful. The Neuropathic Pain Scale (Galer and Jensen 1997),
the Neuropathic Pain Questionnaire (Krause and Backonja 2003), and the
Leeds Assessment of Neuropathic Symptoms and Signs Pain Scale (LANSS;
Bennett 2001; Bennett et al. 2005) are three such tools. Individual pain
qualities and the abnormal sensations reported by patients with neuropathic
pain, as well as general assessment of neuropathic pain symptoms, are the
focus of these tools. Psychometric evaluation in older adults, however, is
limited.

The Functional Pain Scale, a 0–5-point tool that combines pain severity
and function, has been developed with preliminary psychometric evaluation
for use with older adults (Gloth et al. 2001). Pain is rated as tolerable or
intolerable with levels of impairment graded by interference with activity
focusing on ability to watch television, read, and use the telephone. Although the tool might be useful in patients with difficulty using a standard
intensity scale, its grading of intolerability would only be useful for patients
who engage in the three activities defined.

Several comprehensive instruments that assess multiple components of
the pain experience are available and have been used effectively with older
adults, including the Brief Pain Inventory (Cleeland and Ryan 1994), the
Pain Disability Index (Tait et al. 1990), and the Multidimensional Pain

Inventory (Kerns et al. 1985). The Geriatric Pain Measure (Ferrell et al. 2000) is a recent addition to the assessment options developed specifically for use with older adults. A number of other self-report pain/function assessment instruments are available; however, those presented in this chapter were included because they are more commonly used in practice and reflect a variety of approaches to assessment. Comprehensive multidimensional tools can be long, time-consuming, and difficult to score, making them challenging for use in some clinical settings. Three instruments, the Brief Pain Inventory, the Pain Disability Index, and the Geriatric Pain Measure, are relatively short and easy to complete and gather information on the impact of pain that can be used to monitor changes over time as well as response to treatment.

The Brief Pain Inventory (BPI), developed and extensively tested and used with cancer patients, has been validated in 12 foreign languages and has also been validated for use with noncancer chronic pain conditions (Keller et al. 2004) and acute postsurgical pain (Tittle et al. 2003). This 16-item tool gathers information on pain severity (worst pain, least pain, pain on the average, and pain right now) and rates level of pain interference on seven key aspects of function—enjoyment of life, general activity, walking ability, mood, sleep, normal work, and relations with other people. Interference with life activities is scored on a 0–10-point scale. Recently, a modified BPI demonstrated stable and valid assessments in older postoperative patients following coronary artery bypass graft surgery (Mendoza et al. 2004).

The Pain Disability Index (PDI) is a brief, seven-item instrument of pain-related disability that specifically measures perceived interference from pain with the performance of seven areas of daily functioning—family and home responsibilities, recreation, social activity, occupation, sexual behavior, self-care, and life support (e.g., eating and breathing). Pain interference is scored on a 0–10-point Likert scale with "no disability" and "total disability" as anchors. The PDI has good reliability and validity (Tait et al. 1990) and has been used successfully to examine clinical presentation with chronic pain and response to treatment in older persons (Hawk et al. 2000; Cook and Chastain 2001). Although many of the validation studies for the PDI and BPI included older persons, there are limited reports evaluating the psychometric properties of these instruments with older adult samples.

The Geriatric Pain Measure (GPM), a newer tool developed for use specifically by ambulatory older adults experiencing pain, has established preliminary reliability and validity (Ferrell et al. 2000). This tool consists of 22 yes/no questions that assess pain-related physical and psychological function and 2 questions that measure pain severity on a scale of 0–10, scoring factors including pain intensity, disengagement, pain with ambulation, pain with strenuous activities, and pain with other activities. Preliminary use in research suggests that this measure may be a useful addition to the comprehensive assessment toolkit, although additional evaluation is needed (Simmons et al. 2002).

The Multidimensional Pain Inventory (MPI) is a more extensive 61-item instrument that evaluates the impact of and adaptation to chronic pain. It comprises 13 subscales across three sections, including (1) pain severity, perception of how pain interferes with daily life activities, appraisals of the support received from significant others, perceived life control, and affective distress; (2) patients' perceptions of how significant others respond to their displays of pain: negative responses, solicitous responses, and distracting responses; and (3) a checklist of 18 common activities that forms a general activity scale. The MPI has well-established validity, including cross-cultural validity, classifying pain patients into subgroups with unique characteristics that can be used to determine adaptation styles and responses to treatment (Broderick et al. 2004). Preliminary evidence for varying pain profiles in older adults has been demonstrated (Weiner et al. 2001), and a large study to examine the application of the MPI to older adults is ongoing at the University of Pittsburgh.

Pain diaries. The pain diary is an approach to gathering information from patients on a number of aspects of their pain and response to treatment that can be very useful to the primary care provider in monitoring the pain experience over time. Diaries can also educate older adults about their pain experience and identify factors that exacerbate or decrease their pain. A variety of diaries are available, including one downloadable from the American Geriatrics Society (www.healthinaging.org/public_education/pain/), developed as part of a tool kit for use by older patients with persistent pain. Most diaries incorporate at a minimum pain intensity, pain quality, pain relief measures, use of analgesics, and response to intervention, while some include activity, sleep, treatment side effects, and other factors related to the pain experience. Diaries have been shown to be valid and reliable measures of activity and pain severity (Follick et al. 1984). Careful explanation and instructions to the patient and family caregiver are needed to assure consistent use of the diary.

BEHAVIORAL TOOLS

Depending on the setting of care and the specific pain problem, the use of a behavioral observation tool may be useful. Most of the available behavior tools focus on specific pain problems such as back pain and are completed by the health care provider or trained observer based on observations of specific behaviors occurring in response to a prescribed series of activities. The Osteoarthritis Pain Behavior Observation System is an example of an observation approach scoring position, movement, and behavior in those with osteoarthritis of the knee (Keefe and Williams 1992).

Keefe and Block (1982) devised a 10-minute standardized protocol for chronic low back pain involving walking, reclining, and standing that has been adapted for use in elders. However, stronger correlations were found between self-reported pain and disability in a sample of community-dwelling older adults with simulated activities of daily living than with this protocol (Weiner et al. 1996). Activities included long-leg sit, as in bending to put on socks and shoes; bridging, as in lower-body dressing in bed; moving supine to prone, as in turning over in bed; and moving supine to sit, as in getting out of bed.

Another subpopulation of elders that could benefit from the use of direct behavioral observation tools is the older adult with severe dementia who is unable to self-report pain. Several behavioral scales have been developed for assessing pain in this population, and a critique of currently available tools is available at www.cityofhope.org/prc/elderly.asp and in Herr and colleagues (in press). A detailed discussion of nonverbal pain tools and approaches to use of observation in recognizing pain in this vulnerable population is provided in Chapter 7.

PHYSIOLOGICAL MEASURES

Autonomic responses, such as diaphoresis and increased heart rate, blood pressure, or respiratory rate, are typically associated with acute pain. However, the absence of these responses does not indicate the absence of pain (Pasero et al. 1999). In the patient able to communicate and self-report, physiological indicators are of limited use. However, in patients unable to report their discomfort, such as those intubated or unconscious following surgery, these measures may assist in recognizing the presence of pain. Physiological responses to pain are poor indicators of pain in the nonverbal patient with dementia (Farrell et al. 1996; Porter et al. 1996), and thus their place in the assessment process is dubious. There are no reliable objective biological or physiological markers for the presence of pain (American Geriatrics Society 2002).

RECOMMENDATIONS FOR ASSESSMENT
APPROACH IN SPECIFIC SETTINGS

To address the special concerns of pain in older adults, the American Geriatrics Society (2002) has published specific clinical practice guidelines for the assessment and management of persistent pain in older persons, and the American Medical Directors Association (2003) has recently published revised clinical practice guidelines for the management of chronic pain in the long-term care setting. The American Pain Society has been developing clinical practice guidelines for specific pain problems including arthritis (2002), cancer (2004), and fibromyalgia (2005) that include recommendations for older adults. These guidelines provide explicit and useful information on which to base assessment practices across various care settings and are also intended to guide development of policies and procedures that promote routine assessment. Accessing these and other available clinical practice guidelines is an important step in developing evidence-based assessment practices appropriate for the older patient in diverse care settings.

When considering specific recommendations for assessments related to the setting of care, the cognitive and physical condition of the older adult certainly dictates the approach to assessment that can be used. This chapter has focused on the older adult able to self-report pain. For these individuals, factors related to the setting are more dependent on staffing constraints and rapid turnover of unlicensed staff, time for conducting the comprehensive assessment, and overcoming knowledge and attitudinal barriers in patients, families, caregivers, and health care providers. The American Geriatrics Society and the American Medical Directors Association both recommend in their guidelines on chronic and persistent pain in older adults that pain assessment should occur on initial admission; this recommendation seems appropriate for all health care settings. In primary care, presence of pain should be discussed in the initial interview. The frequency and timing of reassessment should be tailored to the individual's pain problem and the setting of care. Persons with persistent pain problems often require regular evaluation and follow-up, such as a weekly telephone call or follow-up appointment. Use of a standardized assessment tool that patients can complete prior to their clinical visit, such as the BPI and/or a pain diary, can be very useful in documenting effectiveness of therapy and guiding treatment decisions.

In the acute care setting, timing of pain assessment and frequency of assessment is dependent on the pain problem. Postsurgical assessment is recommended a minimum of every 2 hours during the first 24 hours and every 4 to 8 hours after the first 24 hours postoperatively if pain is mild or well-controlled, but more often as necessary to monitor for effective pain management (Rakel and Herr 2004). Development of a documentation strategy that keeps assessment and treatment information in a visible place with a user-friendly format, such as a pain flow chart, is needed to monitor and manage acute pain effectively (Arnstein 2002). As noted earlier, use of the NRS is an acceptable approach for older adults, particularly if this scale is an institutional standard for patients in general. Otherwise, the VDS should be considered the tool of choice. Given the individual variability in ability to use and preference for pain scales, other options, such as the Faces Pain Scale, should be available.

A number of challenges complicate the assessment of pain in the nursing home. Pain is often under-recognized, despite the fact that most residents can provide information that would assist in recognizing and treating their pain. Knowledge deficits and biased judgments related to pain in older persons and to strategies for assessing pain in this population are considerable (de Rond et al. 2000; Clark et al. 2004) and contribute to undervaluing of pain and discounting of reports of pain in this population. Many facilities do not have in-house laboratories, radiology, or other resources necessary for accurate diagnosis, and expert consultants are often not readily available, necessitating transports and increasing the potential for iatrogenic illness (Stein 2001). In nursing homes, the Minimum Data Set (MDS) is often used to evaluate and monitor pain and pain-related outcomes (mental status, depression, and personal and instrumental activities of daily living) over time; however, the current structure and procedure of the MDS contributes to underreporting of pain in those with cognitive impairment (Cohen-Mansfield 2004; Feldt 2004). A revised MDS 3.0 is more comprehensive, and when available it may improve pain assessment in the nursing home. Pain flow charts are often not consistently used in the nursing home, yet they provide an excellent mechanism for monitoring changes in the patient's condition that can herald unrecognized pain.

Use of explicit documentation tools in the nursing home setting has shown improvement in the quality of information related to pain assessment that is communicated (O'Connor 2003). Examples of sample tools have been published (Stein 2001). Given the prevalence of cognitive impairment in the nursing home setting, a standard scale that can be completed accurately by most older adults, including those with mild to moderate cognitive impairment, should be standard procedure. A simple VDS that includes none, mild, moderate, and severe as options may be the best choice in this setting. Staffing turnover in nursing homes contributes to inconsistency in assessment procedures. Recommendations to improve pain assessment in the nursing home include assessment on admission, at quarterly reviews, any time there is a change in the MDS, and any time there is a suspicion of pain (American Medical Directors Association 2003). However, every shift screening for pain would be an appropriate goal for the nursing home setting, given the high prevalence of persistent pain problems in this population. Nursing assistants can be educated to follow a simple screening approach, using queries regarding aching, hurting, or discomfort, to regularly monitor for pain.

As care of older patients shifts from hospitals to the home, the family caregiver will continue to play an increasingly important role in pain assessment (Herr and Mobily 1996; Juarez and Ferrell 1996; Kwekkeboom and Herr 2003). Often family caregivers are inadequately prepared to shoulder the challenges of pain assessment and management in their elders. A family education program is essential to dispel misconceptions about pain and its treatment and to prepare caregivers to assess and communicate pain and related issues (Juarez and Ferrell 1996; Wells et al. 2003; Oldham and Kristjanson 2004). Health care providers also must be sensitive to cultural differences that affects pain perception, attitudes, and acceptance of treatment approaches (Juarez et al. 1999).

Establishing institutional standards for assessment procedures based on current best practices, development and use of documentation systems and tools that facilitate assessment and communication of assessment data, and commitment to ongoing education and training of all staff caring for older persons are key strategies to improving pain assessment in older adults in all care settings.

Although data currently exist to support practices for assessing pain in older adults, further research is needed. Testing of most pain scales has occurred primarily with populations without racial or cultural diversity and limited to selected care settings. It is important to study potential differences in assessment practices that affect report and assessment of pain based on diversity of age, gender, education, race, and culture.

Most multidimensional tools currently available have received limited testing in older populations, and continued study and refinement of the most efficient methods for evaluation of pain in the clinical setting are needed. Controlled trials of pain intensity tools that determine sensitivity to detecting changes in pain state are also rare, and further trials are needed. But the most important point is that there are tools that can be used to evaluate pain and its impact in older patients. Although refinements and further validation are warranted, there is no excuse for lack of assessment of pain in this population.

SUMMARY

Thorough and comprehensive assessment of pain in older persons is an essential strategy in improving recognition and management of pain in this growing population. Numerous tools have been developed and validated for use with older adults. These tools can facilitate pain assessment and communication of relevant information across providers and settings. Although adaptation of assessment approaches is often needed based on the individual's comorbid conditions and the setting of care, it is possible to obtain information to guide treatment decision and improve quality of care and quality of life for older persons suffering from pain.

REFERENCES

American Geriatrics Society Panel on Persistent Pain in Older Persons. Clinical practice guidelines: the management of persistent pain in older persons. *J Am Geriatr Soc* 2002; 50:S205–S224.

American Medical Directors Association. *Chronic Pain Management in the Long-Term Care Setting.* San Diego: American Medical Directors Association, 2003.

American Pain Society. *Guideline for the Management of Pain in Osteoarthritis, Rheumatoid Arthritis and Juvenile Chronic Arthritis.* APS Clinical Practice Guideline Series, No. 2. Glenview, IL: American Pain Society, 2002.

American Pain Society. *Principles of Analgesic Use in the Treatment of Acute Pain and Chronic Cancer Pain,* 5th ed. Glenview, IL: American Pain Society, 2003.

American Pain Society. *Guideline for the Management of Cancer Pain in Adults and Children.* APS Clinical Practice Guideline Series, No. 3. Glenview, IL: American Pain Society, 2004.

American Pain Society. *Guideline for the Management of Pain in Fibromyalgia.* APS Clinical Practice Guideline Series, No. 3. Glenview, IL: American Pain Society, 2005.

Arnstein P. Optimizing perioperative pain management. *AORN J* 2002; 76:812–818.

Bennett M. The LANSS pain scale: the Leeds assessment of neuropathic symptoms and signs. *Pain* 2001; 92:147–157.

Bennett M, Smith B, Torrance N, Potter J. The S-LANSS Score for identifying pain of predominantly neuropathic origin: validation for use in clinical and postal research. *J Pain* 2005; 6(3):149–158.

Bergh I, Sjostrom B, Oden A, Steen B. An application of pain rating scales in geriatric patients. *Aging Clin Exp Res* 2000; 12(5):380–387.

Bieri D, Reeve RA, Champion GD, et al. The Faces Pain Scale for the self-assessment of the severity of pain experienced by children: initial validation and preliminary investigation for ratio scale properties. *Pain* 1990; 41:139–150.

Brookoff D. Chronic pain: 1. A new disease? *Hosp Pract* 2000; 35(7):45–52, 59.

Broderick JE, Junghaenel DU, Turk DC. Stability of patient adaptation classifications on the multidimensional pain inventory. *Pain* 2004; 109:94–102.

Chibnall J, Tait R. Pain assessment in cognitively impaired and unimpaired older adults: a comparison of four scales. *Pain* 2001; 92:173–186.

Cipher DJ, Clifford PA. Dementia, pain, depression and behavioral disturbances, and ADLs: toward a comprehensive conceptualization of quality of life in long-term care. *Int J Geriatr Psychiatry* 2004; 19:741–748.

Clark L, Jones K, Pennington K. Pain assessment practices with nursing home residents. *West J Nurs Res* 2004; 26(7):733–750.

Cleeland CS, Ryan KM. Pain assessment: global use of the Brief Pain Inventory. *Ann Acad Med Singapore* 1994; 23:129–138.

Clifford PA, Cipher DJ, Roper KD. Assessing resistance to activities of daily living in long-term care. *J Am Med Dir Assoc* 2003; 4(6):313–319.

Closs SJ, Briggs M. Patient's verbal descriptions of pain and discomfort following orthopaedic surgery. *Int J Nurs Stud* 2002; 39(5):563–572.

Cohen-Mansfield J. The adequacy of the minimum data set assessment of pain in cognitively impaired nursing home residents. *J Pain Symptom Manage* 2004; 27(4):343–351.

Cook AJ, Chastain DC. The classification of patients with chronic pain: age and sex differences. *Pain Res Manage* 2001; 6(3):142–151.

de Rond ME, de Wit R, van Dam FS, Muller MJ. A pain monitoring program for nurses: effect on communication, assessment and documentation of patients pain. *J Pain Symptom Manage* 2000; 20(6):424–439.

Ersek M, Turner JA, McCurry SM, Gibbons L, Kraybill BM. Efficacy of a self-management group intervention for elderly persons with chronic pain. *Clin J Pain* 2003; 19(3):156–167.

Farrell MJ, Katz B, Helme RD. The impact of dementia on the pain experience. *Pain* 1996; 67(1):7–15.

Feldt KS. The checklist of nonverbal pain indicators (CNPI). *Pain Manag Nurs* 2000; 1:13–21.

Feldt K. The complexity of managing pain for frail elders. *J Am Geriatr Soc* 2004; 52:840–841.

Feldt KS, Ryden MB, Miles S. Treatment of pain in cognitively impaired compared with cognitively intact older patients with hip fracture. *J Am Geriatr Soc* 1998; 46:1079–1085.

Ferrell BA. Pain evaluation and management in the nursing home. *Ann Intern Med* 1995; 123:681–687.

Ferrell BA, Ferrell BR, Osterweil D. Pain in the nursing home. *J Am Geriatr Soc* 1990; 38(4):409–414.

Ferrell BA, Ferrell BR, Rivera L. Pain in cognitively impaired nursing home patients. *J Pain Symptom Manage* 1995; 10:591–598.

Ferrell BA, Stein W, Beck JC. The Geriatric Pain Measure: validity, reliability and factor analysis *J Am Geriatr Soc* 2000; 48:1669–1673.

Flor H, Fydrich T, Turk DC. Efficacy of multidisciplinary pain treatment centers: a meta-analytic review. *Pain* 1992; 49:221–230.

Follick MJ, Ahern DK, Laser-Wolsten N. Evaluation of a pain diary for chronic pain patients. *Pain* 1984; 19:373–382.

Gagliese L, Katz J. Age difference in postoperative pain are scale dependent: a comparison of measures of pain intensity and quality in younger and older surgical patients. *Pain* 2003; 103(1–2):11–20.

Gagliese L, Melzack R. Age differences in the quality of chronic pain: a preliminary study. *Pain Res Manag* 1997; 2(3):157–162.

Galer BS, Jensen MP. Development and preliminary validation of a pain measure specific to neuropathic pain: the neuropathic pain scale. *Neurology* 1997; 48:332–338.

Gloth FM, Scheve AA, Stober CV, Chow S, Prosser J. The Functional Pain Scale: reliability, validity and responsiveness in an elderly population. *J Am Med Dir Assoc* 2001; 110–114.

Grafton KV, Foster NE, Wright CC. Test-retest reliability of the Short-Form McGill Pain Questionnaire. Assessment of intraclass correlation coefficients and limits of agreement in patients with osteoarthritis. *Clin J Pain* 2005; 21(1):73–82.

Hawk C, Long CR, Boulanger KT, Morchhauser E, Fuhr AW. Chiropractic care for patients aged 55 and older: report from a practice-based research program. *J Am Geriatr Soc* 2000; 48(5):534–545.

Helme RD, Katz B, Gibson SJ, et al. Multidisciplinary pain clinics for older people: do they have a role? *Clin Geriatr Med* 1996; 12:563–599.

Herr K, Garand L. Assessment and measurement of pain in older adults. In: Ferrell B (Ed). *Clin Geriatr Med* 2001; 17(3):457–478.

Herr K, Mobily P. Comparison of selected pain assessment tools for use with the elderly. *Appl Nurs Res* 1993; 6:39–46.

Herr KA, Mobily PR. Pain management for the elderly in alternative care settings. In: Ferrell BR, Ferrell BA (Eds). *Pain in the Elderly*. Seattle: IASP Press, 1996.

Herr KA, Mobily PR, Kohout FJ, Wagenaar D. Evaluation of the Faces Pain Scale for use with the elderly. *Clin J Pain* 1998; 14:29–38.

Herr K, Spratt K, Mobily P, Richardson G. Pain intensity assessment in older adults: use of experimental pain to compare psychometric properties and usability of selected pain scales with younger adults. *Clin J Pain* 2004; 20:207–219.

Herr K, Bjoro K, Decker S. A state of the science review of nonverbal pain assessment tools for use in patients with dementia. *J Pain Symptom Manage;* in press.

Horgas AL, Dunn K. Pain in nursing home residents. Comparison of residents' self-report and nursing assistants' perceptions. Incongruencies exist in resident and caregiver reports of pain; therefore, pain management education is needed to prevent suffering. *J Gerontol Nurs* 2001; 27(3):44–53.

Juarez G, Ferrell BR. Family and caregiver involvement in pain management. *Clin Geriatr Med* 1996; 12(3):531–547.

Juarez G, Ferrell B, Borneman T. Cultural considerations in education for cancer pain management. *J Cancer Educ* 1999; 14(3):168–173.

Kaasalainen S, Crook J. A comparison of pain-assessment tools for use with elderly long-term-care residents. *Clin J Nurs Res* 2003; 35(4):58–71.

Keefe FJ, Block AR. Development of an observational method for assessing pain behavior in chronic low back pain patients. *Behav Ther* 1982; 13:363–375.

Keefe FJ, Williams DA. Assessment of pain behaviors. In: Turk DC, Melzack R (Eds). *Handbook of Pain Assessment*. New York: Guilford Press, 1992.

Keller S, Bann CM, Dodd SL, et al. Validity of the brief pain inventory for use in documenting the outcomes of patients with noncancer pain. *Clin J Pain* 2004; 20(5):309–318.

Kerns R, Turk D, Rudy T. The West Haven-Yale Multidimensional Pain Inventory (WHYMPI). *Pain* 1985; 23:345–356.

Krause SJ, Backonja M. Development of a neuropathic pain questionnaire. *Clin J Pain* 2003; 19:306–314.

Krulewitch H, London MR, Skakel VJ, et al. Assessment of pain in cognitively impaired older adults: a comparison of pain assessment tools and their use by nonprofessional caregivers. *J Am Geriatr Soc* 2000; 48:1607–1611.

Kwekkeboom K, Herr K. Assisting older clients with pain management in the home. *Home Health Care Manage Pract* 2003; 15(3):237–250.

Lichtenstein MJ, Dhanda R, Cornell JE, Escalante A, Hazuda HP. Disaggregating pain and its effect on physical functional limitations. *J Gerontol A Biol Sci Med Sci* 1998; 53:M361–M371.

Luggen AS. Chronic pain in older adults: a quality of life issue. *J Gerontol Nurs* 1998; 24:48–54.

Manz B, Mosier R, Nusser-Gerlach M, Bergstrom N, Agrawal S. Pain assessment in the cognitively impaired and unimpaired elderly. *Pain Manage Nurs* 2000; 1(4):106–115.

Mendoza TR, Chen C, Brugger A, et al. The utility and validity of the Modified Brief Pain inventory in a multiple-dose postoperative analgesic trial. *Clin J Pain* 2004; 20(5):357–362.

Melzack R. The McGill Pain Questionnaire: major properties and scoring methods. *Pain* 1975; 1:277–299.

Melzack R. The short-form McGill Pain Questionnaire. *Pain* 1987; 30:191–197.

Miller J, Neelon V, Dalton J, et al. The assessment of discomfort in elderly confused patients: a preliminary study. *J Neurosci Nurs* 1996; 28:175–182.

Mobily PR, Herr KA, Clark MK, Wallace RB. An epidemiologic analysis of pain in the elderly. *J Aging Health* 1994; 6:139–154.

Morrison RS, Ahronheim JC, Morrison GR, et al. Pain and discomfort associated with common hospital procedures and experiences. *J Pain Symptom Manage* 1998; 15(2):91–101.

O'Connor M. Pain management: improving documentation of assessment and intensity. *J Healthc Qual* 2003; 25(1):17–21.

Oldham L, Kristjanson LJ. Development of a pain management programme for family carers of advanced cancer patients. *Int J Palliat Nurs* 2004; 10(2):91–99.

Parmelee PA. Pain in cognitively impaired older persons. *Clin Geriatr Med* 1996; 12:473–487.

Pasero C, Reed BA, McCaffery M. Pain in the elderly. In: McCaffery M, Pasero C (Eds). *Pain: Clinical Manual,* 2nd ed. St. Louis: Mosby, 1999; pp 674–710.

Pautex S, Herrmann F, Lelous P, et al. Feasibility and reliability of four pain self-assessment scales and correlation with an observational rating scale in hospitalized elderly demented patients. *J Gerontol Med Sci* 2005; 60A(4):524–529.

Porter FL, Malhotra KM, Wolf CM, et al. Dementia and response to pain in the elderly. *Pain* 1996; 68:413–421.

Rakel B, Herr K. Assessment and treatment of postoperative pain in older adults. *J Perianesth Nurs* 2004; 19(3):194–208.

Roland M, Morris R. A study of the natural history of back pain, part 1: development of a reliable and sensitive measure of disability in low-back pain. *Spine* 1983; 8:141–144.

Scherder E, Bouma A. Acute versus chronic pain experience in Alzheimer's disease—a new questionnaire. *Dement Geriatr Cogn Disord* 2000; 11:11–16.

Simmons SF, Ferrell, BA, Schnelle JF. Effects of a controlled exercise trial on pain in nursing home residents. *Clin J Pain* 2002; 18(6):380–385.

Stein WM. Cancer pain in the elderly. In: Ferrell BR, Ferrell BA (Eds). *Pain in the Elderly.* Seattle: IASP Press, 1996.

Stein WM. Pain in the nursing home. *Clin Geriatr Med* 2001; 17(3):575–594.

Stein WM, Ferrell BA. Pain in the nursing home. *Clin Geriatr Med* 1996; 12:601–613.

Stuppy DJ. The Faces Pain Scale: reliability and validity with mature adults. *Appl Nurs Res* 1998; 11:84–89.

Tait RC, Chibnall J, Krause S. The Pain Disability Index: psychometric properties. *Pain* 1990; 40:171–182.

Taylor LJ, Herr K. Evaluation of the Faces Pain Scale for use with minority elders. *J Gerontol Nurs* 2002; 28(4):15–23.

Taylor LJ, Herr K. Pain intensity assessment: a comparison of selected pain intensity scales for use in cognitively intact and cognitively impaired African American older adults. *Pain Manage Nurs* 2003; 4(2):87–95.

Theiler R, Bischoff HA, Good M, Uebelhart D. Rofecoxib improves quality of life in patients with hip or knee osteoarthritis. *Swiss Med Wkly* 2002; 132(39–40):566–573.

Tittle MB, McMillan SC, Hagan S. Validating the brief pain inventory for use with surgical patients with cancer. *Oncol Nurs Forum* 2003; 30(2):325–330.

Weiner DK. Assessing persistent pain in older adults: practicalities and pitfalls. *Analgesia* 1999; 4:377–395.

Weiner DK, Hanlon JT. Pain in nursing home residents: management strategies. *Drugs Aging* 2001; 18(1):13–29.

Weiner DK, Herr K. Comprehensive interdisciplinary assessment and treatment planning: an integrative overview. In: Weiner D, Herr K, Rudy T (Eds). *Persistent Pain in Older Adults: An Interdisciplinary Guide for Treatment.* New York: Springer, 2002, pp 18–57.

Weiner D, Pieper C, McConnell E, et al. Pain measurement in elders with chronic low back pain: traditional and alternative approaches. *Pain* 1996; 67:461–467.

Weiner DK, Peterson BL, Logue P, Keefe FJ. Predictors of pain self-report in nursing home residents. *Aging* 1998a; 10:411–420.

Weiner D, Peterson B, Keefe F. Evaluating persistent pain in long term care residents: what role for pain maps? *Pain* 1998b; 76:249–257.

Weiner D, Peterson B, Ladd K, McConnell E, Keefe F. Pain in nursing home residents: an exploration of prevalence, staff perspectives, and practical aspects of measurement. *Clin J Pain* 1999; 15:92–101.

Weiner DK, Rudy TE, Gaur S. Are all older adults with persistent pain created equal? Preliminary evidence for a multiaxial taxonomy. *J Pain Research Manage* 2001; 6(3):133–141.

Weiner DK, Rudy TE, Glick RM, et al. Efficacy of percutaneous electrical nerve stimulation for the treatment of chronic low back pain in older adults. *J Am Geriatr Soc* 2003; 51(5):599–608.

Wells N, Hepworth JT, Murphy BA, Wujcik D, Johnson R. Improving cancer pain management through patient and family education. *J Pain Symptom Manage* 2003; 25(4):344–356.

Won A, Lapane K, Gambassi G, et al. Correlates and management of nonmalignant pain in the nursing home. *J Am Geriatr Soc* 1999; 47:936–942.

Wynne CF, Ling SM, Remsburg R. Comparison of pain assessment instruments in cognitively intact and cognitively impaired nursing home residents. *Geriatr Nurs* 2000; 21:20–23.

Correspondence to: Prof. Keela Herr, PhD, RN, FAAN, Adult and Gerontological Nursing, College of Nursing, 452 NB, The University of Iowa, Iowa City, IA 52242, USA. Email: keela-herr@uiowa.edu.

Pain in Older Persons, Progress in Pain
Research and Management, Vol. 35, edited
by Stephen J. Gibson and Debra K. Weiner,
IASP Press, Seattle, © 2005.

7

Assessing Pain in Older Persons with Severe Limitations in Ability to Communicate

Thomas Hadjistavropoulos

*Department of Psychology, University of Regina,
Regina, Saskatchewan, Canada*

The assessment of the pain patient is a comprehensive task that should involve information about a wide variety of areas of functioning including pain intensity, mood, diagnosis, results of physical examinations, social context, personal history, coping strategy usage, and other related domains. This chapter focuses primarily on the aspect of pain assessment that concerns itself with pain detection and pain intensity.

It is widely agreed upon that pain in seniors is undertreated (Ruda 1993; Jones et al. 1996; Kapp 1996; Ferrell et al. 2001; Weiner et al. 2001), and this concern becomes especially salient when one considers seniors who have serious limitations in ability to communicate due to dementia (e.g., Marzinski 1991; Malloy and Hadjistavropoulos 2004). It is believed that the undertreatment of pain among seniors with severe dementia is partly due to difficulties in detecting pain in this population (e.g., Feldt 2000; Hadjistavropoulos et al. 2001; Herr and Garand 2001; Martin et al., in press). Studies have confirmed that pain problems are often missed by physicians when traditional pain evaluation approaches are employed with dementia patients (Cohen-Mansfield and Lipson 2001; Sengstaken and King 1993).

ASSESSMENT THROUGH A COMMUNICATIONS MODEL OF PAIN

The challenges involved in assessing pain among seniors with cognitive impairments can be conceptualized through a communications model of pain (e.g., Prkachin and Craig 1995; Hadjistavropoulos and Craig 2002; Hadjistavropoulos et al. 2004). The model, based on earlier formulations by Rosenthal (1982), describes an A → B → C process whereby the internal state (A; pain) may be encoded in features of expressive behavior (B) that allow an observer to draw inferences (C) about a patient's internal experiences. The model also construes the complex response to tissue injury as varying with respect to reflexive automaticity and cognitive executive mediation (Hadjistavropoulos and Craig 2002). That is, self-report procedures for assessing pain, which are generally easy for an observer to decode, rely on higher mental processes. The ability to comprehend a question and (usually) the ability to respond verbally or in writing are required. Often, the patient must be able to represent the pain along a 10-cm line or through other representational modes. In persons with dementia, such abilities decline along with abstract reasoning, language skills, and other cognitive capacities. In contrast to self-report procedures, observational methods of assessing pain tend to rely on more automatic forms of pain expression and communication (e.g., grimaces or the reflexive withdrawal of a limb). These automatic forms of pain communication are sometimes more difficult to decode and interpret than self-report information. On the other hand, due to their reflexive automaticity, nonverbal behaviors are more likely to be preserved in situations where higher mental processes are compromised. As such, nonverbal behaviors are a primary focus of this chapter.

SELF-REPORT OF PAIN AMONG SENIORS WITH DEMENTIA

During the early to middle stages of the dementing process (i.e., mild to moderate dementia), the patient's communicative abilities tend to remain sufficient for the verbal communication of the pain experience (see Chapter 6 for more information on assessment procedures suitable for seniors who can communicate verbally). In fact, early to mid-stage dementia patients can often provide valid responses to a variety of self-report assessment tools (e.g., Hadjistavropoulos et al. 1998; Scherder and Bouma 2000; Chibnall and Tait 2001). There is little question, however, that as the dementia progresses, patients become less likely to self-report pain complaints (e.g., Parmelee et al. 1993; Hadjistavropoulos et al. 1997), despite a lack of differences in the prevalence of painful conditions between people with and without cognitive impairments (Proctor and Hirdes 2001).

Self-report measures have been found to differ with respect to their psychometric properties when used with seniors suffering from varying degrees of dementia. In attempting to determine the lowest level of impairment that would permit effective use of self-report scales, Weiner et al. (1999) found that seniors with cognitive impairments who could comprehend a 0– 10-point pain assessment scale had a score of 18–22 (out of 30) on the Mini Mental State Examination (MMSE; Folstein et al. 1975), whereas those who could not comprehend the pain scale tended to have MMSE scores that were closer to 12 and 13.

Chibnall and Tait (2001) studied a group of seniors with cognitive impairments (with an average MMSE score of 18) and found good support for the reliability and validity of the 21-point box scale (Jensen et al. 1998) in their sample. The two researchers also demonstrated that the psychometric properties of the 21-point box scale were superior to those of a verbal rating scale (Melzack 1975) and those of the Faces Pain Scale (Bieri et al. 1990). In a related study, Scherder and Bouma (2000) showed that a modified version of the visual analogue scale, the Coloured Analogue Scale (CAS; McGrath et al. 1996), originally developed for young children with marginal self-report skills, was correctly interpreted by patients at the early stages of Alzheimer's disease and by 80% of patients with mid-stage dementia. Scherder and Bouma's (2000) findings are especially significant because these investigators also asked comprehension questions to assess the participants' understanding of the scale's characteristics. Other researchers also showed that the CAS can be used successfully with patients who have mild to moderate dementia (Hadjistavropoulos et al. 1998), although patients with severe dementia tend to provide invalid responses (Hadjistavropoulos et al. 1997).

Based on the findings of Weiner et al. (1999) and Chibnall and Tait (2001), it would be reasonable to suggest that, as a rule of thumb, an MMSE score of 18 or higher would be a good predictor of whether or not a senior is likely to be able to use unidimensional pain measures such as the 21-point box scale and the CAS. Nonetheless, it would always be important to attempt to obtain some form of self-report, even from individuals with lower MMSE scores, because doing so could often provide useful information. For example, Ferrell et al. (1995) showed that 83% of research participants with an average MMSE score of 12 could complete at least one of four unidimensional pain assessment measures, with the Pain Intensity Scale (PPI) of the McGill Pain Questionnaire (Melzack 1975) having the highest completion rate (65%).

In summary, several unidimensional self-report measures of pain (e.g., 21-point box scale, CAS, PPI) seem to be promising in the assessment of pain among seniors with mild to moderate dementia and should be attempted with such populations. Multidimensional scales (e.g., Ferrell et al. 2000) have not been adequately evaluated among patients with dementia, but they are less likely to be useful as they are more difficult to complete than the unidimensional tools discussed here. In all cases, it is useful and important to cross validate self-reports of pain with observational assessment approaches.

OBSERVATIONAL ASSESSMENT PROCEDURES
FOR SENIORS WITH SEVERE DEMENTIA

We can place the methods that have been developed and validated for seniors with serious limitations in ability to communicate into two broad categories: observational assessment procedures that are primarily useful for research and those that would be potentially useful in busy clinical settings.

OBSERVATIONAL PROCEDURES PRIMARILY
SUITABLE FOR RESEARCH

Facial Action Coding System (FACS). Facial expressions are considered to be extremely useful in the assessment of pain because of their flexibility, salience, rapid transmission time, and reflexive nature (Craig et al. 2001). The FACS (Ekman and Friesen 1978; Ekman et al. 2002) was developed to provide objective descriptions of facial activity. It is an atheoretical, comprehensive, anatomically based system that has been used extensively in pain research. Using slow-motion video, qualified coders systematically identify every facial reaction or "action unit" using explicit and rigorous criteria. The application of FACS to the study of pain reactions has led to the identification of a relatively discrete pattern of facial activity that has been observed both in healthy volunteers and pain patients (e.g., Craig 1992; Prkachin 1992; Hale and Hadjistavropoulos 1997). Generally, the findings show that the facial responses of both cognitively intact and cognitively impaired seniors intensify (compared to a baseline period), even in response to very minor pain (Hadjistavropoulos et al. 1997, 1998, 2002). No substantial differences in the facial responses of cognitively intact and cognitively impaired seniors have been detected using FACS (Hadjistavropoulos et al. 1998), although there appears to be a tendency for participants with cognitive impairments to be somewhat more responsive (Hadjistavropoulos et al. 2000a).

The main advantage of FACS is that it minimizes subjective judgments because of its very explicit and rigorous scoring criteria. Moreover, numerous photographs and practice videos accompany the instructions for coding each observable movement of facial muscles. Table I presents an example describing appearance changes due to a facial action unit described as "AU 5—Upper Lid Raiser."

Table I
Facial Action Coding System description of appearance changes associated with Facial
Action Unit 5 (AU 5—Upper Lid Raiser)

1. Widens the eye aperture.
2. Raises the upper eyelid so that some or all of the upper eyelid disappears from view. In some people the upper eyelid is not visible when the face is neutral, and the disappearance of the upper eyelid cannot be used to determine the action of AU 5.
3. As a result of raising of the upper eyelid, more of the upper portion of the eyeball is exposed. How much is exposed depends upon how much of the upper portion of the eyeball is normally exposed in the neutral position and how strong AU 5 is. Sclera above the iris may also be exposed depending upon the position of the upper lid in the neutral face and how strong AU 5 is.
4. As a result of the raising of the upper eyelid, the shape of the upper rim of the eye changes as portions medially and/or laterally are pulled up. This changed shape of the eye usually results in exposure of more sclera adjacent to the iris medially and/or laterally. Thus, AU 5 causes sclera exposure adjacent to the iris laterally and medially.
5. Due to changes described under appearance changes 3 and 4 above, the person seems to be starting in a fixed fashion almost as if the eyeball were protruding.
6. The lower eyelid also raises, very minutely, when there is a strong AU 5. This happens because the strong AU 5 pulls the skin around the eye, including the lower lid, upwards. It is important to note that this small raise of the lower eyelid due to AU 5 does not involve any evidence of tightening of the skin below the lower lid, which is characteristic of AU 7.
7. If the evidence of AU 5 is apparent in only one eye, score it as bilateral, not unilateral.

Source: Ekman and Friesen (2002, p. 24).

Studies using FACS in pain assessment have demonstrated excellent levels of inter-rater reliability (see Craig et al. 2001). Given its strengths, FACS would be a suitable index of pain for research studies (e.g., clinical trials) involving seniors with cognitive impairments. Its main disadvantage is the time-consuming nature of both the required training and the application of the system. Although FACS scores correlate with observers' global ratings of pain, it is important to exercise caution when considering global ratings as these are affected both by the characteristics and background of the observer (Hadjistavropoulos et al. 1998) as well as by stereotypes such as those relating to the patient's physical appearance (Hadjistavropoulos et al. 1996) and age (Hadjistavropoulos et al. 2000b).

Pain Behavior Measurement (PBM). Another observational procedure that has been used to assess pain among seniors with cognitive impairments is PBM. This approach was originally developed and validated by Keefe and Block (1982). Using this procedure, trained coders note the frequency of clearly defined pain behaviors (guarding, bracing, grimacing, sighing, and rubbing the affected area) while the patient undergoes a series of standardized structured activities such as walking and standing. Weiner and colleagues

(1996) found support for the validity of the system among seniors. Specifically, these researchers found that more physically demanding activities (involving the axial skeleton and requiring movements typically needed for the performance of activities of daily living) resulted in more pain behaviors than did less physically demanding activities.

Hadjistavropoulos et al. (2000a) used the PBM with cognitively intact and cognitively impaired seniors who suffered from a variety of musculoskeletal pain conditions. Consistent with Weiner et al. (1996), their study also showed that the number of PBM behaviors increased during more physically demanding activities as compared to more passive ones. More importantly, cognitive status did not seem to substantially affect the occurrence of these behaviors, suggesting that the system represents a suitable approach for assessing pain among persons with cognitive impairments. Although the PBM system is somewhat less labor intensive than FACS, it is still quite time consuming for use in busy clinical settings, since it has requirements such as standardized protocols for patient activity. It remains, however, a promising tool for research studies involving pain in seniors with cognitive impairments.

OBSERVATIONAL ASSESSMENT PROCEDURES
FOR CLINICAL SETTINGS

While several attempts have been made to develop clinically useful tools for assessing pain among seniors with dementia, most studies have failed to provide evidence of adequate validity and reliability for the various instruments. A second concern relates to the small number of items characterizing many of these assessment tools. Dementia can be due to very diverse causes, and no two seniors with this condition are exactly alike. For instance, in the case of multi-infarct dementia, infarcts can occur in very diverse parts of the brain. The diversity in the nature and location of brain damage characterizing dementia has the potential to affect the pain response in varied ways (Farrell et al. 1996). It could be expected, for example, that dementias primarily affecting the frontal lobes of the brain could lead to more disinhibited pain responses than Alzheimer's disease. Moreover, the diversity in brain damage seen in dementia can cause many patients to display relatively idiosyncratic and unusual responses to pain that may not be captured by instruments comprising a small number of items. Nonetheless, clinically useful pain-screening tools that assume the existence of a wide range of possible pain expressions have begun to emerge, and initial validation data are encouraging (e.g., Fuchs-Lacelle and Hadjistavropoulos 2004).

CLINICAL INSTRUMENTS COMPRISING 10 OR FEWER ITEMS

Discomfort Scale. Hurley et al. (1992) developed a non-pain-specific discomfort scale for use with seniors who have communication difficulties (see also Miller et al. 1996). They generated 26 initial items based on interviews with nursing staff and then reduced the number of items to nine (noisy breathing, negative vocalizations, content facial expression, sad facial expression, frightened facial expression, frown, relaxed body language, tense body language, and fidgeting). These items are rated based on the extent to which they are relevant to a given patient. The tool demonstrated satisfactory internal consistency (0.76), but the validity evidence was based on a gold standard of illness involving fever (as opposed to pain per se), which limits potential application in pain intensity assessments.

Checklist of Nonverbal Pain Indicators (CNPI). Feldt (2000) reported on a modification of previously developed observational tools (the University of Alabama Pain Behavior Scale and the Pain Behavior Checklist) for seniors with cognitive impairments. Feldt's observational measure, the CNPI has a yes/no format and includes the following items: nonverbal vocalizations, facial grimacing or wincing, bracing, rubbing, restlessness, and vocal complaints. Feldt found that these behaviors tended to occur less frequently during rest than during periods of movement, that raters can code these behaviors reliably, and that seniors with cognitive impairments do not differ from seniors without cognitive impairments in their pain response. Although the validation information on this tool appears to be promising, the list of behaviors assessed by Feldt had very low internal consistency (0.54–0.64 range). This low consistency score may present a problem for the checklist and may imply that a construct other than pain is being measured by some of the items.

Pain Assessment in Advanced Dementia (PAINAD). The PAINAD (Warden et al. 2003) consists of the following five items (each of which is scored on a scale ranging from 0 to 2): breathing, negative vocalization, facial expression, body language, and consolability. The items are accompanied by detailed descriptors. The psychometric properties of the PAINAD were evaluated among patients with severe dementia (as assessed by the MMSE). The scale demonstrated satisfactory inter-rater reliability, but, like the CNPI (Feldt 2000), it had low internal consistency (at least under some of the administration conditions). In terms of validation, there were differences between scores obtained before and after the patients had received pain medication (although the raters may not have been "blind" with respect to whether or not medication had been administered).

Pain Assessment in the Communicatively Impaired (PACI). Kaasalainen and Crook (2003) used an unpublished measure, the PACI (developed by a group headed by J. Middleton), to assess pain in a group of nursing home residents whose cognitive functioning ranged from intact to severely impaired (no cognitive functioning test scores were reported). The PACI consists of seven items (brow lower, eyelid tighter, cheek raised, guarding, rubbing/touching, and two items referring to sounds and words that are associated with pain). Each item is scored as present or absent, with a possible range of scores from "0 = no pain" to "7 = high pain." The PACI demonstrated good interrater reliability and correlated moderately with cognitively intact residents' self-reports of pain. Nonetheless, the corresponding correlations were not significant for the residents with mild cognitive impairments, nor for the residents with severe impairments. Once the development and initial validation work on this instrument are published, it will become easier to evaluate its properties.

Abbey Scale. More recently, Abbey et al. (2004) published the Abbey Scale, a tool that consists of six items (vocalization, facial expression, change in body language, behavioral change, physiological change, and physical change). Each item is scored on a four-point scale ranging from "Absent = 0" to "Severe = 3." The items were derived from pre-existing scales by Hurley et al. (1992) and Simons and Malabar (1995) and were modified with the aid of a panel of experts in a study using the Delphi technique (e.g., Dalkey 1969), a method of refining and eliciting group opinions. A strength of this scale, relative to other scales with a small number of items (e.g., Feldt 2000; Warden et al. 2003), is its satisfactory internal consistency (0.74 to 0.81). In terms of validity, scores changed significantly following pain interventions by nurses (who filled out the scale and were not blind with respect to whether or not the intervention was administered).

Non-Communicating Patient's Pain Assessment Instrument (NOPPAIN). This instrument, developed by Snow et al. (2004) based on the advice of a multidisciplinary expert panel, emphasizes patient observations during common care tasks. For each task (e.g., bathing or dressing the resident), the person completing the scale provides a "yes" or "no" answer to the question "Did you see pain when you did this?" He or she then indicates along five-point scales the extent to which the patient exhibited each of six reactions (i.e., facial expressions of pain, pain-related words, bracing, pain noises, rubbing, and restlessness). The scale concludes with an overall pain rating ("No pain" to "Pain is almost unbearable") in response to the instruction: "Rate the resident's pain at the highest level you saw it during care." The scale was validated using six video segments of an actress portraying a bed-bound patient and displaying varying degrees of reactivity while basic personal care tasks were being performed. There was satisfactory inter-rater agreement on the ratings, which also corresponded to the pain intensity conditions displayed on the video. These findings must be replicated while assessing real (as opposed to simulated) patients, in order to evaluate this procedure more adequately.

DOLOPLUS-2. Another instrument, used primarily in French-speaking settings, is the DOLOPLUS-2 (Wary 1999), which was developed in French. It consists of five somatic, two psychomotor, and three psychosocial items. The items are scored on 0–3-point scales. Each rating is clearly defined. For example, under the somatic item "sleep pattern," 0 = normal sleep, 1 = difficult to go to sleep, 2 = frequent awakening (restless), and 3 = insomnia. The DOLOPLUS-2 has satisfactory inter-rater reliability (although specific coefficients were not reported) and is significantly correlated with scores on the visual analogue scale (among patients who can complete the scale; Lefebvre-Chapiro and DOLOPLUS 2001). Unlike some of the other brief instruments reviewed in this section, the DOLOPLUS-2 has satisfactory internal consistency of 0.82. Nonetheless, the tool has been criticized for its limited range of items (Gonthier et al. 1999). Overall, the DOLOPLUS-2 approach appears promising, although additional validity evidence is needed. At the time of this writing, an English translation of the scale was available at www.doloplus.com. Investigation of the psychometric properties of the English version is needed. It is worth noting that other groups have also worked on the development and adaptation of French-language pain assessment tools for seniors with limited ability to communicate (e.g., Jean et al. 1998), but validity and reliability evidence is limited.

Pain Assessment Tool in Confused Older Adults (PATCOA). Decker and Perry (2003) developed this nine-item (moaning, quivering, guarding, clenching the jaws, sighing, pointing to where it hurts, reluctance to move, frowning, and grimacing) observational tool to assess pain among "confused older adults." Nonetheless, the PATCOA was investigated among cognitively intact adults undergoing orthopedic surgery, of whom only a very small portion were "confused." Moreover, the internal consistency of the instrument was unsatisfactory. As such, more research (and possibly refinement of the PATCOA items) is needed before clinical use of this tool with older adults who are in a confused state can be recommended with confidence.

Nonverbal Adult Pain Assessment Scale (NVPS). Odhner et al. (2003) developed the NVPS based on a measure (Merkel et al. 1997) that was initially designed for the assessment of children. The NVPS consists of five items (face, activity, guarding, physiologic I, and physiologic II), each of which is rated along a three-point scale. For example, the item "face" is scored as follows: 0 = no particular expression or smile; 1 = occasional grimace, tearing, frowning, or wrinkled forehead; 2 = frequent grimace, tearing, frowning, or wrinkled forehead. The intent of the researchers was to facilitate the assessment of burn unit patients who were intubated and "unable to produce an audible cry." There is no indication in their article that any of the patients, used in a pilot study, had cognitive impairments. The developers demonstrated that, when nurses filled out the tool on the bedside, its internal consistency was good. More research is needed before clinical use of this tool with seniors who have cognitive impairments can be recommended with confidence.

CLINICAL INSTRUMENTS COMPRISING MORE THAN 10 ITEMS

Amy's Guide. Galloway and Turner (1999) developed Amy's Guide, which consists of a list of 36 pain behaviors, for the assessment of pain among elders with cognitive impairments. However, the authors provided no strong evidence of reliability and validity. Essentially, the items were derived from interviews with nurses and were subsequently confirmed in focus groups with nurses. The authors advise that the health professional should select three to four pain indicators (e.g., "frightened facial expression," "feeling grumpy," and "yelling or shouting") that characterize each patient and, if these pain indicators are present, consider the administration of medications.

Scale developed by Simons and Malabar. Simons and Malabar (1995) attempted to validate an observational approach consisting of 25 behaviors (largely derived from the pre-existing literature) grouped into six categories (verbal response, facial expression, body language, physiological change, behavioral changes, and conscious state). However, design limitations limit the usefulness of the work; for example, there were no statistical analyses reported, and raters were not blind to the use of pain interventions. Moreover, a clear scoring scheme was not described.

Pain Assessment in Dementing Elderly (PADE). The PADE (Villanueva et al. 2003) consists of 24 items generated based on a review of the literature. The items are organized into three categories: Physical (posture, facial expression, breathing pattern), Global Assessment (overall pain rating), and Functional (activities of daily living). Many of the items refer to behaviors that are commonly believed to reflect pain and related distress. However, other items are confounded with dementia severity (e.g., eating independently) or seem less relevant to pain (e.g., whether the patient is indicating that he or she wants to leave the facility). The instrument has satisfactory interrater reliability. Some items are scored along visual analogue scales and others using four-point scales (e.g., independence in eating is rated as follows:

1 = independent, 2 = supervision, 3 = limited, and 4 = extensive/total). To assess the validity of the tool, the researchers compared patients with and without pain-related diagnoses and initially did not find any group differences on PADE scores. When they classified the patients with respect to whether pain was a significant clinical factor (which resulted in only two patients shifting groups), the PADE discriminated between these two groups, but so did a measure of verbal agitation. Therefore, it would be important to demonstrate the specificity of the PADE as a measure of pain rather than as an index of agitation. Moreover, the severity of the participating patients' dementia is not entirely clear, especially given that at least some patients were able to provide their own consent for study participation. The authors described the level of dementia as "moderate" to "severe," although no test scores were reported regarding dementia severity.

Pain Assessment Checklist for Seniors with Limited Ability to Communicate (PACSLAC). A more recent effort involved the development of the PACSLAC (Fuchs-Lacelle and Hadjistavropoulos 2004). The scale contains 60 items (organized into four groups: "facial expressions," "activity/body movement," "social/personality/mood indicators," and "physiological indicators/eating/sleeping changes/vocal behavior"), which are scored as present or absent. The vast majority of nurse research participants took less than 5 minutes to complete the checklist, supporting the potential suitability of this tool for busy clinical settings. The PACSLAC items were derived from interviews with experienced professional caregivers of seniors with severe dementia and serious limitations in ability to communicate. The initial internal consistency of the PACSLAC was 0.92, and all items were rated as useful in pain identification by nurses. Moreover, the scale could discriminate among calm events, pain events (for which there was a clear cause for the pain such as a fall), and non-pain-related distress events (such as when a relative was leaving the hospital). The level of dementia severity (i.e., very advanced dementia) of the sample was confirmed through scores on the Present Functioning Questionnaire (Crockett et al. 1989). Although the validation of the tool was based on retrospective nurses' reports about recent pain and non-painful distress events affecting the residents, the initial validation data were encouraging. Moreover, the broad range of pain behaviors covered by the PACSLAC decreases the likelihood of missing less common forms of pain expression that can characterize many residents. Collection of normative data for the PACSLAC is now ongoing (Fuchs-Lacelle and Hadjistavropoulos, in progress). Moreover, the scale has been translated into French, and a validation of the French version is also underway by a group headed by M. Aubin at Laval University, Quebec. Fuchs-Lacelle and Hadjistavropoulos (2004) indicated that until more systematic normative information on the PACSLAC becomes available, clinicians could collect normative information at their specific settings and use it to determine patient deviations from such local norms.

DECIDING WHICH OBSERVATIONAL PROCEDURE
TO USE IN THE CLINICAL SETTING

Over the last few years there has been a proliferation of new pain assessment scales for seniors with dementia. These instruments vary in both length and content. Unless a radically different and valid approach is identified, it would be far more productive for researchers to work toward the further validation and improvement of existing measures than to continue developing new ones.

On the surface, the brief instruments (the Abbey Scale, NOPPAIN, CNPI, PAINAD, PACI, and DOLOPLUS-2) may appeal to clinicians. However, tools with few items may be likely to miss the less common, more idiosyncratic pain expressions that may characterize many patients with dementia. It must be acknowledged, however, that this remains an empirical question. It would be important for future studies of patients with dementia to compare the sensitivity and specificity of briefer versus longer pain assessment tools.

Measures such as the PACSLAC are longer but still take only approximately 5 minutes to complete and show initial promise However, for most of the tools reported here, additional clinical norms are needed in order to facilitate clinical use. Such norms will assist with determinations of pain severity for the individual patient. Until such norms become available, clinicians can collect baseline data on individual patients and examine fluctuations of scores over time as one (but not the only) source of pain-related information. Moreover, the collection of local norms at specific clinical settings could also assist clinicians in evaluating whether a given patient is displaying more pain-related behaviors than other patients. Table II outlines some general recommendations as to how clinicians might wish to approach the pain assessment of seniors with dementia.

Following the normatization and further validation of some of the most promising tools described here, the field must explore other areas relating to pain assessment in the older adult with severe dementia. As we have suggested elsewhere (e.g., Fuchs-Lacelle and Hadjistavropoulos 2004), future research can focus on the more effective detection of pain location in this population. For example, certain behaviors such as limping are more likely to be indicative of pain affecting the leg, foot, or low back. Rubbing an

Table II
Recommendations for the clinician

General Recommendations

Use assessment approaches that include both observational and self-report measures when possible.

Take into account patient history, interview information, and the results of physical examinations.

Self-report measures such as the Coloured Analogue Scale, the 21-point box scale, and a verbal rating scale should be attempted with seniors whose cognitive functioning ranges from intact to mildly or moderately impaired.

The PACSLAC* appears to be a promising tool for assessing pain among persons with cognitive impairments. The initial psychometric findings are encouraging, and the scale can be used with caution. Alternative instruments are also available (e.g., Feldt 2000), but some have significant limitations.

A comprehensive pain assessment should also include evaluations of other related aspects of patient functioning, such as mood, quality of life, coping resources, and social support.

Specific Recommendations Following the Selection of Suitable Assessment Tools

Use an individualized approach, collecting baseline scores for each patient.

Solicit the assistance of caregivers familiar with the patients.

If assessment tools are used to monitor pain levels over time, they must be used under consistent circumstances (e.g., during a structured program of physiotherapy, or over the course of a typical evening).

Most of the assessment tools reviewed in this chapter are screening instruments and, as such, they cannot be considered to represent definitive indicators of pain.

* PACSLAC = Pain Assessment Checklist for Seniors with Limited Ability to Communicate.

affected area is likely to be indicative of pain in that area. Systematic exploration of such behaviors could prove to be a fruitful direction for future studies. Another issue that deserves more research attention is that of specificity. That is, it is important for researchers to demonstrate that the scales reviewed in this chapter are not only sensitive with respect to the identification of pain but can also differentiate pain states from other types of emotional distress. Preliminary work focusing on the ability of the PACSLAC to differentiate pain from general distress is promising (Fuchs-Lacelle and Hadjistavropoulos 2004), but more research in this area is needed.

It must be noted that, given evidence that seniors with mild to moderate dementia can provide valid responses to a variety of unidimensional self-report assessment tools such as the CAS and 21-point box scale, such tools should be used with these patients in conjunction with observational procedures (see Table II). Moreover, scores on pain assessment measures should always be considered in conjunction with patient history, social-contextual factors, results of physical examinations, and the overall functioning of the patient.

CONCLUSIONS

The assessment of pain among seniors with severe limitations in ability to communicate is an area that was largely neglected by researchers for many years. Over the last 5 to 6 years, however, there has been increasing interest in this topic. We have now moved from research that was simply increasing our understanding of the problem of pain assessment in this population to research with direct clinical implications (e.g., the development of useful assessment tools) and potential impact on the lives of suffering patients. While more remains to be done, pain assessment tools are becoming available for clinicians to use in their efforts to increase the well-being and quality of life of seniors who suffer from dementia.

ACKNOWLEDGMENTS

Preparation of this chapter was supported, in part, by a Canadian Institutes of Health Research Investigator Award to Thomas Hadjistavropoulos and by a Canadian Institutes of Health Research New Emerging Team grant. The comments of Jaime Williams are gratefully acknowledged.

REFERENCES

Abbey J, Piller N, De Bellis A, et al. The Abbey pain scale: a 1-minute numerical indicator for people with end-stage dementia. *Int J Palliat Nurs* 2004; 10:6–13.

Bieri D, Reeves R, Champion G, Addicoat L, Ziegler JB. The Faces Pain Scale for the self-assessment of the severity of pain experienced by children: development, initial validation, and preliminary investigation for ratio scale properties. *Pain* 1990; 41:139–150.

Chibnall JT, Tait R. Pain assessment in cognitively impaired and unimpaired older adults: a comparison of four scales. *Pain* 2001; 92:173–186.

Craig KD. The facial expression of pain: better than a thousand words? *Am Pain Soc J* 1992; 1:153–162.

Craig KD, Prkachin KM, Grunau RE. The facial expression of pain. In: Turk DC, Melzack R (Eds). *Handbook of Pain Assessment,* 2nd ed. New York: Guilford Press, 2001, pp 153–169.

Cohen-Mansfield J, Lipson S. Pain in cognitively impaired nursing home residents: how well are physicians diagnosing it? *J Am Geriatr Soc* 2001; 50:1039–1044.

Crockett J, Tuokko H., Koch W, Parks R. The assessment of everyday functioning using the Present Functioning Questionnaire and the Functional Rating Scale in elderly samples. *Clin Gerontol* 1989; 8:3–25.

Dalkey NK. *The Delphi Method: An Experimental Study of Group Opinion.* Santa Monica: Rand, 1969.

Decker SA, Perry AG. The development and testing of the PATCOA to assess pain in older adults. *Pain Manage Nurs* 2003; 4:77–86.

Ekman P, Friesen W. *Investigator's Guide to the Facial Action Coding System.* Palo Alto: Consulting Psychologists Press, 1978.

Ekman P, Friesen W, Hager JC. *Facial Action Coding System.* Salt Lake City: Network Information Research Corporation, 2002.

Farrell MJ, Katz B, Helme RD. The impact of dementia on the pain experience. *Pain* 1996; 67:7–15.

Feldt KS. The checklist of nonverbal pain indicators (CNPI). *Pain Manag Nurs* 2000; 1:13–21.

Ferrell BA, Ferrell BR, Rivera L. Pain in cognitively impaired nursing home patients. *J Pain Symptom Manage* 1995; 10:591–598.

Ferrell BA, Stein WE, Beck JC. The Geriatric Pain Measure: validity reliability and factor analysis. *J Am Geriatr Soc* 2000; 48:1669–1673.

Ferrell BR, Novy D, Sullivan MD, et al. Ethical dilemmas in pain management. *J Pain* 2001; 2:171–180.

Folstein ML, Folstein SE, McHugh PR. Mini-mental state: a practical method for grading the cognitive status of patients for the clinician. *J Psychiatr Res* 1975; 12:189–198.

Fuchs-Lacelle S, Hadjistavropoulos T. Development and preliminary validation of the Pain Assessment Checklist for Seniors with Limited Ability to Communicate (PACSLAC). *Pain Manag Nurs* 2004; 5:37–49.

Galloway S, Turner L. Pain assessment in older adults who are cognitively impaired. *J Gerontol Nurs* 1999; July:34–39.

Gonthier R, Vassal P, Diana MC, Richard A, Navez ML. Sémiologie et evaluation de la douleur chez le sujet dement ou non communicant. *InfoKara* 1999; 53:12–23.

Hadjistavropoulos T, Craig KD. A theoretical framework for understanding self-report and observational measures of pain. *Behav Res Ther* 2002; 40:551–570.

Hadjistavropoulos T, McMurtry B, Craig KD. Beautiful faces in pain: biases and accuracy in the perception of pain. *Psychol Health* 1996; 11:411–420.

Hadjistavropoulos T, Craig KD, Martin N, Hadjistavropoulos H, McMurtry B. Toward a research outcome measure of pain in frail elderly in chronic care. *Pain Clin* 1997; 10:71–79.

Hadjistavropoulos T, LaChapelle D, MacLeod F, Hale C, O'Rourke NO. Cognitive functioning and pain reactions in hospitalized elders. *Pain Res Manage* 1998; 3:145–151.

Hadjistavropoulos T, LaChapelle D, MacLeod F, Snider B, Craig KD. Measuring movement exacerbated pain in cognitively impaired frail elders. *Clin J Pain* 2000a; 16:54–63.

Hadjistavropoulos T, LaChapelle D, Hale C, MacLeod F. Age- and appearance-based stereotypes about patients undergoing a painful medical procedure. *Pain Clin* 2000b; 12:25–34.

Hadjistavropoulos T, von Baeyer C, Craig KD. Pain assessment in persons with limited ability to communicate. In: Turk DC, Melzack R (Eds). *Handbook of Pain Assessment,* 2nd ed. New York: Guilford Press, 2001, pp 134–149.

Hadjistavropoulos T, LaChapelle D, Hadjistavropoulos HD, Green S, Asmundson GJG. Using facial expressions to assess musculoskeletal pain in older adults. *Eur J Pain* 2002; 6:179–187.

Hadjistavropoulos T, Craig KD, Fuchs-Lacelle S. Social influences and the communication of pain. In: Hadjistavropoulos T, Craig KD (Eds). *Pain: Psychological Perspectives.* Mahwah, NJ: Lawrence Erlbaum, 2004, pp 87–112.

Hale C, Hadjistavropoulos T. Emotional components of pain. *Pain Res Manage* 1997; 2:217–225.

Herr KA, Garand L. Assessment and measurement of pain in older adults. *Clin Geriatr Med* 2001; 17:457–478.

Hurley AC, Volicer BJ, Hanrahan PA, Houde S, Volicer L. Assessment of discomfort in Alzheimer patients. *Res Nurs Health* 1992; 15:369–377.

Jean A, Morello R, Alix M. Evaluation de la douleur du sujet très âgé hospitalizé en long séjour. *Revue Gériatrie* 1998; 23:253–256.

Jensen MP, Miller L, Fisher LD. Assessment of pain during medical procedures: a comparison of three scales. *Clin J Pain* 1998; 14:343–349.

Jones JS, Johnson K, McNinch M. Age as a risk factor for inadequate emergency department analgesia. *Am J Emerg Med* 1996; 14:157–160.

Kaasalainen S, Crook J. A comparison of pain-assessment tools for use with elderly long-term-care residents. *Can J Nurs Res* 2003; 35:58–71.

Kapp MB. The ethics of pain management in older adults. In: Woods RT (Ed). *Care of the Aged.* New York: John Wiley and Sons, 2003, pp 267–282.

Keefe FJ, Block AR. Development of an observational method for assessing pain behavior in chronic low back pain patients. *Behav Ther* 1982; 12:63–375.

Lefebvre-Chapiro S, DOLOPLUS. DOLOPLUS®-2: une échelle d' héteroévaluation de la douleur du sujet âgé non communiquant. *J Eur Soins Palliatifs* 2001; 8:191–194.

Malloy DC, Hadjistavropoulos T. The problem of pain management among persons with dementia, personhood and the ontology of relationships. *Nurs Philos* 2004; 5:147–159.

Martin R, Williams J, Hadjistavropoulos T, Hadjistavropoulos HD, MacLean M. A qualitative investigation of seniors' and caregivers' views on pain assessment and management. *Can J Nurs Res;* in press.

Marzinski LR. The tragedy of dementia: clinically assessing pain in the confused nonverbal elderly. *J Gerontol Nurs* 1991; 17:15–28.

McGrath PA, Seifert CE, Speechley KN, et al. A new analogue scale for assessing children's pain. *Pain* 1996; 64:437–443.

Melzack R. The McGill Pain Questionnaire: major properties and scoring methods. *Pain* 1975; 1:191–197.

Miller J, Neelon V, Dalton J, et al. The assessment of discomfort in elderly confused patients: a preliminary study. *J Neurosci Nurs* 1996; 28:175–182.

Odhner M, Wegman D, Freeland, N, Steinmetz A, Ingersol GL. Assessing pain control in nonverbal critically ill adults. *Dimens Crit Care Nurs* 2003; 22:260–267.

Parmelee PA, Smith B, Katz IR. Pain complaints and cognitive status among elderly institution residents. *J Am Geriatr Soc* 1993; 41:517–522.

Prkachin KM. The consistency of facial expressions of pain: a comparison across modalities. *Pain* 1992; 51:297–306.

Prkachin KM, Craig KD. Expressing pain: the communication and interpretation of facial pain signals. *J Nonverb Behav* 1995; 19:191–205.

Proctor WR, Hirdes JP. Pain and cognitive status among nursing home residents in Canada. *Pain Res Manage* 2001; 6:119–125.

Rosenthal R. Conducting judgment studies. In: Scherer K, Ekman D (Eds). *Handbook of Methods in Nonverbal Behavior Research.* New York: Cambridge University Press, 1982, pp 287–361.

Ruda MA. Gender and pain. *Pain* 1993; 53:1–2.

Scherder EJA, Bouma A. Visual analogue scales for pain assessment in Alzheimer's disease. *Gerontology* 2000; 46:47–53.

Sengstaken EA, King SA. The problems of pain and its detection among geriatric nursing home residents. *J Am Geriatr Soc* 1993; 41:541–544.

Simons W, Malabar R. Assessing pain in elderly persons who cannot respond verbally. *J Adv Nurs* 1995; 22:663–669.

Snow AL, Weber JB, O'Malley KJ, et al. NOPPAIN: a nursing assistant-administered pain assessment instrument for use in dementia. *Dement Geriatr Cogn Disord* 2004; 17:240–246.

Villanueva MR, Smith TL, Erickson JS, et al. Pain assessment for the dementing elderly (PADE): reliability and validity of a new measure. *J Am Med Dir Assoc* 2003; 4:1–8.

Warden V, Hurley AC, Volicer L. Development and psychometric evaluation of the Pain Assessment in Advanced Dementia (PAINAD) scale. *J Am Med Dir Assoc* 2003; 4:9–15.

Wary B. Doloplus-2, une échelle pour évaluer la douleur. *Soins Gerontol* 1999; 19:25–27.

Weiner D, Pieper C, McConnell E, Martinez S, Keefe F. Pain measurement in elders with chronic low back pain: traditional and alternative approaches. *Pain* 1996; 67:461–467.

Weiner D, Peterson B, Lad K, McConnell, Keefe F. Pain in nursing home residents: an exploration of prevalence, staff perspectives and practical aspects of measurement. *Clin J Pain* 1999; 15:92–101.
Weiner DK, Rudy TE, Gaur S. Are all older adults with persistent pain created equal? Preliminary evidence for a multi-axial taxonomy. *Pain Res Manage* 2001; 6:133–141.

Correspondence to: Thomas Hadjistavropoulos, PhD, Department of Psychology and Centre on Aging and Health, University of Regina, Regina, SK, Canada S4S 0A2. Email: thomas.hadjistavropoulos@uregina.ca.

Pain in Older Persons, Progress in Pain Research and Management, Vol. 35, edited by Stephen J. Gibson and Debra K. Weiner, IASP Press, Seattle, © 2005.

8

Functional Assessment of Older Adults with Chronic Pain

Thomas E. Rudy[a,b,c,d] and Susan J. Lieber[a,d]

Departments of [a]Anesthesiology, [b]Psychiatry, and [c]Biostatistics and [d]Pain Evaluation and Treatment Institute, University of Pittsburgh, Pittsburgh, Pennsylvania, USA

Chronic pain frequently affects a wide range of parameters relevant to older adults, including mood, physical function, sleep, and appetite. For many, loss of independence related to impaired physical function is of central importance (Leveille et al. 1999). Thus, functional status is a critical component of geriatrics, and is essential for planning treatment, determining efficacy of treatment, maintaining continuity of care, and developing and improving treatment resources. However, the link between chronic pain and function remains unclear. Clinically, older adults with chronic pain often indicate that they experience pain when performing functional activities or that pain curtails their activity involvement (Scudds and Robertson 1998). From a research perspective, however, the relationship between pain and physical function in older adults has not been studied either extensively or comprehensively (Hopman-Rock et al. 1996). Perhaps the most in-depth investigation of the pain-function relationship has occurred in clinical studies of osteoarthritis of the hip, knee, or back. These studies support: (1) a high prevalence of arthritis-related pain (McAlindon et al. 1993), (2) decreases in function associated with pain (Hopman-Rock et al. 1996), (3) pain as a significant predictor of disability (Holm et al. 1998), and (4) the important mediating role of psychological factors on both pain and function (Hopman-Rock et al. 1998; Creamer et al. 1999). Many of the studies on pain and function in the older adult have, however, have used a narrow definition of function (e.g., limited to range of motion).

To understand the true impact of pain on older adults, function needs to be broadly defined. Health care professionals use the term "function" in a multitude of ways, often biased by their specific specialty orientation and training. Functional impact is used to refer to concepts as diverse as a loss or limitation in a body organ or part, restrictions in activities of daily living, restriction in social roles, and disability or handicap.

The framework proposed by the World Health Organization (2001), entitled *International Classification of Functioning, Disability, and Health* (known as ICF), appears to us to be a sufficiently broad conceptual system to guide the assessment of the functional impact of pain in older adults. In the ICF, functioning is seen as an umbrella term encompassing all body functions, activities, and participation; similarly, disability serves as an umbrella term for impairments, activity limitations, or participation restrictions. Within the ICF, the environmental factors interact with functioning and disability. In this way, this framework enables one to develop useful profiles of an individual's functioning, disability, and health in various domains. It should be noted that the ICF has moved away from being a "consequences of disease" classification system to become a "components of health" classification. That is, it classifies health and health-related states. In the ICF, persons are not the units of classification; rather, it describes the situation of each person within an array of health or health-related domains.

Table I provides an overview of the primary components and concepts of the ICF. For the purposes of this chapter, we will focus primarily on the assessment of Activities and Participation component, and to a lesser degree on Contextual Factors (i.e., environmental and personal factors). The ICF defines *activity* as the execution of a task or action by an individual, *participation* as involvement in a life situation, *activity limitations* as the difficulties an individual may have in executing activities, and *participation restrictions* as the problems an individual may experience in involvement in life situations. The nine domains for the Activities and Participation component are designed to cover the full range of life areas, from basic learning and self-care to complex interpersonal and social interactions. These domains are: (1) learning and applying knowledge; (2) general tasks and demands; (3) communication; (4) mobility; (5) self-care; (6) domestic life; (7) interpersonal interactions and relationships; (8) major life areas; and (9) community, social, and civic life. Each of these nine domains is further defined by two important qualifiers, performance and capacity. The *performance* qualifier describes what an individual does in his or her current environment, indicating that the social context also needs to be considered when evaluating performance. The *capacity* qualifier, on the other hand, describes an individual's ability to execute a task or an action. This construct aims to indicate the highest probable level of functioning that a person may reach in a given domain at a given moment.

Table I
Overview of World Health Organization ICF model

	Part 1: Functioning and Disability		Part 2: Contextual Factors	
Components	Body Functions and Structures	Activities and Participation	Environmental Factors	Personal Factors
Domains	Body functions, body structures	Life areas (tasks, actions)	External influences on functioning and disability	Internal influences on functioning and disability
Constructs	Change in body functions (physiological) Change in body structures (anatomical)	Capacity: executing tasks in a standard environment Performance: executing tasks in the current environment	Facilitating or hindering impact of features of the physical, social, and attitudinal world	Impact of attributes of the person
Positive aspect (functioning)	Functional and structural integrity	Participation in activities	Facilitators	Not applicable
Negative aspect (disability)	Impairment	Activity limitation, participation restriction	Barriers/ hindrances	Not applicable

Source: International Classification of Functioning, Disability, and Health (World Health Organization 2001).

Both capacity and performance qualifiers can be evaluated with and without assistive devices or personal assistance. Difficulties or problems in these domains can arise when there is a qualitative or quantitative alteration in the way in which an individual carries out these domain functions. Labeled as *limitations* or *restrictions,* these functional problems should be assessed against a generally accepted population standard. Specifically, the standard or norm against which an individual's capacity and performance is compared should be that of an individual without a similar health condition (such as a disease, disorder, or injury). Later in this chapter we will apply these ICF standards to the functional assessment of older adults with chronic low back pain (LBP).

Contextual factors in the ICF represent the complete background of an individual's life and living, and include two components—environmental factors and personal factors. *Environmental factors* make up the physical, social, and attitudinal environment in which people conduct their lives. These factors are considered external to individuals, but can have a positive or negative influence on their performance, their capacity to execute actions or tasks, and their body function or structure. From this viewpoint, disability is characterized as the outcome or result of a complex relationship between (1) an individual's health condition and personal factors and (2) the external factors that represent the circumstances in which the individual lives. Because of this relationship, different environments may have a very different impact on the same individual with a given health condition.

Personal factors are the particular background of an individual's life and living; they comprise features of the individual that are not part of a given health condition. These factors may include gender, ethnicity, other health conditions, fitness, lifestyle, habits, upbringing, coping styles, social background, education, psychological characteristics, and so forth. Although personal factors are not classified in the ICF, their contribution is considered of central importance because of their potential to significantly affect functional assessment and the outcome of treatment interventions.

The conceptual model of functioning proposed by the ICF seems well suited to guide the functional evaluation of older adults with chronic pain. Some of its many strengths include the integration of diverse factors that may influence performance and disability; its inclusion of psychosocial and environmental factors and the significant impact they can have on functioning; and the use of a standardized, clearly defined, and common language that permits communication about functioning across various disciplines and sciences. With this conceptual model in mind, in the rest of this chapter we will review some of the domains that we believe significantly affect functioning in older adults with chronic pain and review and recommend assessment instruments that clinicians and investigators can use to measure the functional impacts of chronic pain in older adults, highlighting some of the strengths and limitations of these approaches. In keeping with ICF recommendations, we will present some of our norm-referenced research that shows functional assessment differences between older adults with and without chronic LBP, and which measures seem best in detecting these differences. We will also make discipline-specific recommendations for time-efficient functional assessment methods that can be used for older adults with chronic pain.

DOMAINS INFLUENCING FUNCTION IN OLDER ADULTS

The significant prevalence and incidence of chronic pain in older adults reviewed in Chapter 1 highlights the importance of using valid and reliable instruments to measure pain (see Chapters 6 and 7) and its functional impact. It is important for clinicians to bear in mind that the presence of comorbid medical conditions, such as cardiovascular disease, diabetes, and hypertension, often adversely affects function, complicates the presentation of pain, and interferes with treatment interventions.

BIOLOGICAL DOMAIN

Although further research is needed to evaluate the common conception that having pain is part of the natural course of aging, it is important to underscore that pain of any intensity that negatively affects function is not a normal part of aging. Rather, it is reasonable to consider its underlying pathology as a disease process that can potentially accelerate the linear senescence associated with natural aging (Fries and Crapo 1981). Natural aging leads to changes within the biological domain, which may affect functional performance. Within this broad domain lie the neurological and musculoskeletal systems that merit further consideration in older adults with pain conditions. Natural age-associated changes in the neurological system include cerebral atrophy, decreased effectiveness of neurotransmitters, slowing of nerve conduction velocities, loss of motor fibers, and reduced cerebral blood flow. While additional research is needed to determine the extent to which these and other changes are directly linked to functional decline, it appears that these age-related sensory-motor changes contribute to decreased sensation and strength, postural instability, and abnormal gait patterns (Wagner and Kauffman 2001).

Maintenance of balance in static positions and dynamic conditions as well as coordination of movements are two of the key neurologically based components necessary for successful execution of daily activities. Closely linked to balance is the ability to achieve and maintain postural control. In a recent study of older adults conducted by Hirose et al. (2004), abnormal posture was associated with decreased functional performance and with gait disturbances that were not detected in a control group with normal posture. Interestingly, abnormal posture was not correlated with pain reports. Common gait changes associated with aging include decreased step length, stride length, walking velocity, ankle range of motion, and push-off with the toes, as well as increased double stance time.

Widespread changes in the neurochemistry, structure, and function of the central nervous system have the potential to interfere with pain transmission, and as a result influence an individual's pain sensitivity (Gibson and Farrell 2004). Pain associated with osteoarthritis is most often associated with activity and consequently can impact functional performance and ultimately quality of life. For example, decreased proprioception and increased pain intensity have been associated with functional decline in subjects with osteoarthritis of the knee (Sharma et al. 2003).

Although there are common age-related cognitive changes that require adaptation and consequently influence functional performance, they do not necessarily have a significant impact on everyone. Mildly diminished problem-solving, psychomotor, and perceptual skills influence an individual's ability to use and adapt to new information (Riley 2001). However, these changes are not likely to be significant enough to affect the performance of instrumental and basic activities of daily living (ADLs). Changes in memory are often the most feared in older adults. While this area has undergone extensive evaluation by researchers, the memory essential for performing daily life tasks, work, and interpersonal relationships, currently referred to as working memory, has only recently gained scientific attention. For example, Belleville et al. (1998) found that older adults have difficulty processing information contained in working memory, making it harder to perform tasks that require both the retention and manipulation of information, such as following written instructions or solving math problems.

In contrast to the neurological changes, those manifested in the musculoskeletal system, such as the loss of muscle strength and slowing of movement, are more readily apparent both to the individual and his or her clinician (Leveille 2004). A growing body of literature has confirmed a significant relationship between muscle strength and lower extremity function and has detailed the role of loss of strength in predicting future disability in older adults (Visser et al. 2000). In an effort to define the mechanisms that underlie the loss in strength, sarcopenia—the age-related loss of muscle mass—has received increasing scientific attention. Visser et al. (2002) investigated the quantity and quality of lean muscle mass in over 3,000 well-functioning older adults and found that the midthigh muscle area and greater fat infiltration in the muscle were associated with poorer lower-extremity performance. The generalized changes in muscle structure also have been associated with decline in upper-extremity strength and hand function, such as sustained grip and pinch (Raganathan et al. 2001).

In 2001, osteoarthritis was identified as the primary source of chronic joint symptoms in over 50% of adults aged 65 and older (Centers for Disease Control 2002). With the number of older adults increasing in the coming decades, the number of adults reporting arthritis and joint pain is projected to double by the year 2030. Osteoarthritis is most commonly manifested in the hips, knees, and back; not surprisingly, it is frequently associated with complaints of pain. In a recent study conducted in older adults with osteoarthritis by Andersen et al. (2003), the prevalence of knee, hip, and back pain was 21%, 14% and 22%, respectively, and these estimates were significantly related to increasing values on the body mass index. This relationship was stronger for knee pain than for either hip or back pain.

PSYCHOSOCIAL DOMAIN

A growing body of literature reveals that pain and the performance of functional activities can be significantly influenced by many psychosocial variables (Al-Obaidi et al. 2000; Picavet et al. 2002; Woby et al. 2004). Depression is often considered a normal part of aging, yet in reality a minority of older adults experience clinically significant major depression. While depressed symptoms can temporarily occur in response to life stressors, the presence of symptoms less severe than those required for the diagnosis of major depression or dysthymia has led to the classification of subsyndromal or mild depression. It is estimated that the prevalence rate for all depressive disorders in community-dwelling older adults may be as high as 20–25% (Riley 2001). Depression of any type, if left untreated, can lead to inactivity, functional limitations, and ultimately disability. Depressive symptoms appear to have a stronger association with reports of well-being and functioning than other medical conditions, regardless of age (Ormel et al. 1998).

Self-efficacy or the confidence one has in one's ability to successfully complete a task has been linked to disability in persons with pain. Lefebvre et al. (1999) investigated the relationship between daily ratings of pain, mood, and coping efficacy, and found that those who had high self-efficacy reported lower pain levels, lower degrees of negative mood, and higher levels of positive mood and were less likely to seek emotional comfort as a coping method. More recently, Reid et al. (2003) found a modest relationship between self-efficacy and the occurrence of disabling musculoskeletal pain. Other cognitive factors associated with functional performance and self-reported disabilities include fear-avoidance beliefs and perceived control of pain. These factors were more closely related to self-reported disability (Verbunt et al. 2003) than pain intensity, age, or gender in persons with chronic LBP (Woby et al. 2004).

Fear-induced avoidance of activities has received increased attention and is a central construct in cognitive-behavioral models of pain (Rudy and Turk 1991). Several investigations have evaluated the role that the fear of pain plays in pain-related avoidance of activity and subsequent disability. These investigations have resulted in a variety of cognitively based models. Phillips (1987) theorizes that avoidance is determined by a preference to minimize discomfort and pain, plus thoughts and beliefs that re-exposure to certain situations will produce both pain and suffering. A study by Klenerman et al. (1995) of 300 patients with acute LBP suggests that fear-avoidance variables were the most successful in predicting outcome. Similar observations were made by Keen et al. (1999), who found that fear of pain and avoidance of physical activity were two main factors associated with changes in activity level.

CONTEXTUAL FACTORS DOMAIN

The social context and the individual's environment can shape the pain experience and, subsequently, disability and functional limitations. An environment with barriers (e.g., inaccessible housing and other buildings), or without facilitators (e.g., unavailability of assistive devices), can significantly restrict the functioning of older adults with pain. Berkman et al. (2000) recently proposed a framework for examining the impact of social networks on health and well-being. Within this model, the structural aspects include the number and type of social contacts, and the functional aspects include social support and access to material goods and services. Peat et al. (2004) tested the associations between social networks and pain interference in middle-aged and older adults and found that social contacts can impede the development and progression of pain-related disability.

ASSESSMENT OF FUNCTION IN OLDER ADULTS WITH PAIN

Earlier studies suggest that most older adults experience pain of sufficient intensity to adversely impact functional performance. Gagliese and Melzack (1997) suggest that one of the factors potentially limiting effective medical management of pain in this population is the use of inappropriate assessment instruments. Before reviewing functional and psychosocial measures, it is important to consider biomedical factors that may affect function. Many of these are reviewed elsewhere in this volume. At a minimum, comorbidities in pain patients should be noted because they can adversely affect functional performance (Farrell et al. 1995). The Cumulative Illness Rating Scale is a systematic method for recording comorbidities (Linn et al. 1968).

While the primary focus of the clinical practice should dictate the choice of measures, it is fundamental to select psychometrically sound measures that are reliable, valid, and sensitive to change, including being able to detect the effects of common treatment interventions. Whenever possible, measures chosen should have been developed or normed in older adults, should be time efficient, and should not present an excess burden to patients. Standardized performance-based measures and self-report measures augment the customary assessments performed by clinicians because they tap constructs that range from the basic components of function to role function (Sherman and Reuben 1998), much of which is not routinely addressed by many clinical specialties, but is essential when evaluating patients with chronic pain conditions.

PERFORMANCE-BASED MEASURES OF FUNCTION

The recent increase in the use of performance-based measures in the older adult population illustrates a broadening appreciation of their value. Data from these measures can provide realistic functional markers or guideposts that can aid in fine-tuning treatment goals. Assessment of overall physical function has led to the common practice of combining a series of measures to sample upper and lower body function (Reuben and Siu 1990; Berkman et al. 1993; Daltroy et al. 1995). Diagnostically, many of the instruments to date have focused on measuring the impact of a specific impairment, such as lower-extremity weakness (Chandler et al. 1998) or knee osteoarthritis (Dekker et al. 1993; Marks 1994). Ultimately, it is important to choose measures that are both time efficient and sensitive enough to detect subtle changes. We will briefly review some of the functional measures with established psychometric properties that are adequate or better that we have found particularly useful and well suited to older adults with chronic pain conditions, particularly LBP. We also have a strong preference for those measures that are time and cost efficient. These instruments are presented in Table II, listed by domain evaluated, along with the time necessary to complete each instrument.

The Physical Performance Test comprises nine functional tasks that include writing a sentence, simulating eating, lifting a book and placing it on a shelf, donning and doffing a jacket, picking up a penny from the floor, turning 360 degrees, walking, and stair climbing (Reuben and Siu 1990).

Functional reach distance is measured while reaching forward beyond arm's length (in a horizontal plane) while maintaining a fixed base of support in the standing position (Duncan et al 1990; Weiner et al. 1992, 1993). Three trials are completed, and the distance moved is averaged.

Chair rise is measured in the number of seconds it takes the patient to rise from a seated position to standing, averaged for five repetitions. Adaptive behaviors (e.g., pushing off with one's arms) and inability to complete the test are noted (Tinetti 1986).

Gait speed is the time in seconds that it takes a patient to walk on a flat surface 25 feet (7.6 m) at a normal pace, which then is repeated at a fast pace (Bohannon 1997). This test is simple, widely used in research settings, and easily implemented in clinical settings, and is strongly associated with current and future function (Imms and Edholm 1981; VanSwearingen et al. 1998; Guralnik et al. 2000; Studenski et al. 2003). Gait speed is also part of the Short Physical Performance Battery, a summary measure of lower-extremity performance that predicts disability, health care utilization, and mortality (Guralnik et al. 1994, 1995).

Table II
Functional assessment measures by domain

Domain	Functional Assessment Measure	Minutes to Complete
Biological Domain		
Medical comorbidity	Cumulative Illness Rating Scale	8
	SF-36: General health perceptions scale	10*
Psychosocial Domain		
Pain intensity	Visual analogue scale	1
	Pain Thermometer	1
	Verbal descriptor scale	1
Fear-avoidance beliefs	Fear Avoidance Beliefs Questionnaire	5
Self-efficacy	Chronic Pain Self Efficacy Scale	5
Depressive symptoms	Geriatric Depression Scale	5
Self-Report Function		
Functional status	Functional Status Index[1,2]	8
	Physical Activity Scale[1,2,3]	8
	MPI General Activity Scale[2,3]	5
	SF-36: Physical functioning and role limitations-physical composite scale[2,3]	10*
General pain disability	Pain Disability Index[1,2,3]	3
	Human Activity Profile[1,2,3]	15
Site-specific disability	Oswestry Disability Scale (LBP)[1,2,3]	5
	Roland Morris (LBP)[1,2]	5
	WOMAC (hip and knee pain)[1,2]	8
	Neck Pain and Disability Scale[1,2,3]	5
Performance-Based Function		
	Physical performance test	5
	Functional reach	3
	Chair rise	2
	Gait speed	3
	Stair climb	2
	Trunk rotation	2

* This time is to complete the entire SF-36.
Note: Superscript numbers indicate that the instrument measures the following activities of daily living (ADLs): [1]basic ADLs, [2]instrumental ADLs, [3]advanced ADLs.

Stair climb is the time in seconds to ascend and descend one flight of stairs (average is 12 steps), and is a subtest extracted from the physical performance test (Reuben and Siu 1990).

Trunk rotation is an assessment of spinal mobility and endurance. This test was modified from the protocol developed by Lechner (1993). The seated patient is asked to complete 20 rotations without stopping while holding an empty plastic bin (approximately 30 cm by 30 cm) and tapping it on top of stools (45 cm high) positioned at the hip joint and at arm's length to the left and right of the patient. The average time in seconds for a single rotation is computed from the total time and the number of rotations completed.

SELF-REPORT MEASURES OF FUNCTION

The structured interview is the primary self-report measure in the clinical assessment of a patient. Interview questions related to functional abilities are designed to elucidate the impact of pain on activity performance, participation, any adaptations made to sustain performance, and lastly, and perhaps most importantly, the patient's goals for performance and participation. Due to time constraints faced by clinicians and the necessity of addressing other examination findings related to their specific discipline, obtaining information on functional abilities in an interview format can be impractical. These constraints, coupled with the increasing need to demonstrate the efficacy of treatment interventions, have led to the development and use of standardized self-report assessments of function. These measures should be considered an adjunct to clinical assessments because the scope of the questions addressed by these instruments vary and may not be equally relevant to all patient conditions. Additionally, they rely on the patients' perception and interpretation of their pain and on their ability to function, and lastly, they are subject to many influences, including demographic, social, cultural, and psychosocial factors.

Many self-report functional measures evaluate a patient's ability or difficulty in performing activities of daily living (ADLs). Since ADLs are a very broad category, a hierarchy of these activities has been developed to reflect the degree of difficulty or physical resources necessary for their successful completion. Basic ADLs include self-care and basic mobility. Instrumental ADLs are activities associated with independent living in the community. Most recently, the category of advanced ADLs was established to reflect activities that are discretionary and more physically and socially demanding (Reuben et al. 1990).

The instruments we propose below meet criteria for good psychometric properties, time and cost efficiency, and limited patient burden, and we have found them to be particularly useful in our clinical practice and in our research with older adults. This list is by no means exhaustive, but it should provide the clinician with a sound beginning from which to choose when evaluating functional aspects of older adults with persistent pain. Of course, not all measures are relevant for all patients, nor would they necessarily all be used at the same time with a particular patient. Superscript numbers in Table II indicate which ADLs are measured by each instrument.

The Functional Status Index comprises 18 ADL items in five categories and defines function in three distinct but related dimensions: degree of dependence, degree of difficulty, and the amount of pain experienced in performing specific ADLs (Jette 1980).

The Physical Activity Scale is designed to measures the level of physical activity in the past week in the areas of leisure, occupation, and household activities (Washburn et al. 1993).

The MPI General Activity Scale, from the Multidimensional Pain Inventory, is designed to measure the frequency of participation in 19 common activities (Kerns et al. 1985). We believe this type of activity checklist is important because it evaluates the frequency of participation in specific activities, in contrast to most self-report functional measures that only focus on the difficulty or pain related to performing ADLs.

The Medical Outcomes Study 36-Item Short Form Health Survey (SF-36) examines the patient's health over the past 4 weeks in eight different outcome dimensions: energy/fatigue, general health perception, mental health, role limitations due to emotional problems, bodily pain, physical functioning, role limitations due to physical problems, and social functioning. Two higher-order scales have been developed to combine these eight primary dimensions of health, a physical functioning and role limitations-physical composite scale, and a mental health and role limitations-emotional composite scale (McHorney et al. 1993).

The Pain Disability Index is a seven-item questionnaire that measures pain interference with seven social roles: occupation, home and family, recreation, socialization, sex life, self-care, and life support (Tait et al. 1990).

The Human Activity Profile is a 94-item activities questionnaire that covers a wide range of activities, ranging from basic self-care to leisure and exercise. It was specifically developed and normed on community-dwelling older adults in treatment at a chronic pain clinic (Farrell et al. 1996).

The Oswestry Low Back Pain Questionnaire provides an index of perceived disability based upon 10 items assessing level of pain and interference with physical activities, sleep, self care, sex life, social life, and travel. Each area is scored separately and then combined for a total maximal score, which is then doubled and interpreted as a percentage of patient-perceived disability (Fairbank et al. 1980).

The Roland and Morris Disability Index is a 24-item instrument derived from the Sickness Impact Profile in which the phrase "because of my back" was added to each statement, enabling the creation of a disease-specific index. It has been found to have excellent reliability, validity, and responsiveness (Roland and Morris 1983).

The Western Ontario and McMaster Universities Osteoarthritis Index (WOMAC) is a 24-item instrument that assesses pain, disability, and joint stiffness in subjects with hip and knee osteoarthritis (McConnell et al. 2001).

The Neck Pain and Disability Scale is a 20-item instrument designed to measure intensity of neck pain and its interference with vocational, recreational, social, and self-care activities, as well as emotions related to pain (Wheeler et al. 1999).

PSYCHOSOCIAL SELF-REPORT MEASURES RELATED TO FUNCTION

Initial psychosocial interviewing of patients should focus on clarifying pain location, intensity, frequency, and duration. Guidelines for assessment of pain in older adults proposed by Davis and Srivastava (2003) highlight the importance of consistently using a self-report instrument to measure pain severity. Routine and standardized assessment of pain is further supported by the degree that pain affects everyday life, which has been found to increase incrementally with age (Thomas et al. 2004).

Measures of pain intensity are important because pain often can have a direct impact on functional performance. Although our opinion is certainly open to debate, we consider pain intensity a psychosocial measure, rather than a biological one, because of the numerous psychological and social factors that have been demonstrated to influence reports of pain and its intensity. Several common measures have proven to be effective with older adults. (1) The visual analogue scale is a 10-cm line with the descriptive anchors of "no pain" and "worst possible pain" designed to only assess pain intensity (Huskisson 1974); (2) the verbal descriptor scale ranks pain intensity in the range of "no pain," "mild pain," "moderate pain," "severe pain," "very severe pain," and "the most intense pain imaginable" (Herr and Mobily 1993); and (3) the Pain Thermometer presents verbal pain descriptors in a vertical orientation analogous to the thermometer, and its use is appropriate with older adults who have difficulty with abstract concepts or who have mild to moderate cognitive impairment (Weiner et al. 1998).

The Fear Avoidance Beliefs Questionnaire is designed to assess the fear of pain associated with common physical activities and has been found to be highly reliable and valid for patients with chronic LBP patients (Waddell et al. 1993).

Chronic Pain Self-Efficacy is a 22-item questionnaire designed to measure the patient's confidence in performing ADLs (Anderson et al. 1995).

The Geriatric Depression Scale is a brief questionnaire to measure depressed mood, developed and normed for older adults. Patients are asked to respond yes or no to 30 questions in reference to how they felt on the day of testing (Yesavage et al. 1983).

EVALUATING THE DISCRIMINANT VALIDITY OF FUNCTIONAL ASSESSMENT INSTRUMENTS

As noted earlier, the ICF recommends that functional problems be assessed against an accepted population standard. As part of our ongoing research with older adults with chronic pain, we recently examined the impact of chronic LBP on some of the functional assessment measures described above and presented in Table II, that is, those measures relevant to this condition and also applicable to individuals without a chronic pain condition. We will include some preliminary results of this research to highlight how these instruments perform with older adults to provide the reader with additional normative information for older adults and to illustrate the necessity of taking a broader perspective to functional assessment with older adults with chronic pain.

A sample of 298 community-dwelling older adults (155 pain-free controls, 143 with chronic LBP, mean age 73.8, 44% female) had standardized assessments comprising a medical exam, lumbar X-rays, self-report measures, and functional performance tests. Multivariate analysis of variance (MANOVA) and discriminant function analysis were used to evaluate group differences and determine which measures provided the best separation between older adults with chronic LBP and those who were pain free. No group differences were found for age or gender. The results of these analyses are presented in Table III.

A significant MANOVA ($P < 0.0001$), followed by separate ANOVAs, indicated that subjects with chronic LBP and control subjects were significantly different on all 13 of these measures. Effect sizes computed for these group differences (see Table III) indicated that, with the exception of the MPI General Activity Scale and the Physical Activity Scale, these effects were of moderate magnitude (0.50) or greater. Stepwise discriminant function analysis indicated six measures uniquely maximized the separation between the two groups (see Table III). These included comorbidities (Cumulative Illness Rating Scale), depression (Geriatric Depression Scale), self-reported disability (Functional Status Index, SF-36 physical functioning and role limitations physical composite scale), functional reach, and trunk rotation. These six measures produced a classification accuracy of 94% in controls and 84% in those with chronic LBP.

The two performance-based measures, functional reach and trunk rotation, that provided the best unique discrimination between the low back pain

Table III
Evaluating recommended functional assessment measures with individuals
with chronic low back pain (LBP) and control subjects

Domain/Measure	Measure	Means (SD)		Effect Size	DFA* Entry Order
		Controls	LBP		
Biological Domain					
Medical comorbidity	Cumulative Illness Rating Scale	6.63 (2.98)	9.54 (3.51)	–0.90	4
Psychosocial Domain					
Self-efficacy	Chronic Pain Self-Efficacy Scale†	94.50 (7.35)	81.78 (15.09)	1.13	
Depressive symptoms	Geriatric Depression Scale	1.60 (2.15)	4.75 (4.83)	–0.90	5
Self-Report Function					
Functional status	Functional Status Index	0.05 (0.09)	0.39 (0.31)	–1.70	1
	Physical Activity Scale	124.42 (65.02)	105.76 (64.38)	0.29	
	MPI General Activity Scale	3.17 (0.73)	2.84 (0.77)	0.44	
	SF-36: Physical functioning and role limitations physical composite scale	95.05 (9.87)	66.45 (27.66)	1.52	2
Performance-Based Function					
	Functional reach (cm)	31.21 (5.18)	27.81 (5.71)	0.62	6
	Chair rise (s)	2.26 (0.51)	3.10 (1.42)	–0.87	
	Gait speed‡	12.33 (1.60)	14.08 (3.09)	–0.75	
	Stair climb (s)	46.43 (7.11)	54.24 (16.22)	–0.67	
	Trunk rotation (s)	2.31 (0.57)	3.03 (0.84)	–1.02	3

* DFA = discriminant function analysis.
† Fourteen of the 22 self-efficacy items do not contain reference to pain and were completed by controls.
‡ Gait speed is the time in seconds that it takes a patient to walk on a flat surface 25 feet (7.6 m) at a normal pace.

and control groups require less than 5 minutes to administer and easily could be incorporated into the evaluations performed by clinicians. While functional reach has been proven a valid and reliable measure with older adults (Duncan et al. 1990), until now its utility with older adults experiencing chronic LBP had not been investigated. The trunk rotation task, based on a component of the Physical Work Performance Battery for injured workers (Lechner 1993), had not been used previously with older adults. It is noteworthy and not surprising that the performance measures that placed direct stress on the low back had the greatest discriminant power.

While all of the self-report measures were able to detect group differences (Table III), the three measures that had the greatest unique discriminant power encompassed mood and functional status. Clinicians could easily incorporate the Geriatric Depression Scale, the Functional Status Index, and SF-36 into their assessment because they could be completed in the waiting room, clarified during the assessment interview or examination, and scored later.

In summary, these findings indicate that chronic LBP appears to have substantial impact in older adults, including psychosocial measures, self-reported functional measures, and performance-based functional measures. What is particularly encouraging for the purposes of this chapter is that all of these time-efficient measures appear to have discriminant validity and therefore can be used clinically to measure the extent of the functional impact of chronic pain in an older adult. Table III also presents normative information for these measures for community-dwelling older adults with chronic LBP, which may be useful for clinicians to determine the extent of functional impact for a particular patient. Additional research is needed to evaluate the utility of these measures with older adults with other chronic pain conditions, as well as with older adults who are in different social environments (e.g., assisted living facilities or nursing homes).

FUNCTIONAL ASSESSMENT RECOMMENDATIONS FOR PAIN CLINICIANS

Given the wide variety of clinical practice models in existence, we have summarized our recommendations for standardized instrument use by provider in Table IV. For the solo medical practitioner, we feel it is valuable to obtain self-reported function and select psychosocial measures to assess any functional changes associated with the pain. We did not recommend performance-based measures for the primary care practitioner because of likely time constraints, but feel they would be relevant to most, if not all, pain practices and could easily be performed by the pain physician or nursing staff. Comparing the time required (Table II) for the six measures recommended for physicians (Table IV) indicates that only 30 minutes would be needed. Four of these measures are standardized self-report instruments (Chronic Pain Self-Efficacy, Geriatric Depression Scale, Functional Status Index, and MPI General Activity Scale) and would not require any physician

Table IV
Functional assessment measures, recommendations
for use by type of provider

Domain/Measure	Primary Practitioner	OT/ PT*	Psychologist
Biological Domain			
Cumulative Illness Rating Scale	X		
Psychosocial Domain			
Pain intensity	X	X	X
Fear Avoidance Beliefs Questionnaire, Part I		X	X
Chronic Pain Self-Efficacy	X	X	X
Geriatric Depression Scale	X		X
Self-Report Function			
Functional Status Index	X	X	
MPI: General Activity Scale	X	X	X
SF-36: Physical Functioning			
Performance-Based Function			
Functional reach		X	
Trunk rotation		X	
Chair rise		X	
Gait speed		X	
Stair climb		X	

* OT = occupational therapist; PT = physical therapist.

time to complete. They could be given to the patient by one of the office staff in the waiting room prior to the appointment with the physician, if a self-report format is deemed appropriate. Alternately, they could be administered in an interview format by one of the nursing staff. We often prefer the latter option because it seems to yield more reliable and useful data.

In addition to performance-based measures, we also recommend that occupational and physical therapists include in their assessment selected self-report measures of function and pain intensity to augment their routine clinical practice. These measures not only increase their understanding of the functional consequences of pain, but also can serve as useful measures of treatment outcome or as ways to monitor the progress of therapy. Therapists frequently neglect the cognitive components of performance, that is, what patients are saying to themselves about their disability and functional limitations. The inclusion of measures such as the Chronic Pain Self-Efficacy Scale and the Fear-Avoidance Beliefs Questionnaire, which can be completed in 10 minutes or less, provides useful insights into why some patients refuse to comply with the recommended rehabilitation activities. Knowing the breadth and severity of the patient's cognitive distortions is important for therapists so that they can refer patients for psychological or psychiatric help as necessary on a timely basis.

We recommend that pain psychologists focus their assessment on the cognitive and affective consequences of chronic pain, but not to the exclusion of knowledge of functional aspects. They should be aware of the interaction of the psychosocial and functional dimensions and the necessity of using both components in treatment planning. Psychologists of course will select other psychosocial measures in addition to those listed in Table IV for the purposes of their own specific treatment planning (see Chapter 9). Nonetheless, the psychologist should work closely with physicians and therapists so that the team can work together to address the psychological obstacles that frequently are substantial roadblocks to treatment participation and functional restoration.

ACKNOWLEDGMENTS

This work was supported in part by USPHS Research Grant R01AG18299 from the National Institute on Aging, National Institutes of Health.

REFERENCES

Al-Obaidi SM, Nelson RM, Al-Awadhi S, Al-Shuwaie N. The role of anticipation and fear of pain in the persistence of avoidance behavior in patients with chronic low back pain. *Spine* 2000; 25:1126-1131.

Andersen RE, Crespo CJ, Bartlett SJ, Bathon JM, Fontaine KR. Relationship between body weight gain and significant knee, hip, and back pain in older Americans. *Obesity Res* 2003; 11:1159–1162.

Anderson KO, Noel Dowds B, Pelletz RE, Edwards WT, Peeters-Asdourian C. Development and initial validation of a scale to measure self-efficacy beliefs in patients with chronic pain. *Pain* 1995; 63:77–84.

Belleville S, Rouleau N, Caza N. Effect of normal aging on the manipulation of information in working memory. *Mem Cognit* 1998; 26:572–583.

Berkman LF, Seeman TE, ALbert M, et al. High, usual and impaired functioning in community-dwelling older men and women: findings from the MacArthur Foundation Research Network on Successful Aging. *J Clin Epidemiol* 1993; 46:1129–1140.

Berkman LF, Glass T, Brissette I, Seeman TE. From social integration to health: Durkheim in the new millennium. *Soc Sci Med* 2000; 51:843–857.

Bohannon RW. Comfortable and maximum walking speed of adults aged 20–79 years: reference values as determinants. *Age Aging* 1997; 26:15–19.

Centers for Disease Control. Prevalence of self-reported arthritis or chronic joint symptoms among adults—United States 2001. *Morb Mortal Wkly Rept* 2002; 51:948–950.

Chandler JM, Duncan PW, Kochersberger G, Studenski S. Is lower extremity strength gain associated with improvement in physical performance and disability in frail, community-dwelling elders? *Arch Phys Med Rehabil* 1998; 79:24–30.

Creamer P, Lethbridge-Cejku M, Costa P, et al. The relationship of anxiety and depression with self-reported knee pain in the community: data from the Baltimore longitudinal study of aging. *Arthritis Care Res* 1999; 12:3–7.

Daltroy LH, Phillips CB, Eaton HM, et al. Objective measuring physical ability in elderly persons: the physical capacity evaluation. *Am J Public Health* 1995; 85:558–560.

Davis MP, Srivastava M. Demographics, assessment and management of pain the elderly. *Drugs Aging* 2003; 20:23–57.

Dekker J, Tola P, Aufdemkampe G, Winckers M. Negative affect, pain and disability in osteoarthritis patients: the mediating role of muscle weakness. *Behav Res Ther* 1993; 31:203–206.

Duncan PW, Weiner DK, Chandler J, Studenski S. Functional reach: a new clinical measure of balance. *J Gerontol Med Sci* 1990; 45:M192–M197.

Fairbank JC, Couper J, Davies JB, O'Brien J. The Oswestry low back pain disability index. *Physiotherapy* 1980; 66:271–273.

Farrell MJ, Gerontol M, Gibson SJ, Helme RD. The effect of medical status on the activity level of older pain patients. *J Am Geriatr Soc* 1995; 43:102–107.

Farrell MJ, Gibson SJ, Helme RD. Measuring the activity of older people with chronic pain. *Clin J Pain* 1996; 12:6–12.

Fries JF, Crapo LM (Eds). *Vitality and Aging: Implications of the Rectangular Curve.* New York: W.H. Freeman, 1981.

Gagliese L, Melzack R. Chronic pain in elderly people. *Pain* 1997; 70:3–14.

Gibson SAJ, Farrell M. A review of age differences in the neurophysiology of nociception and the perceptual experience of pain. *Clin J Pain* 2004; 20:227–239.

Guralnik JM, Simonsick EM, Ferrucci L, et al. A short physical performance battery assessing lower extremity function: association with self-reported disability and prediction of mortality and nursing home admission. *J Gerontol* 1994; 49:M84–94.

Guralnik JM, Ferrucci L, Simonsick EM, Salive ME, Wallace RB. Lower-extremity function in persons over the age of 70 years as a predictor of subsequent disability. *N Engl J Med* 1995; 332:556–561.

Guralnik JM, Ferrucci L, Pieper CF, et al. Lower extremity function and subsequent disability: consistency across studies, predictive models, and value of gait speed alone compared with the short physical performance battery. *J Gerontol A Biol Sci Med Sci* 2000; 55:M221–231.

Herr KA, Mobily PR. Comparison of selected pain assessment tools for use with the elderly. *Appl Nurs Res* 1993; 6:39–46.

Hirose D, Ishida K, Nagano Y, Takahashi T, Yamamoto H. Posture of the trunk in the sagittal plane is associated with gait in the community-dwelling elderly population. *Clin Biomech* 2004; 19:57–63.

Holm MB, Rogers JC, Kwoh CK. Predictors of functional disability in patients with rheumatoid arthritis. *Arthritis Care Res* 1998; 11:346–355.

Hopman-Rock M, Odding E, Hofman A, Kraaimaat FW, Bijlsma JWJ. Physical and psychosocial disability in elderly subjects in relation to pain in the hip and/or knee. *J Rheum* 1996; 23:1037–1044.

Hopman-Rock M, Kraaimatt FW, Odding E, Bijlsma JWJ. Coping with pain in the hip or knee in relation to physical disability in community-living elderly people. *Arthritis Care Res* 1998; 11:243–252.

Huskisson EC. Measurement of pain. *Lancet* 1974; 2:1127–1131.

Imms F, Edholm OG. Studies of gait and mobility in the elderly. *Age Aging* 1981; 10:147–156.

Jette AM. Functional Status Index: reliability of a chronic disease evaluation instrument. *Arch Phys Med Rehabil* 1980; 61:395–401.

Keen S, Dowell AC, Hurst K, et al. Individuals with low back pain: How do they view physical activity. *Fam Pract* 1999; 16:39–45.

Kerns RD, Turk DC, Rudy TE. The West Haven-Yale Multidimensional Pain Inventory (WHYMPI). *Pain* 1985; 23:345–356.

Klenerman L, Slade PD, Stanley IM, et al. The prediction of chronicity in patients with an acute attack of low back pain in a general practice setting. *Spine* 1995; 20:478–484.

Lechner DE. *Physical Work Performance Evaluation.* Birmingham, AL: University of Alabama Research Foundation, 1993.

Lefebvre JC, Keefe FJ, Affleck B, et al. The relationship of arthritis self-efficacy to daily pain, daily mood, and daily pain coping in rheumatoid arthritis patients. *Pain* 1999; 80:425–435.

Leveille SG. Musculoskeletal aging. *Curr Opin Rheumatol* 2004; 16:114–118.

Leveille SG, Guralnik JM, Hochberg M, et al. Low back pain and disability in older women: independent association with difficulty but not inability to perform daily activities. *J Gerontol* 1999; 54A:M487–M493.

Linn BS, Linn MW, Gurel L. Cumulative Illness Rating Scale. *J Am Geriatr Soc* 1968; 16:622–626.

Marks R. Reliability and validity of self-paced walking time measures for knee osteoarthritis. *Arthritis Care Res* 1994; 7:50–53.

McAlindon TE, Cooper C, Kirwin JR, Dieppe PA. Determinants of disability in osteoarthritis of the knee. *Ann Rheum Dis* 1993; 52:258–262.

McConnell S, Kolopack P, Davis AM. The Western Ontario and McMaster Universities osteoarthritis index (WOMAC): a review of its utility and measurement properties. *Arthritis Care Res* 2001; 45:453–461.

McHorney CA, Ware JE, Raczek AE. The MOS 36-item Short-Form Health Survey (SF-36): II. Psychometric and clinical tests of validity in measuring physical and mental health constructs. *Med Care* 1993; 31:247–263.

Ormel J, Kempen G, Deeg DJH, et al. Functioning, well-being, and health perception in late middle-aged and older people: comparing the effects of depressive symptoms and chronic medical conditions. *J Am Geriatr Soc* 1998; 46:39–48.

Peat G, Thomas E, Handy J, Croft P. Social networks and pain interference with daily activities in middle and old age. *Pain* 2004; 112:397–405.

Phillips H. Avoidance behavior and its role in sustaining chronic pain. *Behav Res Ther* 1987; 25:273–279.

Picavet HS, Vlayeyen JW, Schouten JS. Pain catastrophizing and kinesiophobia: predictors of chronic low back pain. *Am J Epidemiol* 2002; 156:1028–1034.

Raganathan VK, Siemionow V, Sahgal V, Yue GH. Effects of aging on hand function. *J Am Geriatr Soc* 2001; 49:1478–1484.

Reid MC, Williams CS, Gill TM. The relationship between psychosocial factors and disabling musculoskeletal pain in community-dwelling older persons. *J Am Geriatr Soc* 2003; 51:1092–1098.

Reuben DB, Siu AL. An objective measure of physical function of elderly outpatients: the Physical Performance Test. *J Am Geriatr Soc* 1990; 38:1105–1112.

Reuben DB, Laliberte L, Hiris J, Mor V. A hierarchical exercise scale to measure function at the Advanced Activities of Daily Living (AADL) level. *J Am Geriatr Soc* 1990; 38:855–861.

Riley KP. Cognitive development. In: Bonder BR, Wagner MB (Eds). *Functional Performance in Older Adults,* 2nd ed. Philadelphia: F.A. Davis, 2001.

Roland M, Morris R. A study of the natural history of back pain. Part I: Development of a reliable and sensitive measure of disability in low-back pain. *Spine* 1983; 8:141–144.

Rudy TE, Turk DC. Psychological aspects of pain. *Int Anesthesiol Clin* 1991; 29:9–22.

Scudds RJ, Robertson JM. Empirical evidence of the association between the presence of musculoskeletal pain and physical disability in community dwelling senior citizens. *Pain* 1998; 229–235.

Sharma L, Cahue S, Song J, et al. Physical functioning over three years in knee osteoarthritis: role of psychosocial, local mechanical, and neuromuscular factors. *Arthritis Rheum* 2003; 48:3359–3370.

Sherman SE, Reuben DB. Measuring the performance of performance-based measures in community-dwelling elders. *J Gen Int Med* 1998; 13:817–823.

Studenski S, Perera S, Wallace D, et al. Physical performance measures in the clinical setting. *J Am Geriatr Soc* 2003; 51:314–322.

Tait RC, Chibnall JT, Margolis RB. Pain extent: relations with psychological state, pain severity, pain history and disability. *Pain* 1990; 41:295–301.

Thomas E, Peat G, Harris L, Wilkie R, Croft PR. The prevalence of pain and pain interference in a general population of older adults: cross-sectional findings from the North Staffordshire Osteoarthritis Project (NorStOP). *Pain* 2004; 110:361–368.

Tinetti ME. Performance-oriented assessment of mobility problems in elderly patients. *J Am Geriatr Soc* 1986; 95:2.

VanSwearingen JM, Paschal KA, Bonino P, Chen T. Assessing recurrent fall risk of community-dwelling, frail older veterans using specific tests of mobility and the Physical Performance Test of function. *J Gerontol A Biol Sci Med Sci* 1998; 53:M457–464.

Verbunt JA, Seelen HA, Vlaeyen JW, van der Hiejden GJ, Knottnerus JA. Fear of injury and physical deconditioning in patients with chronic low back pain. *Arch Phys Med Rehabil* 2003; 84:1227–1232.

Visser M, Deeg DJH, Lips P, Harris TB, Bouter LM. Skeletal muscle mass and muscle strength in relation to lower extremity performance in older men and women. *J Am Geriatr Soc* 2000; 48:381–386.

Visser M, Kritchevsky SB, Goodpaster BH, et al. Leg muscle mass and composition in relation to lower extremity performance in men and women aged 70 to 79: the health, aging, and body composition study. *J Am Geriatr Soc* 2002; 50:897–904.

Waddell G, Newton M, Henderson I, Somerville D, Main CJ. A fear-avoidance beliefs questionnaire (FABQ) and the role of fear-avoidance beliefs in chronic low back pain and disability. *Pain* 1993; 52:157–168.

Wagner MB, Kauffman TL. Mobility. In: Bonder BR, Wagner MB (Eds). *Functional Performance in Older Adults,* 2nd ed. Philadelphia: F.A. Davis, 2001.

Washburn RA, Smith KW, Jette AM, Janney CA. The Physical Activity Scale for the Elderly (PASE): development and evaluation. *J Clin Epidemiol* 1993; 46:153–162.

Weiner DK, Duncan PW, Chandler J, Studenski SA. Functional reach: a marker of physical frailty. *J Am Geriatr Soc* 1992; 40:203–207.

Weiner DK, Bongiorni DR, Studenski SA, Duncan PW, Kochersberger GG. Does functional reach improve with rehabilitation? *Arch Phys Med Rehabil* 1993; 74:796–800.

Weiner DK, Peterson B, Logue P, Keefe FJ. Predictors of pain self-report in nursing home residents. *Aging (Milano)* 1998; 10:411–420.

Wheeler AH, Goolkasian P, Baird AC, Darden BV. Development of the neck pain and disability scale. *Spine* 1999; 24:1290–1294.

Woby SR, Watson PJ, Roach NK, Urmston M. Are changes in fear-avoidance beliefs, catastrophizing, and appraisals of control predictive of changes in chronic low back pain and disability? *Eur J Pain* 2004; 8:201–210.

World Health Organization. *International Classification of Functioning, Disability, and Health.* Geneva: World Health Organization, 2001.

Yesavage JA, Brink TL, Rose TL, Lum O. Development and validation of a geriatric depression screening scale: a preliminary report. *J Psychiatr Res* 1983; 17:37–49.

Correspondence to: Thomas E. Rudy, PhD, Department of Anesthesiology, University of Pittsburgh School of Medicine, UPMC Pain Medicine at Centre Commons, 5750 Centre Avenue, Suite 400, Pittsburgh, PA 15206, USA. Email: rudyte@anes.upmc.edu.

Pain in Older Persons, Progress in Pain
Research and Management, Vol. 35, edited
by Stephen J. Gibson and Debra K. Weiner,
IASP Press, Seattle, © 2005.

9

Measuring Mood and Psychosocial Function Associated with Pain in Late Life

Patricia A. Parmelee

*Emory Center for Health in Aging, Emory University School of Medicine, and
Birmingham/Atlanta Geriatric Research, Education and Clinical Center,
Atlanta Veterans Affairs Medical Center, Atlanta, Georgia, USA*

Pain is inherently a biopsychosocial phenomenon, involving not just the perception of complex physical stimuli, but also their interpretation and presentation to others. The experience and expression of pain covary and interact with a broad array of intra- and interpersonal factors. The association of pain with well-being is similarly influenced by cognitive, affective, and behavioral processes. Thus, any effort to assess pain comprehensively demands evaluation of psychosocial processes as well. The assessment process is somewhat more complicated in older adults for several reasons. Aging itself affects both basic sensations and perceptions of pain as well as their internal evaluation and presentation to others. Both cohort and maturational effects color older persons' responses to standard tools assessing relevant psychosocial processes. And those processes themselves may differ, or at least be differentially manifested, among older versus younger adults.

In short, assessment of psychosocial influences on and responses to pain is at the very least a different enterprise among older persons as compared with younger adults. It is frequently a more complicated one as well. Nonetheless, we have made good progress over the past two decades in developing assessment tools and techniques appropriate for use with older adults with persistent pain. This chapter offers an overview of the most common of those tools, along with a critique of the current state of the art in assessment of psychosocial factors relevant to pain in older persons.

A WORKING MODEL OF PAIN IN PSYCHOSOCIAL CONTEXT

Fig. 1 offers a shorthand model for organizing psychosocial factors and processes relevant to the experience and assessment of pain in older adults. This figure is not intended as a comprehensive model of causal interrelations among constructs represented. For example, cognitive, affective, and interpersonal processes are all tightly interwoven and mutually influential of one another. Coping, too, interacts with these processes to influence the path from pain to psychological well-being. It is beyond the scope of this chapter to propose a full, integrative model of interrelationships among these variables. Rather, Fig. 1 will serve simply to frame this review of assessment of constructs represented. For more in-depth discussion of age differences in these dynamics, please see Chapter 5 in this volume.

Briefly, the model posits that *personality*—the relatively enduring complex of cognitive, affective, motivational, and behavioral dispositions unique to an individual—is a first, very broad influence on the experience and expression of pain. (This chapter focuses largely on *chronic* pain. Where the term *acute* is not specifically used, chronic pain is implied.) More specific influences derive from three sets of factors: perceptions, attitudes, beliefs, and other *cognitive processes* related to oneself, pain in particular, and the world in general; *affective processes,* which comprise emotional responses that may affect and be affected by pain; and *interpersonal processes*—perceptions of, relationships with, and behavior toward other individuals. Although all these processes may be uniquely associated with psychological well-being, they also affect well-being indirectly, through their effects on

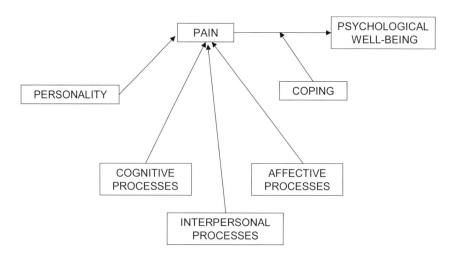

Fig. 1. A working model of mood and psychosocial correlates of pain in older adults.

experienced pain. Coping, defined as cognitive and behavioral attempts to adapt to demands posed by a stressor (in this case, persistent pain), is conceptualized as a moderator of the association of pain with psychological well-being.

Defining *psychological well-being* is no easy task, as there has been considerable debate about the issue (Ryff 1989; Ryff and Keyes 1995; Massee et al. 1998). For current purposes, however, we define it as the absence of emotional distress and maintenance of at least a minimal level of positive morale. Taken in concert with cognitive, affective, and interpersonal processes, as well as pain and physical function (which will not be treated here), psychological well-being is a linchpin of more general quality of life.

The bulk of this chapter will review specific tools and techniques for assessing each of these constructs as they relate to the experience of pain in late life. Before turning to those specifics, however, it will be useful to examine some general issues that may complicate measurement of mood and psychosocial function.

GENERAL ISSUES IN MEASURING MOOD AND PSYCHOSOCIAL FUNCTION

Measurement of any psychosocial construct is usually more difficult than it looks. In the context of pain among older adults, three specific points bear consideration: conceptual distinctions among elements of the model just described, the question of whether assessment of these constructs is really any different among older versus younger adults, and use of single-construct versus multifactorial inventories.

COGNITION, DISPOSITION, DISORDER, AND MORE: WHERE ARE THE DIVIDING LINES?

Even for experts, it can be challenging to distinguish among such closely related constructs as *perception, attitude,* and *belief,* to differentiate motivation from disposition, or to define where personality stops and mental health (or illness) starts. These kinds of distinctions are particularly vexing with respect to psychosocial aspects of pain. This is due in part to the very real interfusion of relevant constructs, as well as to the highly subjective nature of pain itself. However, conceptual difficulties are also traceable to the strongly clinical roots of research in this area. Current empirical work on intra- and interpersonal processes in chronic pain has developed largely from efforts to understand the needs and motives of clinical populations, rather than from theory-based, empirically driven efforts to articulate conceptual models of those processes. As a result, we lack integrative frameworks that would foster clear delineation of subtle differences among, for example, cognitive versus affective components of pain experience, or of coping strategies from their psychological outcomes.

For an example of this conceptual muddiness, consider the (largely nongerontological) literature on catastrophizing. Originally identified as one of a complex of cognitive coping mechanisms (Rosenstiel and Keefe 1983), this tendency to dwell on the most negative possible potential outcome has alternatively been conceptualized as a cognitive bias orthogonal to coping (Turner et al. 2000), as a manifestation of clinical depression (Sullivan and d'Eon 1990), and as a cognitive appraisal preliminary to coping (Thorn et al. 1999). Catastrophizing is also obviously strongly related to neuroticism and other stable dispositions (Affleck et al. 1992; Persson and Sahlberg 2002; Goubert et al. 2004), although we know of no research that has overtly treated it as a personality trait. Instead, the predominant trend has been to reify the construct—catastrophizing is as catastrophizing does, without much concern for where it fits in the larger schema of things (see, however, recent reviews and commentary by Sullivan et al. 2001b; Turner and Aaron 2001).

Lack of clear conceptual differentiation complicates assessment and has slowed elaboration of comprehensive models of psychosocial correlates of pain. Much of the problem lies is the fact that personality, cognition, affect, and even interpersonal processes share common motivational roots in the strong human drive for control—the need to perceive that one is competent to deal effectively with circumstances that befall one (Berlyne 1960; de Charms 1968; Rodin et al. 1990). In fact, I shall use this premise—that psychosocial processes in chronic pain are largely driven by cognitive and behavioral attempts to control pain and one's response to it—as an organizing theme of this chapter. But the fact that dispositions, cognitions, mood states, and social interactions are closely intertwined does not obviate the need for conceptual distinction. In the end, one must take extreme care in choosing assessment domains and tools to avoid muddying results with a set of poorly differentiated, highly intercorrelated measures.

DOES AGE MAKE A DIFFERENCE?

A second concern is whether extant measures of psychosocial concomitants of persistent pain, derived predominantly from work with middle-aged and younger adults, can be translated directly for use with older persons. There is good evidence that, net of real psychophysical differences in pain experience (Gibson and Helme 2001; Helme et al. 2004), psychometric properties of measures of pain itself differ in older and younger populations

(Gagliese and Katz 2003). However, far less attention has been paid to this issue in assessing relevant psychosocial processes—for example, measures of attitudes toward or ways of coping with pain. There are a few documented differences in how older and younger persons score on these measures (e.g., Keefe and Williams 1990; Chipperfield et al. 1999). But we know relatively little about the relative appropriateness and psychometric performance of these kinds of measures in older populations.

What we do know suggests caution both conceptually and methodologically. From a measurement standpoint, many self-report instruments are known to behave quite differently in older versus younger populations. For example, the 36-item Medical Outcomes Study Short Form (SF-36), certainly the most widely used measure of health-related quality of life today, is known to be relatively insensitive to changes in physical functioning among older as compared with younger adults (O'Mahoney et al. 1998; Stadnyk et al. 1998). But for most pain-specific indices, there have been few rigorous age comparisons of either construct validity or psychometric performance.

Conceptually, the notion of perceived control as a driving force behind responses to chronic pain suggests that wholesale extension of assessment approaches directly from younger to older populations may be problematic. The work of Schulz and colleagues (Schulz and Heckhausen 1999; Schulz et al. 2003) indicates that transition to old age is characterized by changes in control strategies that reflect both maturation (learning what one can and cannot expect to control) and adaptation (modifying strategies to accommodate age-related changes). These changes are reflected in turn in such phenomena as increased use of passive coping strategies among older adults (Chipperfield et al. 1999). This, of itself, is not a problem. The problem arises when evaluative norms attending these assessments in younger populations are attached to older persons as well—in this example, the tendency to view passive coping as inferior to or less adaptive than more direct efforts. Thus, the key issue here is not psychometric performance of standard assessment tools—although that may be relevant as well—but interpretation of their results in application to older adults.

SINGLE-CONSTRUCT VERSUS MULTIFACTORIAL TOOLS

A third consideration is use of multidimensional measures versus more specific single-construct indices. There are several good multidimensional measures of pain impact, most notably the Multidimensional Pain Inventory (MPI; Kerns et al. 1985) and the Pain Disability Index (PDI; Tait et al. 1987). The MPI is a widely used instrument that, in its original incarnation, comprised 12 subscales addressing pain experience (e.g., severity, interference with activities, and negative mood), responses of significant others (punishing, solicitous, or distracting), and activities (e.g., household chores or social activities). The much shorter and more general PDI uses a series of anchored numeric rating scales to tap the extent to which pain affects activity in seven domains (e.g., family/home responsibilities, occupation, sexual behavior, and self-care). Disease-specific measures such as the Arthritis Impact Measurement Scales (Meenan et al. 1992) take a similar tack, assessing effects of pain upon a range of physical, interpersonal, and emotional functions.

Other psychosocial influences on and outcomes of pain can similarly be assessed using single-construct as well as multidimensional assessment approaches. For example, cumbersome as it is, the Minnesota Multiphasic Personality Inventory has been used in both research and clinical practice to pinpoint personality correlates of chronic pain (Arbisi and Butcher 2004). But perhaps most controversial is use of multidimensional quality-of-life measures to capture psychosocial outcomes of pain. As already noted, the SF-36 is widely used as a primary measure of quality of life, despite its known drawbacks. Other omnibus quality-of-life measures such as the Sickness Impact Profile (Bergner et al. 1981) and the Quality of Well Being Scale (Kaplan et al. 1989) similarly tap a number of different physical and psychosocial dimensions of well-being that are relevant to pain.

Omnibus tools offer the obvious advantage of yielding a good overview of an individual's status without overburdening the individual or the assessor. Thus, they may well be the measures of choice for initial screening in both clinical and research settings. However, reliance on brief, very general subscales as primary measures of key constructs can cause real problems for more intensive work. Assessment of depression serves as a good example. Many multifactorial tools include a subscale that taps depressive symptoms, and it is tempting to extrapolate from that brief scale to a clinically significant depressive syndrome. To do so, however, is to neglect substantial concerns about the strength and unidimensionality of depressive syndromes—for example, the differentiation of major, minor, and subsyndromal depression (Schneider et al. 2000; Judd et al. 2002) or the intricate association of symptoms of depression and anxiety (Flint 2005). Thus, rather than an "either/or" perspective on this issue, it is crucial to take into consideration one's purposes at each measurement juncture, and to select that instrument—single-construct or omnibus—that will best elucidate the questions at hand.

PSYCHOSOCIAL ASSESSMENT OF PAIN IN OLDER PERSONS: CURRENT STATE OF THE ART

Having laid this general foundation, let us turn now to a brief review of measurement tools, strategies, and issues. Table I summarizes selected measures in each area outlined in our working model (Fig. 1). Because there are so many specific constructs and measures in these areas, I have not compiled a comprehensive list. Rather, those included were chosen to represent the most commonly used, best validated, and most user-friendly tools for assessing key constructs in each of the areas of interest.

INTRAPERSONAL FACTORS: PERSONALITY, COGNITION, AND AFFECT

As noted earlier, there is considerable blurring of conceptual distinctions among the stable dispositional factors we call *personality,* pain-relevant cognitive processes, and concomitant emotional responses. This is due largely to their common motivational basis in the need for control, but also to the relative lack of empirical work aimed directly at delineating their associations and distinctions. Such work is ongoing, and will no doubt shape measurement approaches as the field matures.

Personality factors associated with pain in late life have, surprisingly, not been examined in depth. However, existing knowledge as well as non-age-specific studies suggest that dispositional factors may play an important role in the experience of both chronic and acute pain. From a measurement standpoint, we know that personality is largely (though not completely) stable across the adult lifespan, and can be measured using standardized instruments without much concern for age-related effects (Costa and McCrae 1997).

Table I presents some commonly used personality measures known to perform well with older adults and to predict psychosocial well-being in pain patients. The Revised NEO Personality Inventory (Costa and McCrae 1992) is by far the most parsimonious and least burdensome multidimensional measure for use in both research and clinical settings. Among single traits, neuroticism, hypochondriasis, and dispositional optimism have each been shown to predict pain response in both older and younger populations (Lichtenberg et al. 1986; Affleck et al. 1992; Achat et al. 2000; Meldolesi et al. 2000); each strongly predicts (poor) psychological well-being as well (Brenes et al. 2002). Dispositional hardiness is less extensively studied, but work on other aspects of health suggest that it may be a strong predictor of pain experience as well (Funk 1992; Maddi 1998).

Table I
Common instruments for measuring pain-related mood and psychosocial function among older persons

Domain/Construct	Measure	Source	Brief Description	Validation in Older Adults
Personality				
Multidimensional measures	NEO Personality Inventory	Costa and McCrae 1992	Multi-trait scale tapping the "Big Five" personality dimensions (conscientiousness, extraversion, impulsiveness, neuroticism, and openness to experience). Long and short forms available; subscales may be used separately	Costa and McRae 1986*
Single-item measures	Dispositional Hardiness Scale	Kobasa 1979	36 items comprising commitment, challenge, and control	Lawton et al. 2001
	Hypochondriasis subscale, MMPI	Hathaway and McKinley 1943	33 items assess preoccupation with health; 32-item MMPI-2 subscale now available	Lichtenberg et al. 1984
	Illness Attitudes Scale	Kellner 1986	21 yes-no items assess severity of hypochondriasis	Frazier and Waid 1999
	Life Orientation Test-Revised	Scheier et al. 1994	10-item measure of dispositional optimism	Guarnera and Williams 1987
Cognitive Processes				
Pain-specific	Cognitive Errors Questionnaire	Lefebvre 1981	48 vignettes assessing 4 depression-related cognitive distortions (catastrophizing, overgeneralization, personalization, and selective abstraction). Half use chronic pain as the stimulus situation	Smith et al. 1994 (rheumatoid arthritis version)†
	Inventory of Negative Thoughts in Response to Pain	Gil et al. 1990	21 5-point items comprising 3 subscales: negative self-statements, negative social cognitions, and self-blame	Gil et al. 1990†
	Pain Attitudes Questionnaire	Yong et al. 2001	27 items load on 4 factors representing stoicism (superiority, reticence) and cautiousness (self doubt, reluctance)	Yong et al. 2001
	Pain Beliefs and Perceptions Inventory	Williams and Thorn 1989	16 items measure pain beliefs in the areas of constancy, permanence, self-blame, and mastery	Stroud et al. 2000†

Category	Scale	Source	Description	Reference
	Pain Catastrophizing Scale	Sullivan et al. 1995	13 items comprise 3 subscales describing catastrophic thinking; helplessness, rumination, and magnification	None known
	Survey of Pain Attitudes, Revised	Jensen and Karoly 1989	Separate subscales assess attitudes regarding medical cure (6 items), pain control (8 items), solicitude (6), disability (4), medication, (4), and emotion (7)	Jensen and Karoly 1989†
	Arthritis Helplessness Index	Nicassio et al. 1985	5 items tapping perceived (un)controllability of arthritis symptoms	Stein et al. 1994
	Arthritis Self-Efficacy Scale	Lorig et al. 1989	20 items measuring self-efficacy in 3 domains: pain, function, and other symptoms	Creamer et al. 1999
General	Health Locus of Control Scales	Wallston et al. 1978	18 items tapping perceived locus of control for health items in 3 domains: internal, powerful others, and chance	Buckelew et al. 1990†
	Personal Mastery Scale	Pearlin and Schooler 1978	7-item index of generalized feelings of personal control	Reich and Zautra 1990
Affective Processes *Pain-specific*	Pain Anxiety Symptoms Scale	McCracken et al. 1992	62 items comprising 4 subscales: fear of pain, cognitive anxiety, somatic anxiety, escape and avoidance	None known
	Tampa Scale of Kinesiophobia	Kori et al. 1990	17 items addressing fears about pain and (re)injury	None known
General	Affect-Balance Scale	Bradburn 1969	5 positive and 5 negative affect items	Reich and Zautra 1990
	Philadelphia Geriatric Center (PGC) Positive and Negative Affect Rating Scales	Lawton et al. 1992	5 positive and 5 negative affect items, plus health and pain, rated on 5-point scales	Lawton et al. 1992
	Positive and Negative Affect Scales (PANAS)	Watson et al. 1988	20 5-point scales assess generalized positive and negative affect	Beck et al. 2003
	Profile of Mood States	McNair et al. 1971	65 5-point items tap 6 mood states: depression, anxiety, vigor, anger, fatigue, and confusion	Gibson 1997

Table I *(cont.)*

Domain/ Construct	Measure	Source	Brief Description	Validation in Older Adults
Interpersonal Processes				
Pain-specific	MPI Pain Support	Kerns et al. 1985	14 items address significant others' responses to expressed pain in 3 domains: solicitous, punishing, and distracting	Boothby et al. 2004
General	Interpersonal Support Evaluation List	Cohen and Hoberman 1983	40-item measure assesses perceived support in the areas of appraisal (availability of confidants), belonging, tangible assistance, and self-esteem support	Uchino et al. 2001*
	MOS Social Support Survey	Sherbourne and Stewart 1991	19 items assessing perceived support in 4 areas: emotional/informal, tangible, affectionate, and positive social interaction	Sherbourne and Stewart 1991†
	Social Provisions Scale	Cutrona and Russell 1987	24 4-point items assess perceived functions of close relationships on 4 subscales: intimacy, social integration, reassurance of worth, and opportunity for nurturance	Mancini and Blieszner 1992
Coping				
Pain-specific	Coping Strategies Questionnaire	Rosenstiel and Keefe 1983	42 items assess 7 strategies (making coping self-statements, ignoring pain sensations, reinterpreting pain sensations, praying/hoping, catastrophizing, diverting attention, and increasing activities), but various factor structures have emerged	Keefe et al. 1987
	Chronic Pain Coping Inventory	Jensen et al. 1995	65 items assess behavioral coping strategies in 11 domains	None known
	Vanderbilt Pain Management Inventory	Brown and Nicassio 1987	Separate active (11 items) and passive (7 items) subscales	Brown and Nicassio 1987†; Mercado et al. 2000*

General	Coping with Chronic Illness	Felton and Revenson 1984	54 items comprise 6 subscales: cognitive restructuring, emotional expression, wish-fulfilling fantasy, self-blame, information seeking, and threat minimization	Felton and Revenson 1984*
	Coping Responses Scale	Billings and Moos 1981	19 items on 5-point scale assessing use of attentional and avoidant strategies	None known
	Ways of Coping Scale (Revised)	Folkman and Lazarus 1985	66 items comprise numerous subscales and 2 higher-order factors: problem-focused and emotion-focused coping. Revised by Vitaliano et al. 1985	Kemp and Krause 1999

Psychological Well-Being

Center for Epidemiological Studies Depression Scale	Radloff 1977	20 items on 4-point scale	Radloff and Teri 1986
Geriatric Depression Scale	Yesavage et al. 1983	30 yes/no items; omits somatic and other depressive symptoms possibly confounded with aging; short form available	Yesavage et al. 1983
PGC Morale Scale	Lawton 1975	17 yes/no items assess general emotional well-being; factor analysis yielded agitation, attitude toward own aging, and lonely dissatisfaction subscales	Lawton 1975
Satisfaction with Life Scale	Diener et al. 1985	5-item scale tapping overall life satisfaction	Pavot and Diener 1993
Well-Being Scales	Ryff 1989	6 scales, 9 items each, assess autonomy, environmental mastery, personal growth, positive relations with others, purpose in life, and self-acceptance	Ryff 1989

* Study examined scale in adults ≥65 years old, but did not report psychometric properties separately.

† Sample included adults ≥65 years old, but study did not examine scale properties separately for that group.

Although much work remains to be done, it is clear that these and other stable traits are strong, basic influences upon both responses to pain and overall emotional well-being. Indeed, it is likely that dispositional factors set the stage for other, more specific processes and outcomes. For example, neuroticism is emerging as a general psychological precursor to more specific cognitive-emotional pain responses such as catastrophizing, pain-related anxiety, and passive coping (Persson and Sahlberg 2002; Goubert et al. 2004; Ramirez-Maestre et al. 2004). By going to the "root" of the process—that is, figuring broad dispositional factors into our assessments from the beginning—we may be able more parsimoniously to account for the myriad pain-specific cognitive and affective constructs currently in vogue.

Cognitive processes. There is a growing assortment of pain-specific measures of various cognitive orientations to pain and its effects; the most commonly used are summarized in Table I. With a few notable exceptions (e.g., Yong et al. 2001), these instruments have been applied to older persons sparsely and without much concern for differential psychometric properties in that group. Nonetheless, existing data reveal no obvious problems, and there is no reason at this point to question use of these measures with older adults. However, empirical corroboration of this assumption is obviously needed.

By far the most widely measured cognitive construct relevant to persistent pain is catastrophizing, to which we referred earlier. There is now a tremendous literature on the association of this construct with physical and psychological outcomes of chronic pain (see review by Sullivan et al. 2001b). Originally identified as a coping strategy (Rosenstiel and Keefe 1983), catastrophizing is now treated as a unique cognitive orientation to pain that is characterized by magnification of and preoccupation with threat and perceived inability to cope. Given this definition, it is obvious that catastrophizing is strongly akin to neuroticism, but existing data on its associations with pain and disability net of measured neuroticism are not consistent (Affleck et al. 1992; Martin et al. 1996). Again, more work is needed on this important construct.

A very important set of pain-relevant cognitions, of which catastrophizing may be considered an example, are those directly related to perceived control over pain and its effects. Several generalized measures of perceived control have been shown to perform well among older persons. Perhaps the most straightforward is Pearlin and Schooler's (1978) Personal Mastery scale, a simple seven-item tool that taps generalized perceptions of one's ability directly to deal with life circumstances. More popular lately are measures of Bandura's (1982, 1997, 2001) construct *self-efficacy*, which, generally defined, is one's belief that one can successfully marshal the resources needed to manage the demands of a given situation. Over the past decade or so, the concept of self-efficacy has taken strong hold in work on health, including pain. Process-specific self-efficacy scales have proliferated (Harrison 2004); at least one disease-specific inventory includes a pain self-efficacy scale (Lorig et al. 1989).

Unfortunately, as in much of the literature invoking this concept, pain researchers have tended to take Bandura's definition of self-efficacy at face value, operationalizing it in terms of stated confidence in one's ability to achieve any of several specific desired goals (e.g., Denison et al. 2004; Rokke et al. 2004). This is problematic both conceptually and methodologically. First, it is a highly simplistic translation of his concepts, failing to capture the multiple bases of self-efficacy not only in self-perceptions of one's abilities, but also in direct mastery experiences, vicarious experience of others' successes, and social persuasion. Methodological implications of this approach are even more troublesome. Simply asking persons to rate their certainty or confidence that they can achieve a given end such as pain control or functional independence artificially inflates the correlation of "self-efficacy" with parallel measures of that end as well as other relevant outcomes, such as satisfaction with pain control or actual functional status.

It would be far preferable to use measures that capture the content and complexity of Bandura's formulation a little less literally. In fact, a number of existing instruments, although they may be based in conceptual frameworks other than Bandura's, capture its basic spirit in more subtle fashion than do measures specifically targeting self-efficacy (Kerns et al. 2002; Mezo and Heiby 2004). In addition, several composite measures of pain beliefs and attitudes include subscales regarding perception of control; the Survey of Pain Attitudes (SOPA) is perhaps the best example. The assortment of control-relevant measures that address general health- or disease-specific processes may also be useful in application to pain (see Table I for examples). Whatever the specific approach, it behooves one to return to Bandura's original conceptualization of self-efficacy, and to develop more sophisticated, less literal operationalizations of that construct that can better inform understanding of its role in adaptation to persistent pain.

As a final note, several of the multidimensional pain tools mentioned earlier include measures of pain attitudes and beliefs that may be useful in assessing how older persons think about their pain, its controllability, and its consequences. As with other classes of measures, there has been little direct examination of these tools in older populations. However, they appear on the surface to present few major problems, and should translate fairly well.

Affective aspects of pain have received somewhat less attention in all age groups than have cognitions. However, emerging evidence suggests that pain interacts with affective processes in complex ways across the lifespan (Blalock et al. 1995; Zautra et al. 2001). It is thus important to evaluate available assessment approaches. Again, one may choose between scales tapping pain-specific emotional content, and more general measures of affective states and processes.

Perhaps the most widely used measure of the affective dimension of pain is the McGill Pain Questionnaire (Melzack 1975), which yields an affective subscale based on the emotional content of words respondents select to describe their pain. The MPQ has been widely used and has generated a considerable body of empirical work on the affective component of pain (Fernandez and Turk 1992). However, its length and complexity are problematic in clinical settings, and may pose difficulties with older adult research subjects as well. More useful are scales that directly address emotional responses to pain, such as the Pain Anxiety Symptoms Scale (McCracken et al. 1992), and the Tampa Scale of Kinesiophobia (Kori et al. 1990). Both scales (described in Table I) measure fear of pain, which is by far the most commonly assessed pain-specific emotion. Neither has been evaluated for reliability and validity in older populations, but each should generalize well at least to fairly able older persons.

A range of more general measures of affective tone and process is available; many have proven sound with older adults. The most commonly used of these, summarized in Table I, include multifactorial measures such as the Profile of Mood States (Casten et al. 1995; Gibson 1997), as well as briefer measures of positive and negative mood states (Lawton et al. 1992, 1995). Single-construct instruments such as the State-Trait Anxiety Inventory (Spielberger et al. 1970) are also appropriate for assessing pain-related affective states. These kinds of assessments can provide useful insights into affective concomitants of acute (including experimental) and chronic pain. However, one must again take care clearly to define the limits of underlying concepts.

In particular, the distinction of state from trait—that is, of transient affective tone from more stable underlying temperament or affective disturbances—is crucial. The fact that individuals do have characteristic, relatively enduring patterns of affective response complicates distinctions among personality, affect, and psychological well-being considerably (Watson 2000). We shall consider methodologies aimed at making these distinctions later in this chapter. For the present, it is important to note that individual differences in positive and negative affectivity cannot and should not be confused either with transient affective responses to pain-producing stimuli or with general emotional well-being or pathology. There is a tendency, for example, to use affect checklists such as the Profile of Mood States as substitutes for measures of true emotional dysfunction (e.g., depression or anxiety disorders). Despite clear parallels in terms of general mood states, the majority of affect measures have not been validated for this purpose. Hence, it is unwise to generalize from affect checklists to symptoms of diagnosable affective disorder.

That caveat aside, emotional responses to pain—whether momentary or relatively enduring—are clearly an important aspect of its overall psychosocial impact. This is an important area for further research, again grounded in existing theory, to parse the role of both transient and enduring patterns of affective responses to pain.

COPING WITH PAIN AND ITS EFFECTS

There has been a tremendous amount of research on how persons of all ages cope with persistent pain, including a fair number of studies with older adults. Such studies parallel the more general stress and coping literature (Folkman and Lazarus 1980) in identifying two broad classes of coping strategies, variously labeled problem- versus emotion-focused (Folkman and Greer 2000), cognitive versus emotional (Felton et al. 1984), active versus passive (Brown and Nicassio 1987; Snow-Turek et al. 1996; Covic et al. 2000), or adaptive versus maladaptive (Keefe and Williams 1990). This last terminology reflects the relatively consistent finding that coping strategies aimed at passively monitoring or averting emotional responses to pain or other stressors are associated with poorer psychological adjustment in a number of populations (Felton et al. 1984; Keefe et al. 1987; Snow-Turek et al. 1996; Covic et al. 2000; Smith et al. 2002).

This two-factor model of coping has proven quite robust across widely varying populations and measurement strategies, and it provides a handy shorthand for describing coping efforts in broad strokes. However, it has also rightly been criticized as being overly simplistic (Zautra and Manne 1992). Thus, much recent research has sought to differentiate the elements that make up pain-related coping and to distinguish it from other, related constructs. For example, as discussed earlier, recent work has explored distinctions among coping, catastrophizing, pain beliefs, expectancies, and related constructs (Turner et al. 2000, 2001; Sullivan et al. 2001a; Lefebvre and Keefe 2002). Similarly, there has been considerable work relating various personality factors and psychological dynamics to coping and its outcomes in persons with chronic pain (Keefe et al. 2001; Turk and Okifuji 2002).

As in other areas, coping strategies can be assessed with pain-specific or more generic measures. Several pain-specific tools are available (see Table I). By far the most widely used is Rosenstiel and Keefe's (1983) Coping Strategies Questionnaire. This tool has been used successfully with older adults, particularly those with osteoarthritis (Rapp et al. 2000; Haythornthwaite et al. 2003). Other pain-specific measures, although well validated with younger populations, have been far less extensively applied in older populations. Conversely, general (non-pain-specific) coping inventories known to perform well in older samples have not enjoyed much attention from pain researchers.

An important consideration in selecting a measure of coping is not only the age-relevance and age-appropriateness of various strategies, but also the nature and source of pain involved. For example, the single most common source of pain among older adults is osteoarthritis. My own work with osteoarthritis patients indicates that their pain—and hence the strategies they use to cope with it—is intricately bound up with the resulting activity limitations that pain causes. Although empirical data on the issue are scarce, there can be no doubt that the strategies that these individuals use differ qualitatively as well as quantitatively from those chosen by persons whose pain derives from, say, cancer or disease-related neuropathies. Given this premise, one might further expect that the adaptiveness of active versus passive strategies should vary with the objective controllability of the pain at issue—for example, whether pain responds to direct behavioral strategies such as changing activity patterns. Unfortunately, there has been little investigation of the disease or syndrome specificity of strategies for coping with pain. This, again, is an important area for further investigation with younger and older adults alike. In the meantime, coping measures should be selected with an eye toward the specific dynamics and effects of the disease process in question, in order to ensure that all relevant processes are captured.

INTERPERSONAL PROCESSES

The literature on how other persons affect (and are affected by) the experience and expression of pain has grown rapidly over the past 10 to 15 years. It now encompasses general notions of social support as a moderator of experienced pain and its effects (Evers et al. 2003), as well as pain-specific social influences and dynamics (Newton-John 2002; Smith et al. 2004). Examples of each of these types of measures appear in Table I. Further, thanks mainly to a couple of intervention studies with osteoarthritis sufferers and their spouses (Martire et al. 2003; Keefe et al. 2004), older persons are relatively well represented in this literature. As a result of this work, which is on the cutting edge of studies of marital couples coping with pain, concerns about psychometric adequacy of existing measurement approaches for use with older persons are tempered somewhat.

Perhaps more important in this area is the nature of the relationship being examined. Excluding studies that simply document discrepancies between self- and surrogate ratings of pain, the bulk of work on dyadic processes in pain has been done with married or cohabiting, and overwhelmingly heterosexual, couples. However, many older persons, particularly women, are likely to be unmarried. In particular, the bulk of informal care to frail older adults is provided by adult children, usually daughters, and yet there has been little study of the interpersonal effects of chronic pain in such dyads. To be sure, we have a good sense of the concern of family caregivers about their own ability to manage pain, particularly in the context of cancer or other terminal illnesses (Ferrell and Ferrell 1991). But the vast literature on family caregiving has seldom addressed either care recipients' feelings about expressing their pain or care providers' about how to respond to such expressions. Given the known tendency of the current cohort of older adults to avoid complaining to others (Leventhal and Prohaska 1986; Greenlee 1991), this gap in the literature has tremendous implications for caregiving dynamics. It is to be hoped that existing work on pain-related processes in marital dyads will be extended to this arena in the future.

PSYCHOLOGICAL WELL-BEING: THE EXAMPLE OF DEPRESSION

Emotional effects of chronic pain are well documented in older as well as younger populations (Moldofsky and Chester 1970; Dent et al. 1999; Geerlings et al. 2002). Because the bulk of this work has focused on depression, because of the strong overlap of depression with other affective disorders (Devanand 2002; Lauderdale and Sheikh 2003), and because depression is probably the most common manifestation of dysfunctions of perceived control, this discussion will focus on depression as well. It would, of course, be far preferable to treat that and other psychological dysfunctions in the larger context of quality of life. However, it would take an entire chapter to address that issue alone. Hence, this discussion is limited to depression. Note, though, that Table I offers several measures of general psychological well-being as well, including life satisfaction and morale scales.

Research on the emotional impact of chronic pain has generally been well informed by the large literature on assessment and diagnosis of depressive symptoms and syndromes, and hence meets current measurement standards in that area. Nonetheless, two issues deserve in-depth attention; one is psychometric, the other, conceptual.

On the surface, there would seem to be little debate about the appropriate measurement of depressive symptoms among older adults. The Geriatric Depression Scale (GDS; Yesavage et al. 1983) is widely regarded as the standard for such assessment, as well as for preliminary screening for diagnosable depressive disorder. Previous work leaves little doubt that the GDS is a valid and reliable measure of depressive symptomatology (Koenig et al. 1988; Parmelee et al. 1989). The question is whether it is the best measure for all purposes and for all older adults. Our own work (Parmelee and Katz 1995) indicates that, as with measures of coping, the best instrument for one population may be less than optimal for another. Specifically, we compared the GDS and the Center for Epidemiologic Studies Depression scale (CESD; Radloff 1977) in three populations—very old, very frail long-term care residents; a younger sample of elderly community residents with osteoarthritis of the knee; and older cancer patients. As expected, the GDS performed better than the CESD in the residential care population in terms both of completion rates and of validity vis-à-vis diagnostic interviews designed to yield research parallels of clinical diagnoses. In the more able community samples, however, the CESD proved more robust, yielding fewer missing data and better correspondence to research-diagnosed depression.

Further work is needed to corroborate the results of this study. However, as noted earlier with respect to the utility of the SF-36 with older persons, unquestioning reliance on proven measures can often impede rather than facilitate optimal assessment. This is true not only of generalization from younger to older populations but also—and for our purposes, more importantly—of generalization within the very diverse group of individuals labeled "older persons." As another illustration, there is evidence that depression is differentially manifested among African American as compared with European American elders (Gallo 1998; Baker 2001). Here again, a single measurement approach may becloud rather than clarify dynamics of interest. Rather, investigators need to take the time to explore those dynamics informally in the population of current interest, assuring that they understand subtleties of psychological well-being in that group as well as the measurement approaches that will best capture those subtleties.

A second, conceptual issue is the recurring question of confounding of physical and psychological symptoms. This question was raised in its simplest form a number of years ago, in terms of the possibility that pain and other physical complaints may substitute for, or "mask," symptoms of depression, particularly among older adults (Goldfarb 1974; Williamson 1978). A fair amount of subsequent research has addressed this issue, generally demonstrating that the overlap between physical and psychological symptoms cannot wholly account for the association of pain with depressed mood

(Blalock et al. 1989; Parmelee et al. 1991; Williamson and Schulz 1992). Nonetheless, concerns continue to resurface periodically, particularly regarding the role of somatic symptoms of depression in medical illness generally (Posse and Hallstrom 1998; Sheehan and Bannerjee 1999) and pain syndromes specifically (Dohrenwend et al. 1999).

This is truly a conceptual sticky wicket. Despite our having laid to rest the notion that specific pain complaints may function to mask depression, the links among pain and mood disorders are obviously complex. There is little doubt that chronic pain increases the risk of depression (Romano and Turner 1985; Campbell et al. 2003), or that depressive symptoms heighten the experience of very real pain (Parmelee et al. 1991). But knowledge of cognitive characteristics of depression does raise concerns that its very real correlation with pain may be exaggerated by cognitive biases common to depression (Maxwell et al. 1998). Unfortunately, because of the inherently subjective nature of pain, we do not have the luxury of testing whether such biases are in fact distortions, or whether they represent the heightened accuracy depressives display in self-assessments and causal attributions (Alloy and Abramson 1979; Haaga and Beck 1995).

Part of the difficulty in parsing the association between pain and (impaired) psychological well-being is measurement-related. The subjectivity that inheres in these phenomena requires that we rely heavily on self-reports to capture constructs of interest, yet the cognitive dynamics of depression render those self-reports immediately suspect. Whether it be attributed to decreased inhibitions about complaining, as I and my colleagues have suggested (Parmelee et al. 1991), to differential "mental algebra" in judging pain, or to cognitive distortions such as catastrophizing or filtering (Beck 1963; Persson et al. 1999), the research community tends to distrust the strong correlation between pain and depressive symptoms. Since the problem inheres in the methodology, one way to address it may be to change our methods. The foundation for such a change is offered in the substantial literature on daily or momentary assessment of life processes.

AN ASSESSMENT ALTERNATIVE: REPEATED-MEASURES METHODOLOGIES

Over the past two decades, there has developed a strong literature using multiple repeated measures to assess constructs that are more traditionally captured by generalized, one-time self-reports. These repeated-measures designs are of two general sorts: diary studies and experience sampling, or "ecological momentary assessment" techniques (Stone and Shiffman 1994).

Both approaches sidestep the biases inherent in retrospective, summary self-reports by measuring relevant constructs at multiple time points within a single respondent. The difference lies only in assessment intervals: whereas diary studies ask respondents to summarize experiences over a short time period (usually daily), experience sampling captures behavior, symptoms, and mood states randomly at multiple points within and across days.

A small but growing subset of research using these methods has addressed the associations among pain and various measures of psychosocial function, including transitory mood states (Moldofsky and Chester 1970; Vendrig and Lousberg 1997), activity patterns (Lichter-Kelly et al. 2004), and coping strategies (Tennen et al. 2000). Although the majority of multiple repeated-measures research has sampled younger adults, a handful of studies document both the feasibility of the method with older adults (Larson et al. 1985; Hnatiuk 1991) and its utility in disentangling the dynamics of coping with and emotional responses to chronic pain. For example, Zautra and colleagues, in weekly interviews with older adult arthritis sufferers, found that high levels of positive affect moderated the association of pain with negative affect, essentially buffering against negative moods in persons with high levels of pain (Zautra and Smith 2001; Zautra et al. 2001). Even more intriguing are findings that individual difference variables—including depression—moderate both patterns of associations among pain, mood, and daily activities (Affleck et al. 1992; Vendrig and Lousberg 1997) and the strategies used to cope with chronic pain on a daily basis (Affleck et al. 1999).

Of particular interest are findings that illustrate the methodological implications of diary and experience sampling methods for assessment of pain and its association with psychosocial functioning. For example, Lewis and colleagues (1995), working with osteoarthritis sufferers, found that pain ratings taken four times per day were not strongly correlated with traditional, global ratings of pain, and that at least part of the divergence was explainable in terms of the length of time over which ratings were summated (e.g., pain "right now" versus the past 4 hours versus the past 12 hours). Similar results have been reported for a mixed-age sample (Stone et al. 2004). There is also some evidence that stable personal dispositions—specifically, pain-related catastrophizing—may affect the association between daily measures and summary judgments of pain intensity (Lefebvre and Keefe 2002).

Although such studies are at this point few, they offer exciting insight into the dynamic associations among pain, cognitive and affective processes, coping, and emotional well-being in the context of chronic pain. Further exploration using these kinds of methods may help disentangle these associations in ways that will clarify current conceptual concerns about overlap among constructs. Further, they may help demonstrate the processes by which pain, intra- and interpersonal processes, and psychological well-being interact among older adults.

SUMMARY AND CONCLUSIONS

This chapter has briefly illustrated both the strengths and the weaknesses of current approaches to assessing mood and psychosocial function among older adults with chronic pain. Many choices are available for measuring intrapersonal and interpersonal processes and how these affect and are affected by pain. Measurement properties of such tools are necessarily a concern when one is dealing with very old and/or physically frail older persons; however, the majority of instruments available at this time appear to perform fairly well. The greater challenge is with respect to the conceptual adequacy of extant measurement approaches: the appropriateness of their content and interpretation with respect to the developmental tasks of late life, their adequacy in operationalizing underlying constructs, and their ability to distinguish among convergent, closely intertwined states and processes. It is a matter of debate whether traditional self-report methods are the best means of addressing those points of convergence. The answer will become clear only as more complete conceptual models and more sophisticated measurement approaches are developed and roundly tested.

REFERENCES

Achat J, Kawachi I, Spiro AR, DeMolles DA, Sparrow D. Optimism and depression as predictors of physical and mental health functioning: the Normative Aging Study. *Ann Behav Med* 2000; 22(2):127–130.

Affleck G, Tennen H, Urrows S, Higgins P. Neuroticism and the pain-mood relation in rheumatoid arthritis: insights from a prospective daily study. *J Consult Clin Psychol* 1992; 60(1):119–126.

Affleck G, Tennen H, Keefe FJ, et al. Everyday life with osteoarthritis or rheumatoid arthritis: independent effects of disease and gender on daily pain, mood, and coping. *Pain* 1999; 83(3):601–609.

Alloy LB, Abramson LY. Judgment of contingency in depressed and nondepressed students: sadder but wiser? *J Exp Psychol Gen* 1979; 108:441–485.

Arbisi PA, Butcher JN. Psychometric perspectives on detection of malingering of pain: use of the Minnesota Multiphasic Personality Inventory-2. *Clin J Pain* 2004; 20(6):383–391.

Baker FM. Diagnosing depression in African Americans. *Community Ment Health J* 2001; 37(1):31–38.

Bandura A. Self-efficacy mechanism in human agency. *Am Psychol* 1982; 37:122–147.

Bandura A. *Self-Efficacy: The Exercise of Control.* New York: Freeman; 1997.

Bandura A. Social cognitive theory: an agentic perspective. *Ann Rev Psychol* 2001; 52:1–26.

Beck AT. Thinking and depression I. Idiosyncratic content and cognitive distortions. *Arch Gen Psychiatry* 1963; 14:324–333.

Beck JG, Novy D, Diefenbach GJ, et al. Differentiating anxiety and depression in older adults with generalized anxiety disorder. *Psychol Assess* 2003; 15:184–192.

Bergner M, Bobbit RA, Carter WB, Gilson BS. The Sickness Impact Profile: development and final revision of a health status measure. *Med Care* 1981; 19(787–805).

Berlyne D. *Conflict, Arousal, and Curiosity.* New York: McGraw-Hill; 1960.

Billings AG, Moos RH. The role of coping responses and social resources in attenuating the stress of life events. *J Behav Med* 1981; 4:193–157.

Blalock SJ, DeVellis RF, Brown GK, Wallston KA. Validity of the Center for Epidemiological Studies Depression Scale in arthritis populations. *Arthritis Rheum* 1989; 32(8):991–997.

Blalock SJ, DeVellis RF, Giorgino KB. The relationship between coping and psychological well-being among people with osteoarthritis: a problem-specific approach. *Ann Behav Med* 1995; 17:107–115.

Boothby JL, Thorn BE, Overduin LY, Ward LC. Catastrophizing and perceived partner responses to pain. *Pain* 2004; 109:500–506.

Bradburn N. *The Structure of Psychological Well-Being.* Chicago: Aldine, 1969.

Brenes GA, Rapp SR, Rejeski WJ, Miller ME. Do optimism and pessimism predict physical functioning? *J Behav Med* 2002; 25(3):219–231.

Brown GK, Nicassio PM. Development of a questionnaire for the assessment of active and passive coping strategies in chronic pain patients. *Pain* 1987; 31:53–64.

Buckelew SP, Shutty MSJ, Hewett J, et al. Health locus of control, gender differences and adjustment to persistent pain. *Pain* 1990; 42:287–294.

Campbell LC, Clauw DJ, Keefe FJ. Persistent pain and depression: a biopsychosocial perspective. *Biol Psychiatry* 2003; 54:399–409.

Casten R, Parmelee PA, Kleban MH, Lawton MP, Katz IR. The relationships among anxiety, depression and pain in a geriatric institutional sample. *Pain* 1995; 61:271–276.

Chipperfield JG, Perry RP, Menec VH. Primary and secondary control-enhancing strategies: implications for health in later life. *J Aging Health* 1999; 11(4):517–539.

Cohen S, Hoberman H. Positive events and social supports as buffers of life change stress. *J Appl Soc Psychol* 1983; 13:99–125.

Costa PT Jr, McCrae RR. Cross-sectional studies of personality in a national sample: 1. Development and validation of survey measures. *Psychol Aging* 1986; 1(2):140–143.

Costa P, McCrae R. *Revised NEO Personality Inventory (NEO PI-R) and NEO Five-Factor Inventory (NEO-FFI): Professional Manual.* Odessa, FL: Psychological Assessment Resources, 1992.

Costa PTJ, McCrae RR. Longitudinal stability of adult personality. In: Hogan R, Johnson J, Briggs S (Eds). *Handbook of Personality Psychology.* San Diego: Academic Press, 1997, pp 269–290.

Covic T, Adamson B, Hough M. The impact of passive coping on rheumatoid arthritis pain. *Rheumatology* 2000; 39:1027–1030.

Creamer P, Lethbridge-Cejku M, Hochberg MC. Determinants of pain severity in knee osteoarthritis: effect of demographic and psychosocial variables using 3 pain measures. *J Rheumatol* 1999; 26(8):1785–1792.

Cutrona CE, Russell D. The provisions of social relationships and adaptation to stress. In: Jones WH, Perlman D (Eds). *Advances in Personal Relationships,* Vol. 1. Greenwich, CT: JAI Press, 1987, pp 37–67.

de Charms R. *Personal Causation: The Internal Affective Determinants of Behavior.* New York: Academic Press; 1968.

Denison E, Asenlof P, Lindberg P. Self-efficacy, fear avoidance, and pain intensity as predictors of disability in subacute and chronic musculoskeletal pain patients in primary health care. *Pain* 2004; 111(3):245–252.

Dent OF, Waite LM, Bennett HP, et al. A longitudinal study of chronic disease and depressive symptoms in a community sample of older people. *Aging Ment Health* 1999; 3(4):351–357.

Devanand DP. Comorbid psychiatric disorders in late life depression. *Biol Psychiatry* 2002; 52(3):236–242.

Diener E, Emmons R, Larsen J, Griffin S. The Satisfaction with Life Scale. *J Pers Assess* 1985; 49(1):71–75.

Dohrenwend BP, Raphael KG, Marbach JJ, Gallagher RM. Why is depression comorbid with chronic myofascial face pain? A family study test of alternative hypotheses. *Pain* 1999; 83(2):183–192.

Evers AW, Kraaimaat FW, Geenen R, Jacobs JW, Bijlsma JW. Pain coping and social support as predictors of long-term functional disability and pain in early rheumatoid arthritis. *Behav Res Ther* 2003; 41(11):1295–1310.

Felton BJ, Revenson TA, Hinrichsen GA. Stress and coping in the explanation of psychological adjustment among chronically ill adults. *Soc Sci Med* 1984; 18:889–898.

Fernandez E, Turk DC. Sensory and affective components of pain: separation and synthesis. *Psychol Bull* 1992; 112(2):205–217.

Ferrell BA, Ferrell BR. Pain management at home. *Clin Geriatr Med* 1991; 7(4):765–776.

Flint AJ. Generalised anxiety disorder in elderly patients: epidemiology, diagnosis and treatment options. *Drugs Aging* 2005; 22(2):101–114.

Folkman S, Greer S. Promoting psychological well-being in the face of serious illness: when theory, research and practice inform each other. *Psycho-oncology* 2000; 9:11–19.

Folkman S, Lazarus RS. An analysis of coping in a middle-aged community sample. *J Health Soc Behav* 1980; 21:219–239.

Folkman S, Lazarus RS. If it changes it must be a process: study of emotion and coping during three stages of a college examination. *J Pers Soc Psychol* 1985; 48:150–170.

Frazier LD, Waid LD. Influences on anxiety in later life: the role of health status, health perceptions, and health locus of control. *Aging Ment Health* 1999; 3(3):213–230.

Funk SC. Hardiness: a review of theory and research. *Health Psychol* 1992; 11(5):335–345.

Gagliese L, Katz J. Age differences in postoperative pain are scale dependent: a comparison of measures of pain intensity and quality in younger and older surgical patients. *Pain* 2003; 103(1–2):11–20.

Gallo JJ. Depressive symptoms of whites and African Americans aged 60 years and older. *J Gerontol B Psychol Sci* 1998; 53(5):277–286.

Geerlings S, Twisk JWR, Beekman ATF, Deeg DJH, van Tilburg W. Longitudinal relationship between pain and depression in older adults: sex, age and physical disability. *Soc Psychiatry Psychiatr Epidemiol* 2002; 37:23–30.

Gibson SJ. The measurement of mood states in older adults. *J Gerontol Psychol Sci* 1997; 52:(167–174).

Gibson SJ, Helme RD. Age-related differences in pain perception and report. *Clin Geriatr Med* 2001; 17(3):433–456, v–vi.

Gil KM, Williams DA, Keefe FJ, Beckham JC. The relationship of negative thoughts to pain and psychological distress. *Behav Ther* 1990; 21(349–362).

Goldfarb AI. Masked depression in the elderly. In: Lesse S (Ed). *Masked Depression.* New York: Jason Aronson, 1974, pp 236–249.

Goubert L, Crombez G, Van Damme S. The role of neuroticism, pain catastrophizing and pain-related fear in vigilance to pain: a structural equations approach. *Pain* 2004; 107(3): 234–241.

Greenlee KK. Pain and analgesia: considerations for the elderly in critical care. *AACN Clin Issues Crit Care Nurs* 1991; 2:720–728.

Guarnera S, Williams RL. Optimism and locus of control for health and affiliation among elderly adults. *J Gerontol* 1987; 42(6):594–595.

Haaga DA, Beck AT. Perspectives on depressive realism: implications for cognitive theory of depression. *Behav Res Ther* 1995; 33(1):41–48.

Harrison AL. The influence of pathology, pain, balance, and self-efficacy on function in women with osteoarthritis of the knee. *Phys Ther* 2004; 84(9):822–831.

Hathaway SR, McKinley JC. *Minnesota Multiphasic Personality Inventory.* New York: Psychological Corporation, 1943.

Haythornthwaite JA, Clark MR, Pappagallo M, Raja SN. Pain coping strategies play a role in the persistence of pain in post-herpetic neuralgia. *Pain* 2003; 106(3):453–460.

Helme RD, Meliala A, Gibson SJ. Methodologic factors which contribute to variations in experimental pain threshold reported for older people. *Neurosci Lett* 2004; 361(1–3):144–146.

Hnatiuk SH. Experience sampling with elderly persons: an exploration of the method. *Int J Aging Hum Dev* 1991; 33(1):45–64.

Jensen MP, Karoly P. *Revision and Cross-Validation of the Survey of Pain Attitudes (SOPA).* Presented at: Annual Meeting of the Society of Behavioral Medicine, San Francisco, March 1989.

Jensen MP, Turner JA, Romano JM, Strom SE. The Chronic Pain Coping Inventory: development and preliminary validation. *Pain* 1995; 60:203–216.

Jensen MP, Turner JA, Romano JM. Changes in beliefs, catastrophizing, and coping are associated with improvement in multidisciplinary pain treatment. *J Consult Clin Psychol* 2001; 69(4):655–662.

Judd LL, Schettler PJ, Akiskal HS. The prevalence, clinical relevance, and public health significance of subthreshold depressions. *Psychiatry Clin North Am* 2002; 25(4):685–698.

Kaplan RM, Anderson JP, Wu AW, et al. The Quality of Well-Being Scale: applications in AIDS, cystic fibrosis, and arthritis. *Med Care* 1989; 27(Suppl 3):S27–S43.

Keefe FJ, Williams DA. A comparison of coping strategies in chronic pain patients in different age groups. *J Gerontol Psychol Sci* 1990; 45:P161–P165.

Keefe FJ, Caldwell DS, Queen KT, et al. Pain coping strategies in osteoarthritis patients. *J Consult Clin Psychol* 1987; 55, 208–212.

Keefe FJ, Lumley MA, Anderson T, Lynch T, Carson KL. Pain and emotion: new research directions. *J Clin Psychol* 2001; 57:587–607.

Keefe FJ, Blumenthal J, Baucom D, et al. Effects of spouse-assisted coping skills training and exercise training in patients with osteoarthritic knee pain: a randomized controlled study. *Pain* 2004; 110(3):539–549.

Kellner R. *Somatization and Hypochondriasis.* New York: Prager, 1986.

Kemp B, Krause S. Depression and life satisfaction among people ageing with post-polio and spinal cord injury. *Disabil Rehabil* 1999; 21;241–249.

Kerns RD, Turk DC, Rudy TE. The West Haven-Yale Multidimensional Pain Inventory (WHYMPI). *Pain* 1985; 23:4.

Kerns RD, Rosenberg R, Otis JD. Self-appraised problem solving and pain-relevant social support as predictors of the experience of chronic pain. *Ann Behav Med* 2002; 24(2):100–105.

Kobasa SC. Stressful life events, personality and health: an inquiry into hardiness. *J Pers Soc Psychol* 1979; 37:1–11.

Koenig HG, Meador KG, Cohen HJ, Blazer DG. Self-rated depression scales and screening for major depression in the older hospitalized patient with medical illness. *J Am Geriatr Soc* 1988; 36(8):609–706.

Kori SH, Miller RP, Todd DD. Kinesiophobia: a new view of chronic pain behavior. *Pain Manage* 1990; 3:35–43.

Larson R, Zuzanek J, Mannell R. Being alone versus being with people: disengagement in the daily experience of older adults. *J Gerontol* 1985; 40(3):375–381.

Lauderdale SA, Sheikh JL. Anxiety disorders in older adults. *Clin Geriatr Med* 2003; 19(4):721–741.

Lawton MP. The Philadelphia Geriatric Center Morale Scale: a revision. *J Gerontol* 1975; 30:85–89.

Lawton MP, Kleban MH, Dean J, Rajagopal D, Parmelee PA. The factorial generality of brief positive and negative affect measures. *J Gerontol Psychol Sci* 1992; 47(4):P228–P237.

Lawton MP, De Voe MR, Parmelee P. Relationship of events and affect in the daily life of an elderly population. *Psychol Aging* 1995; 10(3):469–477.

Lawton MP, Moss M, Hoffman C, et al. Valuation of life: a concept and a scale. *J Aging Health* 2001; 13:3–31.

Lefebvre MF. Cognitive distortion and cognitive errors in depressed psychiatric and low back pain patients. *J Consult Clin Psychol* 1981; 49:517–525.

Lefebvre JC, Keefe FJ. Memory for pain: the relationship of pain catastrophizing to the recall of daily rheumatoid arthritis pain. *Clin J Pain* 2002; 18:56–63.

Leventhal EA, Prohaska TR. Age, symptom interpretation and health behavior. *J Am Geriatr Soc* 1986; 34:185–191.

Lewis B, Lewis D, Cumming G. Frequent measurement of chronic pain: an electronic diary and empirical findings. *Pain* 1995; 60:341–347.

Lichtenberg PA, Skehan MW, Swensen CH. The role of personality, recent life stress and arthritic severity in predicting pain. *J Psychosom Res* 1984; 28(3):231–236.

Lichtenberg PA, Swensen CH, Skehan MW. Further investigation of the role of personality, lifestyle and arthritic severity in predicting pain. *J Psychosom Res* 1986; 30(3):327–337.

Lichter-Kelly L, Stone AA, Broderick JE, Schwartz JE. Associations among pain intensity, sensory characteristics, affective qualities, and activity limitations in patients with chronic pain: a momentary, within-person perspective. *J Pain* 2004; 5(8):433–439.

Lorig K, Chastain RL, Ung E, Shoor S, Holman HR. Development and evaluation of a scale to measures self-efficacy in people with arthritis. *Arthritis Rheum* 1989; 32(1):37–44.

Maddi SR. Dispositional hardiness in health and effectiveness. In: Friedman HS (Ed). *Encyclopedia of Mental Health.* San Diego: Academic Press, 1998.

Mancini JA, Blieszner R. Social provisions in adulthood: concept and measurement in close relationships. *J Gerontol Psychol Sci* 1992; 41(1):P14–P20.

Martin MY, Bardley LA, Alexander RW, et al. Coping strategies predict disability in patients with primary fibromyalgia. *Pain* 1996; 68(1):45–53.

Martire LM, Schulz R, Keefe FJ, et al. Feasibility of a dyadic intervention for management of osteoarthritis: a pilot study with older patients and their spousal caregivers. *Aging Mental Health* 2003; 7(1):53–60.

Massee R, Poulin C, Dassa C, et al. The structure of mental health: higher-order confirmatory factor analyses of psychological distress and well-being measures. *Soc Indicators Res* 1998; 45:475–504.

Maxwell TD, Gatchel RJ, Mayer TG. Cognitive predictors of depression in chronic low back pain: toward an inclusive model. *J Behav Med* 1998; 21(2):131–143.

McCracken LM, Zayfert C, Gross RT. The Pain Anxiety Symptoms Scale: development and validation of a scale to measure fear of pain. *Pain* 1992; 50(1):67–73.

McNair DM, Lorr M, Droppleman LF. *Manual for the Profile of Mood States.* San Diego: Educational and Industrial Testing Services, 1971.

Meenan RF, Mason JH, Anderson JJ, Guccione AA, Kazis LE. AIMS2. The content and properties of a revised and expanded Arthritis Impact Measurement Scales Health Status Questionnaire. *Arthritis Rheum* 1992; 35(1):1–10.

Meldolesi G, Picardi A, Accivile E, Toraldo di Francia R, Biondi M. Personality and psychopathology in patients with temporomandibular joint syndrome: a controlled investigation. *Psychother Psychosom* 2000; 69(6):322–328.

Melzack R. The McGill Pain Questionnaire: major properties and scoring methods. *Pain* 1975; 1:277–299.

Mercado AC, Carroll LJ, Cassidy JD, Cote P. Coping with neck and low back pain in the general population. *Health Psychol* 2000; 19(4):333–338.

Mezo PG, Heiby EM. A comparison of four measures of self-control skills. *Assessment* 2004; 11(3):238–250.

Moldofsky H, Chester WJ. Pain and mood patterns in patients with rheumatoid arthritis. A prospective study. *Psychosom Med* 1970; 32(3):309–318.

Newton-John TRO. Solicitousness and chronic pain: a critical review. *Pain Rev* 2002; 9(1):7–21.

Nicassio PM, Wallston KA, Callahan LF, Herbert M, Pincus T. The measurement of helplessness in rheumatoid arthritis. The development of the arthritis helplessness index. *J Rheumatol* 1985; 12(3):462–467.

O'Mahoney PG, Rodgers H, Thomson RG, Dobson R, James OFW. Is the SF-36 suitable for assessing health status of older stroke patients? *Age Ageing* 1998; 27(1):19–22.

Parmelee P, Katz IR. *Differential Utility of the GDS and the CES-D with Diverse Groups of Frail Older Persons.* Presented at: Annual Meeting of the Gerontological Society of America, Los Angeles, 1995.

Parmelee PA, Lawton MP, Katz IR. Psychometric properties of the Geriatric Depression Scale among institutionalized aged. *Psychol Assess* 1989; 1:331–338.

Parmelee PA, Katz IR, Lawton MP. The relation of pain to depression among institutionalized aged. *J Gerontol Psychol Sci* 1991; 46(1):P15–P21.

Pavot W, Diener E. Review of the Satisfaction with Life Scale. *Psychol Assess* 1993: 5(2);164–172.

Pearlin LI, Schooler C. The structure of coping. *J Health Soc Behav* 1978; 19(1):2–21.

Persson LO, Sahlberg D. The influence of negative illness cognitions and neuroticism on subjective symptoms and mood in rheumatoid arthritis. *Ann Rheum Dis* 2002; 61(11):1000–1006.

Persson LO, Berglund K, Sahlberg D. Psychological factors in chronic rheumatic diseases—a review. The case of rheumatoid arthritis, current research and some problems. *Scand J Rheumatol* 1999; 28(3):131–136.

Posse M, Hallstrom T. Depressive disorders among somatizing patients in primary health care. *Acta Psychiatr Scand* 1998; 98(3):187–192.

Radloff LS. The CES-D Scale: a self-report depression scale for research in the general population. *Appl Psychol Measure* 1977; 1:385–401.

Radloff LS, Teri L. Use of the CESD with older adults. *Clin Gerontol* 1986; 5:119–135.

Ramirez-Maestre C, Lopez Martinez AE, Zarazaga RE. Personality characteristics as differential variables of the pain experience. *J Behav Med* 2004; 27(2):147–165.

Rapp SR, Rejeski WJ, Miller ME. Physical function among older adults with knee pain: the role of pain coping skills. *Arthritis Care Res* 2000; 13(5):270–279.

Reich JQ, Zautra AJ. Dispositional control beliefs and the consequences of a control-enhancing intervention. *J Gerontol Psychol Sci* 1990; 45(2):P46–P51.

Rodin J, Schooler C, Schaie KW. *Self-Directedness: Cause and Effects Throughout the Life Course.* Hillsdale, NJ: Erlbaum, 1990.

Rokke PD, Fleming-Ficek S, Siemens NM, Hegstad HJ. Self-efficacy and choice of coping strategies for tolerating acute pain. *J Behav Med* 2004; 27(4):343–360.

Romano JM, Turner JA. Chronic pain and depression: does the evidence support a relationship? *Psychol Bull* 1985; 97(1):18–34.

Rosenstiel AK, Keefe FJ. The use of coping strategies in chronic low back pain patients: relationship to patient characteristics and current adjustment. *Pain* 1983; 17(1):33–44.

Ryff CD. Happiness is everything, or is it? Explorations on the meaning of psychological well-being. *J Pers Soc Psychol* 1989; 57:1069–1081.

Ryff CD, Keyes CLM. The structure of psychological well-being revisited. *J Pers Soc Psychol* 1995; 69:719–727.

Scheier MF, Carver CS, Bridges MW. Distinguishing optimism from neuroticism (and trait anxiety, self-master, and self-esteem): a re-evaluation of the Life Orientation Test. *J Pers Soc Psychol* 1994; 67:1063–1078.

Schneider G, Kruse A, Nehen HG, Senf Q, Heuft G. The prevalence and differential diagnosis of subclinical depressive syndromes in inpatients 60 years and older. *Psychother Psychosom* 2000; 69(5):251–260.

Schulz R, Heckhausen J. Aging, culture and control: setting a new research agenda. *J Gerontol Psychol Sci* 1999; 54B(3):P139–145.

Schulz R, Wrosch C, Heckhausen J. The life span theory of control: issues and evidences. In: Zarit SH, Pearlin LI, et al. (Eds). *Personal Control in Social and Life Course Contexts: Societal Impact on Aging.* New York: Springer, 2003, pp 233–262.

Sheehan B, Bannerjee S. Somatization in the elderly. *Int J Geriatr Psychiatry* 1999; 14(12):1044–1049.

Sherbourne CD, Stewart AL. The MOS Social Support Survey. *Soc Sci Med* 1991; 32(6):705–714.

Smith JA, Lumley MA, Longo DJ. Contrasting emotional approach coping with passive coping for chronic myofascial pain. *Ann Behav Med* 2002; 24:326–335.

Smith SJA, Keefe FJ, Caldwell DS, Romano JM, Baucom D. Gender differences in patient-spouse interactions: a sequential analysis of behavioral interactions in patients having osteoarthritic knee pain. *Pain* 2004; 112(1–2):183–187.

Smith TW, Christensen AJ, Peck JR, Ward JR. Cognitive distortion, helplessness, and depressed mood in rheumatoid arthritis: a four-year longitudinal analysis. *Health Psychol* 1994; 13(3):213–217.

Snow-Turek AL, Norris MP, Tan G. Active and passive coping strategies in chronic pain patients. *Pain* 1996; 64:455–462.

Spielberger CD, Gorsuch RL, Lushene RE. *Manual for the State-Trait Anxiety Inventory.* Palo Alto, CA: Consulting Psychologists Press, 1970.

Stadnyk K, Calder J, Rockwood K. Testing the measurement properties of the Short Form-36 Health Survey in a frail elderly population. *J Clin Epidemiol* 1998; 51(10):827–835.

Stein CA, Wallston KA, Nicassio PM. Predictors of attrition in health intervention research among older subjects with osteoarthritis. *Health Psychol* 1994; 13:421–431.

Stone AA, Shiffman S. Ecological momentary assessment (EMA) in behavioral medicine. *Ann Behav Med* 1994; 16(3):199–202.

Stone AA, Broderick JE, Shiffman SS, Schwartz JE. Understanding recall of weekly pain from a momentary assessment perspective: absolute agreement, between- and within-person consistency, and judged change in weekly pain. *Pain* 2004; 107(1–2):61–69.

Stroud MW, Thorn BE, Jensen MP, Boothby JL. The relation between pain beliefs, negative thoughts, and psychosocial functioning in chronic pain patients. *Pain* 2000; 84:347–352.

Sullivan MJ, d'Eon JL. Relationship between catastrophizing and depression in chronic pain patients. *J Abnorm Psychol* 1990; 99:260–263.

Sullivan MJL, Bishop SR, Pivik J. The Pain Catastrophizing Scale: development and validation. *Psychol Assess* 1995; 7:524–532.

Sullivan MJ, Rodgers WM, Kirsch I. Catastrophizing, depression and expectancies for pain and emotional distress. *Pain* 2001a; 91(1–2):147–54.

Sullivan MJ, Thorn B, Haythornthwaite JA, et al. Theoretical perspectives on the relation between catastrophizing and pain. *Clin J Pain* 2001b; 17:52–64.

Tait RC, Pollard CA, Margolis RB, Duckro PN, Krause SJ. The Pain Disability Index: psychometric and validity data. *Arch Phys Med Rehabil* 1987; 68(7):438–441.

Tennen H, Affleck G, Armeli S, Carney MA. A daily process approach to coping: linking theory, research, and practice. *Am Psychol* 2000; 55(6):626–636.

Thorn B, Rich MA, Boothby JL. Pain beliefs and coping attempts: conceptual model building. *Pain Forum* 1999; 8:172–175.

Turk DC, Okifuji A. Psychological factors in chronic pain: evolution and revolution. *J Consult Clin Psychol* 2002; 70:678–690.

Turner JA, Aaron LA. Pain-related catastrophizing: what is it? *Clin J Pain* 2001; 17(65–71).

Turner JA, Jensen MP, Romano JM. Do beliefs, coping, and catastrophizing independently predict functioning in patients with chronic pain? *Pain* 2000; 85:115–125.

Turner JA, Dworkin SF, Mancl L, Huggins KH, Truelove EL. The roles of beliefs, catastrophizing, and coping in the functioning of patients with temporomandibular disorders. *Pain* 2001; 92(1–2):41–51.

Vendrig AA, Lousberg R. Within-person relationships among pain intensity, mood, and physical activity in chronic pain: a naturalistic approach. *Pain* 1997; 73:71–76.

Vitaliano PP, Russo J, Carr JE, Maiuro RD, Becker J. The Ways of Coping Checklist: revision and psychometric properties. *Multivariate Behav Res* 1985; 20:3–26.

Wallston KA, Wallston BS, DeVellis R. Development of the Multidimensional Health Locus of Control (MHLC) scales. *Health Educ Monogr* 1978; 6(160–170).

Watson D. *Mood and Temperament.* New York: Guilford Press, 2000.

Watson D, Clark LA, Tellegen A. Development and validation of brief measures of positive and negative affect: the PANAS scales. *J Pers Soc Psychol* 1988; 54:1063–1070.

Williams DA, Thorn BE. An empirical assessment of pain beliefs. *Pain* 1989; 36:351–358.

Williamson J. Depression in the elderly. *Age Ageing* 1978; 7(Suppl):35–40.

Williamson GM, Schulz R. Pain, activity restriction, and symptoms of depression among community-residing elderly adults. *J Gerontol Psychol Sci* 1992; 47(6):P367–P372.

Yesavage JA, Brink TL, Rose TL, et al. Development and validation of a geriatric depression screening scale: a preliminary report. *J Psychiatr Res* 1983; 17(1):37–49.

Yong H-H, Gibson SJ, de L. Horne DJ, Helms RD. Development of a pain attitudes questionnaire to assess stoicism and cautiousness for possible age differences. *J Gerontol Psychol Sci* 2001; 56B(5):279–284.

Zautra AJ, Manne SL. Coping with rheumatoid arthritis: a review of a decade of research. *Ann Behav Med* 1992; 14:31–39.

Zautra AJ, Smith BW. Depression and reactivity to stress in older women with rheumatoid arthritis and osteoarthritis. *Psychosom Med* 2001; 63(4):687–696.

Zautra AJ, Smith B, Affleck G, Tennen H. Examinations of chronic pain and affect relationships: applications of a dynamic model of affect. *J Consult Clin Psychol* 2001; 69(5):786–795.

Correspondence to: Patricia A. Parmelee, PhD, Emory Center for Health in Aging, 1841 Clifton Road NE, Atlanta, GA 30329, USA. Email: pparmel@emory.edu.

Part IV

Pain Treatment Modalities

Pain in Older Persons, Progress in Pain
Research and Management, Vol. 35, edited
by Stephen J. Gibson and Debra K. Weiner,
IASP Press, Seattle, © 2005.

10

Oral Analgesics: Efficacy, Mechanism of Action, Pharmacokinetics, Adverse Effects, Drug Interactions, and Practical Recommendations for Use in Older Adults

Joseph T. Hanlon,[a,b,c] David R.P. Guay,[d,e] and Timothy J. Ives[f]

[a]Division of Geriatric Medicine, Department of Medicine, School of Medicine, [b]Department of Pharmacy and Therapeutics, School of Pharmacy, University of Pittsburgh, and [c]Center for Health Equity Research and Promotion, Veterans Administration Pittsburgh Health Care System, Pittsburgh, Pennsylvania, USA; [d]Institute for the Study of Geriatric Pharmacotherapy, Department of Experimental and Clinical Pharmacology, College of Pharmacy, University of Minnesota, and [e]Partnering Care Senior Services, Health Partners Inc., Minneapolis, Minnesota, USA; [f]Division of Pharmacotherapy, School of Pharmacy, University of North Carolina, Chapel Hill, North Carolina, USA

Older persons living in the community often develop pain disorders that lead to the prescribing of analgesics. In one study nearly 60% of community-dwelling elders reported use of analgesics, with the most common drug class being nonsteroidal anti-inflammatory drugs (NSAIDs), followed by acetaminophen (paracetamol) and then opioids (Hanlon et al. 1996). Another study reported that 49% of nursing home residents reported persistent nonmalignant pain, with the most common analgesics used being acetaminophen, propoxyphene, hydrocodone, and tramadol (Won et al. 2004). In one study propoxyphene use was nearly twice as great in nursing home residents as compared with community-dwelling older adults (15.5% versus 6.8%, respectively) (Kamal-Bahl et al. 2003). Despite the prevalence of pain across multiple settings of care, there is considerable evidence that chronic pain in older adults, whether due to malignant or nonmalignant causes, is undertreated (Bernabei et al. 1998; Pahor et al. 1999; Chodosh et al. 2004; Won et al. 2004).

This chapter will address three major types of agents used for analgesia in the older adults (1) non-opioid analgesics (NSAIDs and acetaminophen), (2) opioids and tramadol, and (3) adjunctive agents (antiepileptics, mexiletine, and baclofen) (American Geriatric Society 2002). Each major section will provide information about mechanisms of action, pharmacokinetics, efficacy, adverse effects, and selected drug interactions. Recommended agents and starting doses for older adults will also be discussed, and agents that should be avoided in this population will be mentioned. A number of other chapters in this volume discuss analgesics for specific disorders. For a discussion of the prescription of tricyclic antidepressants, topical capsaicin, lidocaine patches, pregabalin, duloxetine, tramadol, and venlafaxine for the treatment of postherpetic neuralgia and other forms of neuropathic pain, see Chapter 17. For a discussion of the prescription of glucosamine chondroitin for the treatment of pain associated with knee osteoarthritis, the reader is referred to Chapter 14. Chapter 19 discusses the use of corticosteroids, bisphosphonates, and other agents for the treatment of cancer-related pain.

NON-OPIOID ANALGESICS

NONSTEROIDAL ANTI-INFLAMMATORY DRUGS

Mechanism of action. NSAIDs are divided into two major categories: nonselective cyclooxygenase (COX) inhibitors and COX-2-selective inhibitors. The acetylated (aspirin) and non-acetylated salicylates (magnesium, choline, and sodium salicylate salt forms) and other NSAIDs primarily produce analgesia through reversible inhibition of COX, the enzyme that catalyzes the conversion of arachidonic acid to prostaglandin precursors (Nikolaus and Zeyfang 2004). At low doses, aspirin is a selective inhibitor of platelet COX-1, whereas NSAIDs cause reversible inhibition of both COX-1 and COX-2 isoenzymes (Crofford et al. 2000). Prostaglandins are inflammatory mediators that sensitize peripheral nociceptors (Vane 1971; Vane and Botting 2003). Inhibition of COX-2 is believed to be responsible for the anti-inflammatory and analgesic effects of NSAIDs.

Pharmacokinetic considerations. In general, NSAIDs are well absorbed after oral administration, exhibit low non-flow-dependent hepatic clearance and low to nonexistent first-pass metabolism, have small distribution volumes, and are highly bound to plasma proteins, principally to albumin (~95%) (Barkin 2001). The drug-free fraction of NSAIDs may be increased in patients with hypoalbuminemia (Weiner and Hanlon 2001). Protein binding is saturable in the usual dose range for some NSAIDs (salicylates, naproxen, and ibuprofen), so that increasing daily doses may lead to a less-than-proportional increase in steady-state serum concentrations; in contrast, free drug concentrations increase proportionally with dose (Workman 1998). Factors that have been assessed for their effect on NSAID plasma protein binding include gender and age; female gender has been linked to a decrease in naproxen binding, and increasing age has been associated with variable effects on plasma protein binding of different NSAIDs: decreased binding for diflunisal, salicylate, ketorolac but no change for etodolac, ibuprofen, oxaprozin, while data are conflicting for piroxicam and naproxen. Hepatic and renal disease may be associated with reduced NSAID plasma protein binding as well, in the latter case primarily due to the presence of small-molecular-weight endogenous binding inhibitors. The plasma protein binding of salicylate, diflunisal, naproxen, oxaprozin, and sulindac (and their metabolites) is reduced in patients with renal disease.

All NSAIDs except indomethacin and oxaprozin are virtually entirely dependent on hepatic metabolism for elimination, either through oxidation or glucuronidation. The isozymes of cytochrome P-450 requisite for NSAID metabolism and the possibility of phenotypic differences in NSAID metabolism have not been explored. Limited data are available regarding enterohepatic circulation of NSAIDs, but it may occur with indomethacin and sulindac due to an extensive degree of biliary excretion. Celecoxib, the longest-used COX-2 inhibitor, undergoes extensive liver metabolism via the cytochrome P450 system, with the CYP2C9, 2C19, and 2D6 isoenzymes (Bell and Schnitzer 2001).

Renal elimination of the parent compound constitutes only a small proportion of the clearance mechanism of most NSAIDs. The clearance of agents such as ketoprofen, fenoprofen, naproxen, and indomethacin may be decreased to a variable degree in patients with renal impairment, due to the retention of unstable acyl-glucuronide metabolites that may hydrolyze to reform the parent compound. This recycling is one reason for caution in the use of these agents in patients with renal impairment. Urine pH plays a major role in the elimination of salicylates, as renal clearance increases markedly when urine pH exceeds 6.5 (Proudfoot et al. 2003).

Efficacy. NSAIDs are indicated for short-term use in inflammatory arthritic conditions such as gout, pseudogout, and other acute rheumatic disorders. They are also useful in combination with opioids for treating bone pain from cancer. Anti-inflammatory activity, potency, analgesic efficacy, metabolism, excretion, and adverse effects vary widely among NSAIDs. Failure of response to one NSAID may not predict response to another (Bjordal et al. 2004). One advantage of NSAIDs is their lack of sedation,

respiratory depression, or tolerance/addiction effects. All NSAIDs have a
ceiling effect (a level at which increased dose results in no increase in
analgesia). These agents can be used alone or in combination with opioids
(e.g., oxycodone/aspirin) or with other analgesics. NSAIDs should be used
with caution, as they are no better than acetaminophen for many cases of
mild-to-moderate non-inflammatory pain (e.g., osteoarthritis of the knee and
perhaps other chronic pain syndromes). Also, the incidence of adverse reactions is extremely high in older patients. With respect to analgesic efficacy,
COX-2 inhibitors have no advantage over nonselective NSAIDs. There is a
very high degree of interpatient variability in response with all NSAIDs.

   Adverse drug effects/drug interactions. Potentially serious adverse effects of salicylates and other NSAIDs include renal impairment, peripheral
edema, precipitation of heart failure, hyperkalemia, gastrointestinal (GI) disorders, cardiovascular disorders, cerebrovascular accidents, and central nervous system (CNS) disturbances such as cognitive dysfunction (Griffin et al.
2000; Page and Henry 2000; Brater et al. 2001). The risk of GI bleeding due
to NSAIDs is about 1% in the general population and 3–4% in persons more
than 60 years old, but almost 10% in persons over 60 with a previous history
of GI bleeding. The risk of GI bleeding can be reduced but not eliminated
with concomitant use of either misoprostol or a proton pump inhibitor such
as omeprazole (Silverstein et al. 1995; Dubois et al. 2004). In addition, the
adverse effects of these gastroprotective drugs must be weighed against their
limited benefits; moreover, these drugs do not reverse other adverse reactions of NSAIDs (e.g., renal impairment, sodium retention, and bleeding
diathesis from platelet dysfunction). Limited short-term data suggest that
use of COX-2-selective agents reduces the incidence of serious GI outcomes. Stratification of patients by GI risk is generally recommended in
selecting an agent. One of the COX-2 inhibitors, rofecoxib (now withdrawn
from the market), appears to increase the risk of cardiovascular events after
long-term use (Solomon et al. 2004). Inhibition of COX-2 also inhibits the
production of systemic prostacyclin, which may have a prothrombotic effect. COX-2 inhibitors are thought to cause more cardiovascular thrombotic
events than nonselective NSAIDs. The risk of cardiovascular events with
COX-2 inhibitors is undergoing evaluation, but preliminary evidence indicates a class effect, and there have been several warnings and withdrawals
from the market (see the U.S. Food and Drug Administration Web site,
www.fda.gov).

   A number of NSAID-related drug-drug interactions are of clinical significance. NSAIDs can increase the plasma concentrations and toxicity of
lithium and methotrexate, so concurrent therapy should be avoided. If these
drugs are used concurrently, more careful clinical and therapeutic drug

monitoring is recommended. The concomitant use of NSAIDS with diuretics and other antihypertensives may decrease their effectiveness. The use of NSAIDs with corticosteroids increases the risk of peptic ulcer disease. Alteration of platelet function or coagulation can occur when warfarin and NSAIDs are taken concomitantly (Sam et al. 2004).

Contraindications, drug-disease state interactions, and precautions. Patients hypersensitive to aspirin or other NSAIDs may experience severe bronchospasm and anaphylactic reactions with any member of this drug class. Nonacetylated salicylates are less likely to precipitate these reactions, and acetaminophen infrequently cross-reacts with NSAIDs, causing mild bronchospasm in less than 5% of cases. Celecoxib contains a cross-reactive sulfonamide moiety and may cause reactions in patients allergic to sulfonamides. In cases with several significant disease states (i.e., chronic renal failure, heart failure, hypertension, and peptic ulcer), NSAIDs should be used with caution. In particular, the risk of NSAID-induced renal impairment and fluid retention is enhanced in individuals whose renal homeostasis is markedly prostaglandin-dependent. Such individuals include those who have blood volume contraction (e.g., following overly aggressive diuresis or hemorrhage), a functional decrease in circulating blood volume (e.g., congestive heart failure, pre-existing renal impairment, or cirrhosis), or diabetes mellitus. All NSAIDs, including COX-2 agents, can worsen congestive heart failure (Mamdani et al. 2004).

Dosing and administration. Recommended starting to maximum daily doses for selected NSAIDs are shown in Table I. Of the NSAIDs listed, only ibuprofen is available over the counter without a physician prescription in the United States. Other NSAIDs are not recommended for use in older patients because of their potential for toxicity, including ketorolac, mefenamic acid, piroxicam, oxaprozin, and naproxen (McLeod et al. 1997; Fick et al. 2003). In general, short-acting agents (half-life <5 hours) are preferred, due to a decreased risk of renal toxicity (Gloth 2001; Davis and Srivastava 2003). For chronic pain that is associated with musculoskeletal disorders such as osteoarthritis and rheumatoid arthritis a 2–3-week trial should be initiated followed by dose titration or a change to an alternate agent. Efficacy is highly variable from person to person. Some authorities advocate waiting 24 hours after an injury or contusion that may cause bleeding into tissue; use of a non-acetylated salicylate in the interim may be indicated. Utilization of a proton pump inhibitor in combination with a traditional NSAID agent can improve tolerance and may decrease risk of serious GI events (Dubois et al. 2004). Indeed, a trial looking at this combination showed no disadvantage over the use of a COX-2 inhibitor in patients with NSAID-induced GI bleeding (Chan et al. 2004). Based upon optimal pricing for a proton pump inhibitor or H_2-antagonist, this combination can be a low-cost alternative to a COX-2 agent. For further discussion of the prescribing of nonacetylated salicylates for the older adult with persistent nonmalignant pain, the reader is referred to Chapter 16.

ACETAMINOPHEN

Mechanism of action. Acetaminophen is a weak, reversible, nonspecific COX inhibitor (very limited inhibition). Acetaminophen exerts its analgesic activity through inhibition of COX and related prostaglandin synthesis, but it has essentially no anti-inflammatory activity.

Pharmacokinetic considerations. Acetaminophen is well absorbed and is metabolized via glucuronidation. The half-life ($t_{1/2}$) of acetaminophen may be prolonged in older adults, but not enough to warrant routine dosage adjustment (Triggs et al. 1975; Divoll et al. 1982). It may be possible, however, to achieve adequate analgesia with a lower total daily dosage by extending the dosing interval to at least 6 hours in individuals with a creatinine clearance of 10–50 mL/minute.

Efficacy. Acetaminophen is considered the analgesic of choice for most older persons with mild to moderate pain, especially those with musculoskeletal disorders. Acetaminophen appears to be as effective as ibuprofen for chronic osteoarthritis of the knee (Courtney and Doherty 2002; van den Bemt et al. 2002).

Adverse effects, drug-drug and drug-disease interactions, and precautions. Acetaminophen can cause irreversible hepatic necrosis following the acute ingestion of more than 10 g or chronic use of more than 4 g/day. The known risk factors for toxicity from chronic use include alcoholism or regular and heavy use of alcohol, use of hepatic enzyme inducers (e.g., rifampin, phenytoin, carbamazepine, and barbiturates) and other hepatotoxic drugs, malnourishment or recent fasting, dehydration, and pre-existing liver disease. The risk of hepatotoxicity from chronic use is decreased by using the lowest effective dose, or a maximum daily dose of 4 g, including multi-ingredient products (e.g., acetaminophen and opioid combinations), assuring adequate nutrition and hydration, and avoiding concurrent hepatotoxic drugs. The chronic use of acetaminophen also appears to be an independent, dose-dependent risk factor for nephropathy, but it is unknown whether the use of acetaminophen alone increases the extent or rate of progression of renal impairment (Matzke 1997). Acetaminophen in doses exceeding 2 g/day for more than 1 week may potentiate the effect of warfarin. Routine prothrombin time (PT/INR) monitoring is recommended in patients receiving both agents.

Dosing and administration. Acetaminophen is relatively safe and is available over the counter in many countries. Dosage regimens vary and should be individualized (see Table I). In dosages of 650 to 1000 mg by mouth four times a day, acetaminophen is safer for most patients than NSAIDs and other analgesics.

OPIOIDS AND RELATED ANALGESICS

Mechanism of action. The mechanism of action for most opioid analgesics is binding to mu receptors in the CNS (Weiner and Hanlon 2001; Davis and Srivastava 2003). Tramadol, a non-opioid, shares this mechanism of action as well as blocking the reuptake of norepinephrine (Davis and Srivastava 2003).

Pharmacokinetics. There is limited specific information about the pharmacokinetics and pharmacodynamics of opioids in older adults. Methadone is well absorbed, binds extensively to alpha-1 acid glycoprotein, and is metabolized by at least two hepatic isoenzymes (CYP3A4 and 2D6). While there are no specific data about the pharmacokinetics of methadone in older adults, because of its lipophilicity and age-related increases in fat body mass, it is believed that the half-life of this agent is further prolonged from its average of 30 hours seen in younger adults (Davis and Srivastava 2003). Fentanyl is another lipophilic agent, but it is not well absorbed orally and is metabolized by CYP3A4. A study of parenteral fentanyl found no difference in its hepatic clearance in older as compared to younger individuals (Scott and Stanski 1987). There is conflicting information about the existence of age-related changes in the transdermal absorption of fentanyl (Holdsworth et al. 1994; Thompson et al. 1998). In a recent pharmacokinetic study of transmucosal fentanyl, no differences were found between young and old subjects (Kharasch et al. 2004).

Table I
Recommended non-opioid analgesics

Chemical Class: Agents	Min. to Max. Daily Dose (mg)	Dosing Interval*	$t_{1/2}$ (hours)‡
Non-acetylated salicylates: salsalate	1500 to 3000	b.i.d to t.i.d.	2–20
NSAIDs: propionic acid class, ibuprofen	1200 to 2400	t.i.d. to q.i.d.	1–3
Acetaminophen†	2000 to 4000	q.i.d.	1–3

* b.i.d. = twice a day; t.i.d. = three times a day; q.i.d. = four time a day.
† Drug of choice for non-inflammatory disorders.
‡ $t_{1/2}$ = terminal disposition half-life.

Many other oral analgesics (i.e., hydrocodone, oxycodone, codeine, and tramadol) are hepatically metabolized by CYP2D6. Of these four agents there are only age-specific pharmacokinetic data for oxycodone. Kaiko et al. (1996), in a study comparing the pharmacokinetics of oral oxycodone in 28 young and old men and women, determined that there are no age-related differences in the peak plasma concentration or area under the curve. Both codeine and tramadol are pro-drugs that must first be metabolized from the parent compound to become active analgesics (Davis and Srivastava 2003). It has been shown that the half-life of both codeine and oxycodone is prolonged in patients with advanced chronic kidney disease (Kurella et al. 2003). Morphine given orally is well absorbed, but it is subject to a significant first-pass effect that is reduced with advanced age. Therefore, older individuals exhibit significantly higher initial and maximum plasma morphine concentrations after oral administration (Baillie et al. 1989). Morphine, a hydrophilic drug, has a high hepatic extraction ratio and undergoes hepatic glucuronidation. Considerable evidence suggests that the clearance of morphine is significantly reduced in older versus younger individuals (Stanski et al. 1978; Owen et al. 1983; Baillie et al. 1989). Two active metabolites, morphine-6 glucuronide and morphine-3-glucuronide, are primarily renally cleared and thus can accumulate in older patients with age-related decline in renal function.

Efficacy. Most opioid analgesics are equally efficacious for persistent pain when given in equianalgesic doses. For example, while codeine is thought to be a weak opioid, a meta-analysis clearly demonstrated that it is more effective than acetaminophen; other data show that its efficacy is comparable to that of other oral opioid analgesics (Moertel et al. 1972; de Craen et al. 1996). Recent studies have shown tramadol to be effective in neuropathic pain and pain due to osteoarthritis (Harati et al. 1998; Babul et al. 2004).

Adverse effects, drug-drug and drug-disease interactions, and precautions. Clear evidence shows that older adults have an increased pharmacodynamic sensitivity to opioid analgesics (Bellville et al. 1971; Kaiko 1980; Scott and Stanski 1987). Therefore, older adults taking opioids may be at greater risk for experiencing opioid side effects including sedation, nausea, vomiting, constipation, urinary retention, and respiratory depression (Weiner and Hanlon 2001). Sedation can be problematic when initiating opioids, but it usually dissipates after a few days. In end-of-life situations, some clinicians have used methylphenidate or donepezil to reduce opioid sedation (Walsh 2000; Bruera et al. 2003). Opioid analgesics when first initiated can cause nausea and vomiting, but these effects, like sedation, are usually transient (Weiner and Hanlon 2001). Practitioners should anticipate constipation with opioids and make sure that patients are vigilant about watching out for this side effect. At the first sign of constipation, a stimulant laxative such as senna extract should be started. Some practitioners advocate the prophylactic prescription of a regularly scheduled stimulant laxative (i.e., senna extract) at the same time that the opioid is started. Respiratory depression is rarely seen in elders receiving oral opioids chronically. The exceptions are reports of respiratory depression occurring 5–10 days after initiating long-acting agents such as either methadone or fentanyl (Weiner and Hanlon 2001; Regnard and Pelham 2003). Opioids can also decrease detrusor contractility, and in some older adults this may result in urinary retention (Andersson 2004). Theoretically, tramadol, which is a weaker mu-receptor agonist, may be less likely to cause urinary retention. Alternatively, the use of short-acting immediate-release opioids that result in lower serum levels may also lessen the problem with urinary retention (Andersson 2004).

Both tolerance and physical dependence can occur with regular use of opioids. However, psychological dependence is not usually exhibited with chronic use. Typically the need for higher opioid doses represents a progression of the underlying painful condition. Pain can be easily controlled by increasing the opioid dose. Finally, few patients have true allergies to opioids. In those cases where patients have had an idiosyncratic allergic reaction to a naturally occurring opioid (e.g., morphine), switching to methadone, fentanyl, or tramadol can circumvent the problem.

There are few clinically significant drug-drug interactions involving opioids (Drug Facts and Comparisons 2004). Propoxyphene has been shown to increase the plasma concentration of carbamazepine. Meperidine should never be given in a patient receiving a monoamine oxidase inhibitor. Phenytoin may decrease methadone concentrations. Quinidine and perhaps other cytochrome P450 isozyme 2D6 inhibitors (e.g., paroxetine) can inhibit the analgesic effect of codeine and tramadol by blocking their metabolism into active agents.

There are several clinically significant drug-disease state interactions to consider with opioids (McLeod et al. 1997; Fick et al. 2003). The use of opioids may increase the risk of falls in patients with a preexisting history of dysmobility (Weiner et al. 1998; Ensrud et al. 2003). Opioids can also exacerbate preexisting constipation and urinary retention in older men with benign prostatic hypertrophy. Finally, preexisting dementia may be worsened as well (Kotylar et al. 2005). However, recent data suggest that the risk of delirium is higher with undertreated pain than with opioid treatment (Morrison et al. 2003). Discontinuing other drugs associated with cognitive impairment (e.g., benzodiazepines, anticholinergics) can help in situations where opioids are required.

Dosing and administration. Several agents can be recommended for use in older adults with persistent pain. Because of age-related changes in pharmacokinetics and pharmacodynamics, the initial daily dosage in opioid-naive older patients needs to be lower. Table II outlines equianalgesic recommended starting doses of preferred analgesics for older patients. In older patients who are concerned about the stigma of addiction associated with taking morphine and similar agents, tramadol may be a reasonable alternative. It is recommended that patients receiving an opioid should also receive a non-opioid (e.g., acetaminophen). Although all opioids can be used as monotherapy, combination therapy with a non-opioid (e.g., acetaminophen or an NSAID) provides additive analgesia and can decrease the opioid dose given on a regularly scheduled basis to relieve persistent pain (Stockler et al. 2004).

Several agents should be avoided in older adults (Fick et al. 2003). Specifically due to enhanced risk of toxicity, pentazocine and meperidine are not recommended for use in older adults (Fick et al. 2003). Propoxyphene, although widely prescribed, has been shown in a meta-analysis to be no more effective than acetaminophen alone (Li Wan Po and Zhang 1997). This fact, in combination with propoxyphene's retention of all the side effects of other opioids, recommends against its use in older adults (Fick et al. 2003). While combination products containing hydrocodone (e.g., Vicodin) are commonly prescribed, their use cannot be recommended due to insufficient evidence-based data regarding their pharmacokinetics and efficacy in older adults. While methadone is not absolutely contraindicated in older adults, its long and variable half-life make it difficult to use, so its prescription should probably be limited to experienced pain practitioners. For further information about individual agents, including dose titration and switching between opioids, please refer to more comprehensive reviews of this subject (Weiner and Hanlon 2001; American Geriatric Society 2002; Guay et al. 2002).

Table II
Recommended opioid analgesic starting regimens*

Drug	Dosage Regimen†	$t_{1/2}$ (hours)‡
Codeine	30 mg orally every 6 hours	3–4
Oxycodone	5 mg orally every 6 hours	3–4
Morphine	2.5 mg orally every 4 hours	2–3.5

* Dosage regimens are approximately equianalgesic, and it is assumed that the patient is opioid naive.
† It is assumed that the agent is given with a non-opioid analgesic (i.e., acetaminophen).
‡ $t_{1/2}$ = terminal disposition half-life.

ADJUNCTIVE ANALGESICS

As mentioned in the introduction to this chapter, several other chapters in this book discuss adjunctive agents as they apply to the treatment of specific pain disorders. Those that have not already been covered in these chapters are discussed in detail below.

ANTIEPILEPTIC DRUGS

Mechanism of action. The precise mechanism(s) of analgesic activity for antiepileptic drugs (AEDs) are not known but may be related to their anti-seizure activity. Traditionally, carbamazepine has been the most commonly used AED, and its efficacy in trigeminal neuralgia has been well documented (Sidebottom and Maxwell 1995). However, much interest today surrounds the use of gabapentin and lamotrigine, as well as the newest AEDs.

Pharmacokinetics. Table III illustrates the effects of aging, renal disease, and hepatic disease on AED pharmacokinetics. The majority of agents are primarily hepatically metabolized. The notable exception is gabapentin, which is primarily renally excreted without prior metabolism. Moreover, the systemic clearance of most AEDs is reduced with increasing age. The notable exception is lamotrigine, which is primarily metabolized by glucuronidation (Cloyd et al. 1994; Bernus et al. 1997; Graves et al. 1998; Boyd et al. 1999; Guay 2001a,b, 2003a,b).

Efficacy. The use of carbamazepine (in trigeminal neuralgia) and gabapentin as analgesics for neuropathic pain are reasonably well-supported by clinical trials data (Sidebottom and Maxwell 1995; Guay 2001a, 2003a). Lamotrigine is less well supported, with the exception of human immunodeficiency virus-associated painful sensory neuropathy due to antiretroviral drugs (Guay 2001b). At present, there is a paucity of randomized controlled trial data for oxcarbazepine, levetiracetam, zonisamide, and topiramate as analgesics (Guay 2003b). Until such data become available, it may be prudent to consider carbamazepine and gabapentin as first-line AEDs for neuropathic pain, followed by lamotrigine as the second-line AED, and then the others as third-line (salvage) options.

Adverse effects/drug-interactions/precautions. The most common adverse effects of the AEDs involve the CNS and include sedation, fatigue, drowsiness, dizziness, lightheadedness, and ataxia. One randomized controlled trial demonstrated fewer cognitive effects with lamotrigine compared to carbamazepine (Brodie et al. 1999). In a prospective cohort study by Ensrud et al. (2002), the association between falls and AEDs was evaluated in older women utilizing multivariate analyses that controlled for epilepsy as an indication. Subjects that took any AED were at significantly increased risk of a single fall (adjusted odds ratio [adj. OR] = 1.75, 95% confidence interval [CI] = 1.1–2.7) and multiple falls (two or more) (adj. OR = 2.56, 95% CI = 1.5–4.4) compared with non-users (Ensrud et al. 2002).

Serious, even life-threatening adverse effects may also occur. Bone marrow suppression and hepatotoxicity due to carbamazepine are rare but recognized effects that warrant occasional complete blood count (with differential) and liver function panel monitoring during therapy. Carbamazepine and oxcarbazepine may cause the syndrome of inappropriate antidiuretic hormone secretion (SIADH), thus warranting occasional monitoring of serum sodium levels during therapy. The appearance of any type of skin rash in a lamotrigine recipient is justification for immediate drug discontinuation because the rash may otherwise progress rapidly to life-threatening forms in a small proportion of affected patients. Rechallenge should never be considered. The risk of skin rash is reduced by avoidance of concurrent valproate therapy and by use of slow dose-escalation strategies.

Topiramate has been associated with systemic (metabolic) acidosis, acute myopia with secondary angle closure glaucoma, oligohidrosis and hyperthermia, kidney stones, paresthesias, and cognitive and neuropsychiatric problems (a complex of psychomotor slowing, difficulty with attention and concentration, and speech or language problems, particularly word-finding difficulty). Some of these reactions are a result of its carbonic anhydrase inhibitor activity (with the exception of ocular, CNS, and temperature dysregulation effects). Zonisamide is also a carbonic anhydrase inhibitor and may cause kidney stones as well.

Table III lists clinically relevant AED drug-drug interactions. Most important are those involving carbamazepine, a drug with a narrow therapeutic range drug. In particular, diltiazem, propoxyphene, and verapamil all significantly reduce the systemic clearance and increase the half-life of carbamazepine. Table III also provides information about the recommended AED dosing regimens for analgesia.

Abbreviations for Table III: AUC = area under the plasma concentration-versus-time curve; b.i.d. = twice daily; CCB = calcium channel blockers; CL/F = apparent systemic body clearance; C_{max} = peak plasma concentration; conc. = concentration; CrCl = creatinine clearance; CYP450 = cytochrome P450 drug-metabolizing enzymes; e.o.d. = every other day; F = bioavailability; INH = isoniazid; Mg/Al = magnesium/aluminum; Pb = phenobarbital; PHT = phenytoin; q.d. = once daily; q.i.d. = four times daily; RCL = renal clearance; SS = steady-state; $t_{1/2}$ = terminal disposition half-life; t.i.d. = thrice daily. →

Table III

Antiepileptic drugs for neuropathic pain

Drug	Effect of Aging on Kinetics	Effect of Renal or Hepatic Impairment on Kinetics	Clinically Relevant Drug-Drug Interactions	Recommended Dosing Regimens for Analgesia (Normal Renal Function)
Carbamazepine (CBZ)	CL/F at SS decreases 25–40%	Hepatic: no data; renal: no data (possible effect on active epoxide metabolite?)	CBZ is a potent inducer of CYP450 activity, decreasing the therapeutic effects of many drugs. Propoxyphene, valproate, CCBs (diltiazem, verapamil), cimetidine, INH, and macrolide antimicrobials decrease CBZ metabolism, leading to CBZ toxicity	50–100 mg b.i.d. to start, then increase dose by 100 mg/d per week to max. 1200 mg/d
Gabapentin (GP)	CL/F decreases with increasing age (36% for age 70+ vs. age <30 y)	Hepatic: none; renal: CL/F decreases as CrCl decreases (mandates change in approach to dosing re. initial dose, dose increments, and intervals between dose increments)	Mg/Al antacids simultaneously decrease GP bioavailability	100–300 mg q.d. to start, then increase to b.i.d., then to t.i.d., then increase slowly to max. 3600 mg/d (give t.i.d. or q.i.d.)
Lamotrigine (LTG)	None	Hepatic: decreased CL/F in moderate to severe hepatic disease (lower dose 50–75%); renal: decreased CL/F when CrCl < 30 mL/min (dosing ramifications unclear)	Enzyme inducers decrease LTG conc. up to 50%; valproate increases LTG conc. about 50%; LTG decreases valproate conc. about 25%	(1) Patient on enzyme inducer(s) and valproate: 25 mg e.o.d. for 2 wk, then 25 mg q.d. for 2 wk, then increase in 25–50 mg/d increments every 1–2 wk to max. 600 mg/d. (2) Patient on enzyme inducer(s) *not* taking valproate: 50 mg q.d. for 2 wk, then increase in 100 mg/d increments every 1–2 wk to max. 600 mg/d. (3) Patient on *no* enzyme inducer and *no* valproate: 25 mg q.d. for 2 wk, then increase to 50 mg/d for 2 wk, then to 100 mg/d for 1 wk, then increase in 100 mg/d increments per week to max. 400 mg/d.

Mexiletine. An oral congener of lidocaine, mexiletine has been reported effective in neuropathic pain including diabetic neuropathy and central post-stroke pain (Galer 1995). Like lidocaine, mexiletine is a sodium channel blocker and acts as a membrane stabilizer. Two studies have demonstrated that the single-dose and steady-state pharmacokinetics of mexiletine are not altered by advanced age (el Allaf et al. 1986; Grech-Belanger et al. 1989). However, one study did report a statistically significant reduction in systemic clearance of 0.3% per year from the age of 40 years onwards (Ueno et al. 1993).

Mexiletine's most common adverse effects involve the CNS (dizziness, tremor, irritability, nervousness, and headache). Gastrointestinal distress can be reduced by taking the drug with food and escalating the dose slowly over several weeks. Mexiletine should not be used in individuals with second- or third-degree heart block. Patients with any preexisting cardiac pathology should be referred to a cardiologist before mexiletine is prescribed. An initial dose of 150 or 300 mg once or twice daily should be used, titrated upwards based on response to a maximum of 1200 mg/day. The usual effective dosage range is 150 to 300 mg three times daily.

Baclofen. The only pain disorder for which baclofen has a role is trigeminal neuralgia, achieving its effect by inhibiting the release of presynaptic excitatory amino acids (Sidebottom and Maxwell 1995). Baclofen is felt to be less effective than carbamazepine and should be considered second-line therapy due to its tolerability profile (Fromm 1994; Sidebottom and Maxwell 1995). Addition of baclofen may be useful in patients failing carbamazepine monotherapy. There is no clinically important effect of aging on single-dose baclofen pharmacokinetics.

Common adverse effects include drowsiness, dizziness, ataxia, confusion, nausea, and vomiting (Sidebottom and Maxwell 1995). About 1 in 10 patients cannot tolerate baclofen due to adverse effects (Fromm 1994). Combination therapy with baclofen and carbamazepine may augment some adverse effects (particularly drowsiness, nausea, and vomiting) (Sidebottom and Maxwell 1995). Slowing the rate of dose escalation may minimize these effects, but the severity of the pain may limit how slowly the dose is escalated (Fromm 1994). Baclofen should be discontinued gradually after chronic use because acute withdrawal results in a syndrome characterized by hallucinations, seizures, anxiety, and/or tachyarrhythmias that may last up to 2 months. If a withdrawal reaction does occur, baclofen should be reinstituted at the previous dose and decreased by 5 to 10 mg/d at weekly intervals until it has been completely withdrawn. Baclofen should be initiated at a dosage of 5 to 10 mg two or three times daily, increasing the dose by 5 to 10 mg/d every 2 to 3 days based on response to the usual effective dosage range of 50 to 60 mg/day. A dose of 80 mg/day should not be exceeded.

SUMMARY

Numerous agents are safe and effective for treating pain in older adults. Acetaminophen for mild to moderate acute or chronic pain and gabapentin for specific types of neuropathic pain are preferred agents. If an NSAID or opioid is required, preference should be given to agents with a short half-life (e.g., ibuprofen, morphine) to reduce the risk of adverse effects in older adults. Further research is needed regarding the pharmacokinetics, pharmacodynamics, efficacy, and safety of medications used to treat pain in this population.

REFERENCES

American Geriatric Society Panel on Persistent Pain in Older Persons. The management of persistent pain in older adults. *J Am Geriatr Soc* 2002; 50:S205–224.

Andersson KE. New pharmacologic targets for the treatment of the overactive bladder: an update. *Urology* 2004; 63(3 Suppl 1):32–34.

Babul N, Noveck R, Chipman H, et al. Efficacy and safety of extended-release, once-daily tramadol in chronic pain: a randomized 12-week clinical trial in osteoarthritis of the knee. *J Pain Symptom Manage* 2004; 28:59–71.

Baillie SP, Bateman DN, Coates PE, et al. Age and the pharmacokinetics of morphine. *Age Aging* 1989; 18(4):258–262.

Barkin RL. Acetaminophen, aspirin, or ibuprofen in combination analgesic products. *Am J Ther* 2001; 8:433–442.

Bell GM, Schnitzer TJ. COX-2 inhibitors and other non-steroidal anti-inflammatory drugs in the treatment of pain in the elderly. *Clin Geriatr Med* 2001; 17:489–502.

Bellville JW, Forrest WH, Miller E, et al. Influence of age on pain relief from analgesics. *JAMA* 1971; 217:1835–1841.

Bernabei R, Gambassi G, Lapane K, et al. Management of pain in elderly patients with cancer. SAGE Study Group: systematic assessment of geriatric drug use via epidemiology. *JAMA* 1998; 279(23):1877–1836.

Bernus I, Dickinson RG, Hooper WD, et al. Anticonvulsant therapy in aged patients: clinical pharmacokinetic considerations. *Drugs Aging* 1997; 10:278–289.

Bjordal JM, Ljunggren AE, Klovning A, Slordal L. Non-steroidal anti-inflammatory drugs, including cyclo-oxygenase-2 inhibitors, in osteoarthritis knee pain: meta-analysis of randomized placebo controlled trials. *BMJ* 2004; 329:1317–1322.

Boyd RA, Turck D, Abel RB, et al. Effects of age and gender on single-dose pharmacokinetics of gabapentin. *Epilepsia* 1999; 40:474–479.

Brater DC, Harris C, Redfern JS, Gertz B. Renal effects of COX-2 selective inhibitors. *Am J Nephrol* 2001; 21:1–15.

Brodie MJ, Overstall PW, Giorgi L. Multicentre, double-blind, randomized comparison between lamotrigine and carbamazepine in elderly patients with newly diagnosed epilepsy. The UK Lamotrigine Elderly Study Group. *Epilepsy Res* 1999; 37:81–87.

Bruera E, Strasser F, Shen L, et al. The effect of donepezil on sedation and other symptoms in patients receiving opioids for cancer pain: a pilot study. *J Pain Symptom Manage* 2003; 26:1049–1054.

Chan FK, Hung LC, Suen BY, et al. Celecoxib versus diclofenac plus omeprazole in high-risk arthritis patients: results of a randomized double-blind trial. *Gastroenterology* 2004; 127:1038–1043.

Chodosh J, Solomon DH, Roth CP, et al. The quality of medical care provided to vulnerable older patients with chronic pain. *J Am Geriatr Soc* 2004; 52:756–761.

Cloyd JC, Lackner TE, Leppik IE. Antiepileptics in the elderly. *Arch Fam Med* 1994; 3:589–598.

Courtney P, Doherty M. Key questions concerning paracetamol and NSAIDs for osteoarthritis. *Ann Rheum Dis* 2002; 61:767–773.

Crofford L, Lipsky P, Brooks P, et al. Basic biology and clinical application of specific cyclooxygenase-2 inhibitors. *Arthritis Rheum* 2000; 43:4–13.

Davis MP, Srivastava M. Demographics, assessment and management of pain in the elderly. *Drugs Aging* 2003; 20:23–57.

de Craen AJ, Di Giulio G, Lampe-Schoenmaeckers JE, Kessels AG, Kleijnen J. Analgesic efficacy and safety of paracetamol-codeine combinations versus paracetamol alone: a systematic review. *BMJ* 1996; 313:321–325.

Divoll M, Ameer B, Abernethy DR, et al. Age does not alter acetaminophen absorption. *J Am Geriatr Soc* 1982; 30:240–244.

Drug Facts and Comparisons. St. Louis: Wolters Kluwer, 2004.

Dubois RW, Melmed GY, Henning JM, Laine L. Guidelines for the appropriate use of non-steroidal anti-inflammatory drugs, cyclo-oxygenase-2-specific inhibitors and proton pump inhibitors in patients requiring chronic anti-inflammatory therapy. *Aliment Pharmacol Ther* 2004; 19:197–208.

el Allaf D, Carlier J, Dresse A. Effects of age on the pharmacokinetics of mexiletine. *Int J Clin Pharmacol Res* 1986; 6:303–307.

Ensrud KE, Blackwell T, Mangione CM, et al. Central nervous system active medications and risk for falls in older women. *J Am Geratr Soc* 2002; 50:1629–1637.

Fick DM, Cooper JW, Wade WE, et al. Updating the Beers criteria for potentially inappropriate medication use in older adults: results of a US consensus panel of experts. *Arch Intern Med* 2003; 63:2716–2724.

Fromm GH. Baclofen as adjuvant analgesic. *J Pain Symptom Manage* 1994; 9:500–509.

Galer BS. Neuropathic pain of peripheral origin: advances in pharmacologic treatment. *Neurology* 1995; 45(Suppl 9):S17–S25.

Gloth FM. Pain management in older persons: prevention and treatment. *J Am Geriatr Soc* 2001; 49:188–199.

Graves NM, Brundage RC, Wen Y, et al. Population pharmacokinetics of carbamazepine in adults with epilepsy. *Pharmacotherapy* 1998; 18:273–281.

Grech-Belanger O, Barbeau G, Kishka P, et al. Pharmacokinetics of mexiletine in the elderly. *J Clin Pharmacol* 1989; 29:311–315.

Griffin MR, Yared A, Ray WA. Nonsteroidal anti-inflammatory drugs and acute renal failure in elderly persons. *Am J Epidemiol* 2000; 151:488–496.

Guay DRP. Adjunctive agents in the management of chronic pain. *Pharmacotherapy* 2001a; 21:1070–1081.

Guay DRP. Lamotrigine in the treatment of neuropathic pain. *Consult Pharm* 2001b; 16:1057–1067.

Guay DRP. Oxcarbazepine, topiramate, zonisamide, and levetiracetam: potential use in neuropathic pain. *Am J Geriatr Pharmacother* 2003a; 1:18–37.

Guay DRP. Update on gabapentin therapy of neuropathic pain. *Consult Pharm* 2003b; 17:158–170, 173–178.

Guay D, Lackner T, Hanlon JT. Pharmacologic management: non-invasive modalities. In: Weiner DK, Herr K, Rudy TE (Eds). *Persistent Pain in Older Adults: An Interdisciplinary Guide for Treatment.* New York: Springer, 2002; pp 160–187.

Hanlon JT, Fillenbaum GG, Studenski SA, Ziqubu-Page T, Wall WE. Suboptimal analgesic use in community dwelling elderly. *Ann Pharmacother* 1996; 30:739–744.

Harati Y, Gooch C, Swenson J, et al. Double-blind randomized trial of tramadol for the treatment of the pain of diabetic neuropathy. *Neurology* 1998; 50(6):1842–1846.

Holdsworth MT, Forman WB, Killilea TA, et al. Transdermal fentanyl disposition in elderly subjects. *Gerontology* 1994; 40:32–37.

Kaiko RF. Age and morphine analgesia in cancer patients with postoperative pain. *Clin Pharmacol Ther* 1980; 28:823–826.

Kaiko RF, Benziger DP, Fitzmartin RD, et al. Pharmacokinetic-pharmacodynamic relationships of controlled-release oxycodone. *Clin Pharmacol Ther* 1996; 59:52–61.

Kamal-Bahl SJ, Doshi JA, Stuart BC, Briesacher BA. Propoxyphene use by community-dwelling and institutionalized elderly Medicare beneficiaries. *J Am Geriatr Soc* 2003; 51:1099–1104.

Kharasch ED, Hoffer C. Whittington D. Influence of age on the pharmacokinetics and pharmacodynamics of oral transmucosal fentanyl citrate. *Anesthesiology* 2004; 101:738–743.

Kotylar M, Gray SL, Lindblad CI, Hanlon JT. Psychiatric manifestations of medications in the elderly. In: Malletta G, Agronin M (Eds). *Principles and Practice of Geriatric Psychiatry,* 1st ed. Philadelphia: Lippincott Williams and Wilkins, 2005, in press.

Kurella M, Bennett WM, Chertow GM. Analgesia in patients with ESRD: a review of available evidence. *Am J Kidney Dis* 2003; 42:217–228.

Li Wan Po A, Zhang WY. Systematic overview of co-proxamol to assess analgesic effects of addition of dextropropoxyphene to paracetamol. *BMJ* 1997; 315:1565–1571.

Mamdani M, Juurlink DN, Lee DS, et al. Cyclo-oxygenase-2 inhibitors versus non-selective non-steroidal anti-inflammatory drugs and congestive heart failure outcomes in elderly patients: a population-based cohort study. *Lancet* 2004; 363:1751–1756.

Matzke GR. Clinical consequences of nonnarcotic analgesic use. *Ann Pharmacother* 1997; 31:245–248.

McLeod PJ, Huang AR, Tamblyn RM, et al. Defining inappropriate practices in prescribing for elderly people: a national consensus panel. *CMAJ* 1997; 156:385–391.

Moertel G, Ahmann DL, Taylor WF, et al. A comparative evaluation of marketed analgesic drugs. *N Engl J Med* 1972; 286:813–815.

Morrison RS, Magaziner J, Gilbert M, et al. Relationship between pain and opioid analgesics on the development of delirium following hip fracture. *J Gerontol* 2003; 58:M76–M81.

Nikolaus T, Zeyfang A. Pharmacological treatments for persistent non-malignant pain in older persons. *Drugs Aging* 2004; 21:19–41.

Owen JA, Sitar DS, Berger L, et al. Age-related morphine kinetics. *Clin Pharmacol Ther* 1983; 34:364–368.

Page J, Henry D. Consumption of NSAIDs and the development of congestive heart failure in elderly patients: an under-recognized public health problem. *Arch Intern Med* 2000; 160:777–784.

Pahor M, Guralnik JM, Wan JY, et al. Lower body osteoarticular pain and dose of analgesic medications in older disabled women: the Women's Health and Aging Study. *Am J Public Health* 1999; 89:930–934.

Proudfoot AT, Krenzelok EP, Brent J, et al. Does urine alkalinization increase salicylate elimination? If so, why? *Toxicol Rev* 2003; 22:129–136.

Regnard C, Pelham A. Severe respiratory depression and sedation with transdermal fentanyl: four case studies. *Palliat Med* 2003; 17:714–716.

Sam C, Massaro JM, D'Agostino RB Sr, et al. Warfarin and aspirin use and the predictors of major bleeding complications in atrial fibrillation (the Framingham Heart Study). *Am J Cardiol* 2004; 94:947–951.

Scott JC, Stanski DR. Decreased fentanyl and alfentanil dose requirements with age: a simultaneous pharmacokinetic and pharmacodynamic evaluation. *J Pharmacol Exp Ther* 1987; 240:159–165.

Sidebottom A, Maxwell S. The medical and surgical management of trigeminal neuralgia. *J Clin Pharm Ther* 1995; 20:31–35.

Silverstein FE, Graham DY, Senior JR, et al. Misoprostol reduces serious gastrointestinal complications in patients with rheumatoid arthritis receiving non-steroidal anti-inflammatory drugs. *Ann Intern Med* 1995; 123:241–249.

Solomon DH, Schneeweiss S, Glynn RJ, et al. Relationship between selective cyclooxygenase-2 inhibitors and acute myocardial infarction in older adults. *Circulation* 2004; 109:2068–2073.

Stanski DR, Greenblatt DJ, Lowenstein E. Kinetics of intravenous and intramuscular morphine. *Clin Pharmacol Ther* 1978; 24:52–59.

Stockler M, Vardy J, Pillai A, Warr D. Acetaminophen (paracetamol) improves pain and well-being in people with advanced cancer already receiving a strong opioid regimen: a randomized, double-blind, placebo-controlled cross-over trial. *J Clin Oncol* 2004; 22:3389–3394.

Thompson JP, Bower S, Liddle AM, et al. Perioperative pharmacokinetics of transdermal fentanyl in elderly and young adult patients. *Br J Anaesth* 1998; 81(2):152–154.

Triggs EJ, Nation RL, Long A, Ashley JJ. Pharmacokinetics in the elderly. *Eur J Clin Pharmacol* 1975; 8:55–62.

Ueno K, Kawaguchi Y, Tanaka K. Pharmacokinetics of mexiletine in middle-aged and elderly patients. *Clin Pharm* 1993; 12:768–770.

van den Bemt PM, Geven LM, Kuitert NA. The potential interaction between oral anticoagulants and acetaminophen in everyday practice. *Pharm World Sci* 2002; 24:201–204.

Vane JR. Inhibition of prostaglandin synthesis as a mechanism of action for aspirin-like drugs. *Nat New Biol* 1971; 231:232–235.

Vane JR, Botting RM. The mechanism of action of aspirin. *Thrombosis Res* 2003; 110:255–258.

Walsh D. Pharmacological management of cancer pain. *Semin Oncol* 2000, 27:45–63.

Weiner DK, Hanlon JT. Pain in nursing home residents: management strategies. *Drugs Aging* 2001; 18:13–29.

Weiner D, Hanlon JT, Studenski S. CNS drug-related falls liability in community dwelling elderly. *Gerontology* 1998; 44:217–221.

Won AB, Lapane KL, Vallow S, et al. Persistent nonmalignant pain and analgesic prescribing patterns in elderly nursing home residents. *J Am Geriatr Soc* 2004 52:867–874.

Workman BS. Management of chronic pain in older people. *Aust J Hosp Pharm* 1998; 28:361–367.

Correspondence to: Prof. Joseph T. Hanlon, PharmD, MS, Department of Medicine (Geriatrics), University of Pittsburgh, Kaufman Medical Building, Suite 514, 3471 5th Avenue, Pittsburgh, PA 15213, USA. Tel: 412-692-2364; Fax: 412-692-2370; email: hanlonj@dom.pitt.edu.

Pain in Older Persons, Progress in Pain
Research and Management, Vol. 35, edited
by Stephen J. Gibson and Debra K. Weiner,
IASP Press, Seattle, © 2005.

11

Physical Therapy Approaches to the Management of Pain in Older Adults

Rhonda J. Scudds and Roger A. Scudds

*Department of Rehabilitation Sciences, Faculty of Health and Social Sciences,
Hong Kong Polytechnic University, Hong Kong*

The medical practitioner who cares for older adults with persistent pain conditions usually reaches for pharmacological therapies as the first line of treatment. Often, however, nonpharmacological modalities such as those used in physical therapy are just as effective, or even more effective, and less toxic. These modalities should almost always be considered as a first-line treatment, or at the very least as adjunctive therapies for the vast majority of older adults with persistent musculoskeletal pain. Although many standard physical therapy treatments are used to manage pain in older adults, some do not yet have adequate scientific evidence to support their use in this population. Throughout this chapter, evidence of the effectiveness of specific physical therapy modalities for older adults with pain will be presented. It should be recognized, at the outset, that the strength of the evidence is limited for many such treatment modalities, apart from exercise. However, recommendations will be made based on the best available evidence and on good clinical practice.

The majority of the older people who are seen by physical therapists are those with musculoskeletal conditions, with many suffering from persistent pain associated with osteoarthritis of the hips or knees. Persistent back and neck pain from a variety of causes such as lumbar spinal stenosis, osteoarthritis, rheumatoid arthritis, and osteoporosis are also common. Peripheral neuropathies may occur in the context of these disorders or independently. Myofascial pain syndrome and fibromyalgia tend to be thought of as pain conditions affecting younger individuals, but in fact they also occur commonly in older adults, as discussed in Chapter 16. Much of the discussion of physical therapy approaches to pain management in this chapter will focus on strategies for the management of persistent musculoskeletal pains common in older adults. With the description of each physical therapy approach, musculoskeletal conditions known or thought to benefit from each will be discussed.

WHY OLDER ADULTS REQUIRE A DIFFERENT PHYSICAL THERAPY APPROACH: SPECIALIZED NEEDS AND GOALS

As with all approaches to the management of persistent pain in the older adult, certain precautions must be taken when incorporating specific physical therapy approaches into the overall management of the older individual. These precautions will also be discussed for each approach mentioned in this chapter. They include such concerns as increased frailty, deconditioning, and the potentially greater number of comorbid conditions that are associated with pain. Before using particular modalities, the therapist should also consider the cognitive ability of older patients along with their potential impairments in vision, hearing, touch, and pain perception, as well as changes to the skin and altered thermoregulation. Additional psychosocial barriers to physical therapy treatment must also be considered when working with older people (Lansbury 2000). Wide variability exists in the expectations, beliefs, and capabilities of older people with persistent pain.

When working with older adults who have persistent pain, the main goal of the physical therapist is not purely to reduce pain, but also to optimize function and prevent disability, improving quality of life and allowing patients to maintain their functional independence. Management strategies in older adults must be very individualized. Physical therapy is rarely the only approach to the management of persistent pain in older adults, but it should be incorporated into the overall biopsychosocial management approach in order to minimize the number of invasive treatments required. It provides a conservative alternative or adjunct to pharmacological pain management. Recommendations from the American Geriatrics Society Panel on Persistent Pain in Older Persons (2002) include the use of evidence-based pharmacological and nonpharmacological approaches to the management of persistent pain in older adults.

ROLE OF THE PHYSICAL THERAPIST IN THE MANAGEMENT OF PERSISTENT PAIN

Physical therapists are important members of the health care team because they can provide a comprehensive evaluation of pain and can expertly assess the impairments, disabilities, and handicaps associated with conditions of the musculoskeletal system. Before a physical therapy program can be developed for pain management for an older individual, a thorough medical examination should be completed and a medical history taken. A comprehensive assessment of physical, psychological, and social functioning is also recommended. Pain assessment should focus on all aspects of the pain experience, including intensity, duration, location, and frequency as well as the impact of the pain on overall physical and psychological function. In addition to conducting standard physical, functional, and pain assessments, the physical therapist must take special care to understand the older person's social and family support systems and the impact of pain on the patient's functional activities. The therapist must understand the patient's cognitive abilities, mental status, beliefs about pain and pain management, and his or her overall goals, and must learn the details of the patient's medication use. Based on a thorough assessment, the physical therapist can work with the patient to develop short-term and long-term goals for the management of pain. Physical-therapy-directed pain management may involve passive and active approaches, as described below. The physical therapist also plays a critical role in educating the patient about the musculoskeletal condition, about the importance of adherence to the management plan, and about self-management for ongoing benefits, including how to protect the body or minimize the chance of further damage and how to handle an acute flare-up of the condition.

PHYSICAL-THERAPY-DIRECTED PAIN MANAGEMENT APPROACHES

Common physical therapy treatments and approaches to persistent pain fall into one of two main categories: passive treatments and active treatments (Table I). Passive treatments—those applied to the patient—include superficial and deep heating modalities, ultrasound, transcutaneous electrical nerve stimulation, interferential current, acupuncture, and manual techniques such as joint mobilization and soft tissue massage. In general, the literature offers less evidence for the effectiveness of passive as compared with active pain management. Active approaches include a variety of exercises aimed at increasing strength, endurance, flexibility, and balance. As discussed below, good scientific evidence exists to support the benefits of exercise for older people with persistent pain.

Table I
Common physical therapy approaches to pain management

Passive Treatments
Electro-physical Modalities
  Transcutaneous electrical nerve stimulation (TENS)
  Interferential current therapy
  Ultrasound
  Low-power laser
  Short-wave diathermy
  Superficial heating
  Pulsed electromagnetic field therapy
  Acupuncture
  Electroacupuncture
Manual Techniques
  Joint mobilization
  Joint manipulation
  Massage/soft tissue techniques

Active Treatments (Therapeutic Exercise)
Types
  Progressive strengthening exercises
  Aerobic (endurance) exercises
  Stretching/flexibility exercises
Location
  Land-based
  Water-based (aquatic therapy)

Other Approaches to Pain Management
Education (e.g., disease, posture, exercise adherence,
  biomechanics, joint protection)
Assistive device prescription

PASSIVE TREATMENTS

Superficial heat. Superficial heat, either applied by the physical therapist or self-applied, is a common modality in the management of persistent pain in older persons. Superficial heating over the area of pain can be applied either as dry heat, such as with an electric heating pad, or as moist heat. Moist heat is commonly used for the treatment of persistent low back pain or neck pain and is thought to deliver slightly deeper heating compared with dry heat. Paraffin wax treatment is mostly used for conditions such as osteoarthritis and rheumatoid arthritis that involve small joints, for example in the hand and fingers, when the condition is not in an acute stage. Lastly, hydrotherapy, in which a body part or the whole body is immersed in warm water, can also be used to treat persistent musculoskeletal pain in older adults. Superficial heating modalities can increase joint temperature (Oosterveld et al. 1992) and should not be applied in situations where joint heating is not a desired result, for example during an acute flare-up of rheumatoid arthritis.

The effect of superficial heating is temporary and is based on relaxing the soft tissue and increasing circulation to the area. It may also enhance general relaxation. When applying heat to an older person, special precautions must be addressed. Pain perception in older adults may be altered, and most notably, pain thresholds may be increased (Gibson and Helme 2001). As a result, special care must be taken to avoid the potentially damaging effect of excessive heat if the patient cannot feel whether the application is too hot. A mild warmth is all that is required to achieve the beneficial effect of temporary heating, and it is important to educate the patient in this regard.

The second precaution that must be taken when using heating modalities focuses on the vitality of the older person's peripheral circulation and thermoregulatory system and on the presence of any cardiopulmonary disease. The local thermoregulatory system must be adequate to dissipate the heat that is being applied, but in older people it may be compromised by age-related changes to the skin or by peripheral vascular disease. If cardiac function is deficient, the body's ability to cope with full immersion in warm water may be impaired (Gloth and Matesi 2001). These conditions are not absolute contraindications to the application of heat. However, knowledge of the patient's skin condition and cardiovascular health allows the therapist to determine whether heat treatment is advisable and whether to monitor the patient's condition more frequently and use precautions such as providing an extra layer of towelling between a hot pack and the skin. A mottled red and white appearance on the skin may suggest overheating due to the skin's inability to properly dissipate the heat.

Deep heat. Deeper heating modalities such short-wave diathermy and continuous therapeutic ultrasound are also used by physical therapists to treat persistent pain in deeper-lying joints or tissues that superficial heating modalities cannot reach. Ultrasound or soft-wave diathermy can reduce chronic pain that persists after tissue healing is presumed to have occurred, but the mechanism of action remains unclear. However, an increase in the cellular metabolism of the tissues involved may provide some explanation (Belanger 2002). There is very little high-quality evidence from randomized controlled trials for the use of deep heat to manage pain in conditions common to older adults. There is some evidence, of varying quality, for the benefits of ultrasound for musculoskeletal conditions such as lateral epicondylitis, herpes zoster, and postherpetic neuralgia (Garrett and Garrett 1982; Payne 1984; Trudel et al. 2004). Early studies examining the effects of short-wave diathermy on osteoarthritis were mostly positive, but recent evidence has been more contradictory, with studies showing no benefits of the treatment outweighing those showing benefit (Marks et al. 1999).

Electrical nerve stimulation. Electrical nerve stimulation is used extensively to treat persistent pain in both younger and older individuals and is usually used as an adjunct to other pharmacological and physical therapy treatments. The most research has focused on transcutaneous electrical nerve stimulation (TENS), the most common form of electrical stimulation used by physical therapists. As its name implies, TENS involves electrical current that is passed through the skin via electrodes attached to the surface of the skin. Small, portable TENS devices are available for purchase by older patients to use at home after adequate education and training.

Although many different forms of TENS are available, the two main modes of TENS are considered to be "conventional TENS" and "acupuncture-like TENS." Conventional TENS is described as high-frequency (>80 Hz), low pulse width (<150 microseconds), low-intensity (comfortable) stimulation, whereas "acupuncture-like TENS" is described as low-frequency (<10 Hz), high pulse width (>150 microseconds), high-intensity (tolerable) stimulation (Belanger 2002). Other types of TENS are basically variations of these two main modes that provide variable pulse widths or variable frequencies in an attempt to prevent accommodation. The placement of the TENS electrodes depends on experimentation to find what is most effective for each individual patient. Most commonly, two to four electrodes are placed over the area of pain, over the nerve roots, or over the peripheral nerves that innervate the area of pain. Combinations of these electrode placements can also be used.

The theoretical mechanisms by which TENS reduces pain are mainly twofold. The gate control theory of pain may explain its short-acting effects (lasting for a few hours), and stimulation of the endogenous opioid system may underlie its longer-acting effects (Sluka et al. 1999). Conventional TENS stimulates large-diameter sensory fibers, supposedly blocking the transmission of nociceptive information in the substantia gelatinosa in the dorsal horn of the spinal cord (Melzack and Wall 1965). Acupuncture-like TENS, on the other hand, is suggested to reduce pain primarily by stimulating smaller-diameter sensory fibers, which in turn stimulate a descending inhibitory feedback loop, mediated by endogenous opioids, through the periaquaductal gray area back down to the dorsal horn of the spinal cord (Mayer and Price 1995; Sluka and Walsh 2003).

Controlled experimental studies have yielded controversial results regarding the benefits of TENS in the management of persistent pain. The benefits for pain reduction in rheumatoid arthritis are disputed (Brosseau et al. 2003b). Controlled studies indicate the beneficial effects of TENS for the management of pain in osteoarthritis of the knee (Philadelphia Panel 2001; Osiri et al. 2000). Although many uncontrolled studies report the benefits of TENS for low back pain, a greater proportion of controlled studies report negative results (Milne et al. 2000). The use of TENS for other forms of persistent pain, for example neuropathic pain, show promising results (Thorsteinsson et al. 1977; Armstrong et al. 1997; Kumar and Marshall 1997; Thorsen and Lumsden 1997).

Special considerations must be taken when applying TENS to older adults because they are more likely to present with conditions for which TENS is contraindicated and may require close monitoring during treatment. One contraindication is the presence of a cardiac pacemaker if no cardiac monitoring equipment is available (Johnson 2002). Placement of the electrodes over the anterior cervical region, over the carotid sinus, over the vagus or phrenic nerves, or over the heart is also contraindicated (Belanger 2002). Several precautions should also be observed when using TENS with older people: (1) Any implanted electrical devices in the person's body must be noted because the electric signal from the TENS has the potential to interfere with the proper functioning of the implanted device. (2) Impaired skin sensation in the treated area, for any reason, or any skin conditions must also be assessed prior to treatment with TENS so that skin irritation due to an allergic reaction to the electrode gel or due to a high intensity of current can be avoided. (3) Any undiagnosed pain should be treated with caution because acupuncture-like TENS can increase local blood flow to the area being stimulated. Although TENS is now being used to treat neuropathic pain, special care must be taken to avoid stimulation over areas where the skin is unhealthy or has a tendency to break down easily, as with peripheral neuropathy.

Miscellaneous electrical and physical modalities. Several other electrical and physical modalities are used by physical therapists to treat pain. These include interferential current therapy, low power (helium neon and gallium arsenide) laser therapy, pulsed electromagnetic fields, acupuncture, and electroacupuncture. Acupuncture and electroacupuncture are discussed in Chapter 14. Little scientific evidence is available to support the beneficial effects of many of these modalities for the management of pain. Some evidence for the use of laser is available for short-term pain relief, predominantly in hand and finger joints affected by rheumatoid arthritis (Brosseau et al. 2000). Evidence is mixed for the effects of low-power laser for trigger point treatment (Snyder-Mackler et al. 1989; Thorsen et al. 1992; Hakguder et al. 2003). Conflicting evidence has also been reported for the use of low-power laser for the management of peripheral neuralgia (Moore et al. 1988; Eckerdal and Bastian 1996) and for pain accompanying osteoarthritis (Bjordal et al. 2003; Brosseau et al. 2004). Pulsed electromagnetic field therapy has been shown to produce a statistically significant improvement in the symptoms of knee osteoarthritis (Hulme et al. 2002). However, the small improvements found may not necessarily be clinically important. Additional research must be conducted to determine whether any of these modalities provide important pain-relieving effects.

Manual therapy. Physical therapy also involves a large amount of manual therapy that involves stretching of soft tissue and mobilization of peripheral and spinal joints. Joint manipulation, joint mobilization, massage, and other soft tissue manual techniques are regularly used by physical therapists to treat pain. Joint manipulation can be described as a high-velocity, low-amplitude movement of a joint, either vertebral or peripheral, beyond the limits of its passive range of motion. Joint mobilization involves a variety of grades of low-velocity, oscillatory passive movements of a joint performed by the physical therapist, who may use both small- and large-amplitude movements with the goal of reducing pain and improving joint range of motion. The primary aim of Grade I and Grade II joint mobilizations is pain reduction, while Grade III and IV mobilizations are also aimed at increasing joint range of motion by stretching the surrounding soft tissue that is thought to be limiting the joint's normal full range of motion (Edmond 1993). The evidence in younger adults suggests that these treatments may have a short-term effect in reducing chronic low back pain. However, research evidence is lacking for the benefits of manipulation and mobilization techniques or to elucidate their mode of action in reducing persistent pain in older adults. In addition, the use of high-velocity manipulation with older adults, where joints and bones may show the degenerative effects of aging, is questionable.

Massage therapy is a general term that can encompass many different forms of manual therapy used by physical therapists and massage therapists, such as classical massage, myofascial release, craniosacral therapy, and Swedish massage techniques. For a discussion of myofascial pain syndrome treatment, see Chapter 16. A recent review by the Cochrane collaboration concluded that massage, particularly when combined with exercise and education, may be beneficial in the management of chronic low back pain (Furlan et al. 2002). However, the subjects in the studies included in the review were predominantly young. The effects that massage techniques may have on chronic pain in older adults are unknown. Massage is thought to reduce pain through general relaxation and by increasing blood flow to a painful area that may correspond with vasoconstriction. Massage may also relieve inflammatory pain by reducing chronic inflammation in the extremities.

ACTIVE TREATMENTS: EXERCISE

Exercise has long been known to have numerous health benefits, and physical therapists have always incorporated exercise into their treatment planning. However, only relatively recently have the benefits of exercise for persistent pain in older adults been published and emphasized (Gloth and Matesi 2001). Persistent pain is associated with a decrease in physical activity and subsequent deconditioning. These effects might be more detrimental in older people, where muscle strength, flexibility, and cardiovascular and pulmonary function tend to gradually decline with increasing age. Older adults report more pain-related disability. Whether for prevention or management of disability and pain, older adults must be strongly encouraged to maintain some sort of exercise program, given adequate medical clearance to do so. Active exercise not only can help prevent pain-related disability in older people, but can also improve physical functioning and reduce pain, even in the very old. There is no evidence that participating in mild to moderate strength or endurance exercise programs or a combination of both types of exercises produces any negative effects on pain in older people with long-standing arthritis symptoms (Coleman et al. 1996). Detailed guidelines regarding exercise prescription for older adults with osteoarthritis have been published by the American Geriatrics Society's Panel on Exercise and Osteoarthritis (2001).

Although the benefits of exercise are well established, barriers still exist that make the older patient's participation in active exercise and the maintenance of the exercise program a challenge for the physical therapist. A recent qualitative research study in Australia revealed that exercise and physical therapy were the least preferred coping mechanisms used by older people in chronic pain management (Lansbury 2000). This preference may not be as apparent in the West as in other societies, such as in China, where older people are regularly seen exercising in the early morning as either individuals or in groups. With more education and publicity about the positive effects of exercise, future cohorts of older people may be much more inclined to participate in some sort of regular exercise.

A physical examination by a physician is recommended before the start of any exercise program. Different types of exercise programs can be designed to help reduce pain in a variety of chronic, painful musculoskeletal conditions that are common in the older population. The types of exercises that are prescribed to older people are dependent on the condition itself and its relevant precautions and on the individual and his or her abilities and goals. As a result, exercise prescription is very individualized. Group exercise programs, when combined with individual home exercise programs, provide a greater degree of pain reduction and physical improvement than home exercise alone (McCarthy et al. 2004). The inclusion of group exercise programs has the added advantage of providing older people with social support and may enhance their motivation to continue to exercise.

Older people with persistent pain tend to be deconditioned, so one goal of the physical therapy pain management program is to improve patients' overall fitness, addressing both the cardiopulmonary and musculoskeletal systems. Strengthening exercises for specific muscle groups are also recommended in order to improve the dynamic stability of painful joints, thus potentially reducing pain. The addition of some form of weight-bearing activities is also recommended, not only to prevent osteoporosis and related fractures, but to manage persistent pain in those already living with osteoporosis (Bravo et al. 1996; Malmros et al. 1998). For patients with spinal osteoporosis, special precautions, such as avoidance of spinal flexion exercises, must be taken in order to prevent further detrimental effects in already weakened bones.

The use of strengthening and aerobic exercises has best been shown to be effective in pain reduction for older people with osteoarthritis in the lower limbs, especially in the knees (Kovar et al. 1992; Ettinger et al. 1997; Petrella and Bartha 2000; Baker et al. 2001; Fransen et al. 2001; Philadelphia Panel 2001; Evcik and Sonel 2002). For aerobic exercise, both low- and high-intensity exercise has beneficial results on pain (Brosseau et al. 2003a). Aerobic exercise alone, strengthening exercises alone, and combinations of aerobic, strengthening, and stretching activities have all been shown to be beneficial for older people with persistent musculoskeletal pain (Fransen et al. 2001).

More recently, physical therapy exercise programs consisting of combinations of progressive resistance training, aerobic exercise, joint flexibility exercises (stretching), manual therapy, and education about exercise have been shown to have pain-reducing effects in older people with lower-extremity osteoarthritis (Deyle et al. 2000; Hopman-Rock and Westhoff 2000; Hughes et al. 2004).

A comprehensive exercise program that includes stretching, strengthening, aerobic fitness, and education can also be recommended in the management of older adults with mild to moderate spinal stenosis (Bodack and Monteiro 2001), despite a current lack of scientific evidence to support its use. This conservative approach to the management of this condition is suggested prior to more invasive surgical approaches. Stretching focuses on tight musculature around the hips and spine, strengthening focuses on the anterior trunk muscles, and general aerobic conditioning can take many forms, but hydrotherapy exercises may be the most tolerable to begin with.

The program should also include education about posture and proper biomechanics (Bodack and Monteiro 2001). Combinations of aerobic exercise, hydrotherapy, education, and cognitive-behavioral therapy may also be beneficial for seniors diagnosed with fibromyalgia (Busch et al. 2002; Sim and Adams 2002).

Although Tai Chi, a Chinese system of exercise designed for self-defense and meditation, has been practiced for many years in Eastern societies, it is only relatively recently that its popularity has grown in the West. Studies relating to its therapeutic effects have also commenced, mostly focusing on its effects on cardiorespiratory, physical, and psychosocial functioning. However, a recent critical review of the therapeutic effects of Tai Chi supports its beneficial effects on low back pain and lower-extremity osteoarthritis (Klein and Adams 2004).

Hydrotherapy or aquatic therapy is a popular approach used by physical therapists to conduct individual or, more often, group exercise programs to enhance stretching, strengthening, and endurance in older adults with persistent pain. The warmth and buoyancy of the water provide a comfortable environment in which weight is taken off painful joints. While aquatic exercise groups are frequently run by physical therapists, this type of exercise is regarded as a long-term self-management approach to pain management. Such programs can be started up in a community setting, and interested participants can be trained to be leaders of maintenance classes. Research evidence supports the use of aquatic therapy as an approach to the management of persistent pain for older people with rheumatoid arthritis (Hall et al. 1996; Templeton et al. 1996; Wong 2004), ankylosing spondylitis (van Tubergen et al. 2001), fibromyalgia (Mannerkorpi et al. 2002), and low back pain (Geytenbeek 2002). Medical screening for contraindications to aquatic therapy is necessary prior to entering into an aquatic exercise program. Contraindications include severe cardiovascular disease, uncontrolled seizures, incontinence, severe hypotension, and hypertension.

PRESCRIPTION OF ASSISTIVE AMBULATORY DEVICES

Physical therapists often assess the need for ambulatory aids, which are sometimes recommended to older adults in the management of pain. Relieving some force on a painful extremity or joint may produce profound analgesic effects. One important role for ambulatory aids, therefore, is as analgesic modalities whose purpose is assistance with optimal functional restoration. Prescription of these aids should not, however, occur in isolation. Continued efforts to improve strength, endurance, range of motion, and posture should be ongoing in the attempt to reduce pain and reduce the need for an assistive ambulatory aid. Another important role for ambulatory aids in older adult pain patients is improving postural stability. The disuse atrophy that can accompany pain-related inactivity, or the opioids and other medications that are often prescribed, may heighten the risk of falls, and so prescribing an assistive device may be a critical part of pain rehabilitation. Ambulatory aids include standard canes, quadruped canes, crutches, and walkers. The type of device that is prescribed is based on the amount of weight relief needed and on the individual's ability to balance.

SUMMARY AND RECOMMENDATIONS FOR CLINICIANS

Physical therapists play a central role in the treatment of older adults with painful musculoskeletal disorders. Many of the disorders from which older adults suffer, particularly soft tissue disorders (e.g., myofascial pain, and fibromyalgia syndrome), have a more robust response to active and passive physical therapy techniques than to pharmacological interventions. The role that physical therapists play in educating older adults about how to pace their exercises and how to self-manage exacerbations of pain is critical in promoting compliance with recommended programs, leading to more positive outcomes and decreasing expenditure of health care resources. Failure of response to prior physical therapy efforts should be viewed not as inherent lack of responsiveness of the patient or the painful disorder, but as an indication that ineffective techniques or unrealistic treatment goals may have been previously employed. Treating patients with chronic pain requires a different orientation and set of skills than treating patients with acute sports-related injuries. Further, treating frail older adults may require formulating treatment goals that are very different from those of younger pain patients. When prescribing physical therapy for the older adult pain patient, therefore, it is important for physicians to refer patients to a specialist with expertise in treating older adults and in treating patients with chronically painful disorders.

REFERENCES

American Geriatrics Society Panel on Exercise and Osteoarthritis. Exercise prescription for older adults with osteoarthritis pain: consensus practice recommendations—a supplement to the AGS clinical practice guidelines on the management of chronic pain in older adults. *J Am Geriatr Soc* 2001; 49:808–823.

American Geriatrics Society Panel on Persistent Pain in Older Persons. The management of persistent pain in older persons. *J Am Geriatr Soc* 2002; 50:S205–S224.

Armstrong DG, Lavery LA, Fleischli JG, Gilham KA. Is electrical stimulation effective in reducing neuropathic pain in patients with diabetes? *J Foot Ankle Surg* 1997; 36:260–263.

Baker KR, Nelson ME, Felson DT, et al. The efficacy of home based progressive strength training in older adults with knee osteoarthritis: a randomized controlled trial. *J Rheumatol* 2001; 28:1655–1665.

Belanger A-Y. Transcutaneous electrical nerve stimulation. In: Belanger A-Y (Ed). *Evidence-Based Guide to Therapeutic Physical Agents*. Philadelphia: Lippincott Williams & Wilkins, 2002, pp 26–65.

Bjordal JM, Couppe C, Chow RT, Tuner JM, Ljunggren EA. A systematic review of low level laser therapy with location-specific doses for pain from chronic joint disorders. *Aust J Physiother* 2003; 49:107–116.

Bodack MP, Monteiro M. Therapeutic exercise in the treatment of patients with lumbar spinal stenosis. *Clin Orthop* 2001; 384:144–152.

Bravo G, Gauthier P, Roy PM, et al. Impact of a 12-month exercise program on the physical and psychological health of osteopenic women. *J Am Geriatr Soc* 1996; 44:756–762.

Brosseau L, Welch V, Wells G, et al. Low level laser therapy for osteoarthritis and rheumatoid arthritis: a meta-analysis. *J Rheumatol* 2000; 27:1961–1969.

Brosseau L, MacLeay L, Robinson V, Wells G, Tugwell P. Intensity of exercise for the treatment of osteoarthritis. *Cochrane Database Syst Rev* 2003a; 2:CD004259.

Brosseau L, Yonge KA, Robinson V, et al. Transcutaneous electrical nerve stimulation (TENS) for the treatment of rheumatoid arthritis in the hand. *Cochrane Database Syst Rev* 2003b; 2:CD004377.

Brosseau L, Welch V, Wells G, et al. Low level laser therapy (Classes I, II and III) for treating osteoarthritis. *Cochrane Database Syst Rev* 2004; 3:CD002046.

Busch A, Schachter CL, Peloso PM, Bombardier C. Exercise for treating fibromyalgia syndrome. *Cochrane Database Syst Rev* 2002; 3:CD003786.

Coleman EA, Buchner DM, Cress ME, Chan BK, de Lateur BJ. The relationship of joint symptoms with exercise performance in older adults. *J Am Geriatr Soc* 1996; 44:14–21.

Deyle GD, Henderson NE, Matekel RL, et al. Effectiveness of manual physical therapy and exercise in osteoarthritis of the knee: a randomized, controlled trial. *Ann Intern Med* 2000; 132:173–181.

Eckerdal A, Bastian HL. Can low reactive-level laser be used in the treatment of neurogenic facial pain? A double-blind, placebo-controlled investigation of patients with trigeminal neuralgia. *Laser Ther* 1996; 8:247–252.

Edmond SL (Ed). *Manipulation and Mobilization: Extremity and Spinal Techniques*. St. Louis: Mosby, 1993.

Ettinger WH Jr, Burns R, Messier SP, et al. A randomized trial comparing aerobic exercise and resistance exercise with a health education program in older adults with knee osteoarthritis. The Fitness Arthritis and Seniors Trial (FAST). *JAMA* 1997; 277:25–31.

Evcik D, Sonel B. Effectiveness of a home-based exercise therapy and walking program on osteoarthritis of the knee. *Rheumatol Int* 2002; 22(3):103–106.

Fransen M, McConnell S, Bell M. Exercise for osteoarthritis of the hip or knee. *Cochrane Database Syst Rev* 2001: 2:CD004376.

Furlan AD, Brosseau L, Imamura M, Irvin E. Massage for low-back pain. *Cochrane Database Syst Rev* 2002; 2:CD001929.

Garrett AS, Garrett M. Ultrasound therapy for herpes zoster pain. *J R Coll Gen Pract* 1982; 32:709, 711.

Geytenbeek J. Evidence for effective hydrotherapy. *Physiotherapy* 2002; 88(9):514–529.

Gibson SJ, Helme RD. Age-related differences in pain perception and report. *Clin Geriatr Med* 2001; 17:433–456.

Gloth MJ, Matesi AM. Physical therapy and exercise in pain management. *Clin Geriatr Med* 2001; 17:525–535.

Hakguder A, Birtane M, Gurcan S, Kokino S, Turan FN. Efficacy of low level laser therapy in myofascial pain syndrome: an algometric and thermographic evaluation. *Lasers Surg Med* 2003; 33:339–343.

Hall J, Skevington SM, Maddison PJ, Chapman K. A randomized and controlled trial of hydrotherapy in rheumatoid arthritis. *Arthritis Care Res* 1996; 9:206–215.

Hopman-Rock M, Westhoff MH. The effects of a health educational and exercise program for older adults with osteoarthritis for the hip or knee. *J Rheumatol* 2000; 27:1947–1954.

Hughes SL, Seymour RB, Campbell R, et al. Impact of the fit and strong intervention on older adults with osteoarthritis. *Gerontologist* 2004; 44:217–228.

Hulme JM, Judd MG, Robinson VA, et al. Electromagnetic fields for the treatment of osteoarthritis. *Cochrane Database Syst Rev* 2002; 1:CD003523.

Johnson M. Transcutaneous electrical nerve stimulation (TENS). In: Kitchen S (Ed). *Electrotherapy: Evidence-Based Practice,* 11th ed. Edinburgh: Churchill Livingstone, 2002, pp 259–286.

Klein PJ, Adams WD. Comprehensive therapeutic benefits of Taiji. A critical review. *Am J Phys Med Rehabil* 2004; 83:735–745.

Kovar PA, Allegrante JP, MacKenzie CR, et al. Supervised fitness walking in patients with osteoarthritis of the knee. A randomized, controlled trial. *Ann Intern Med* 1992; 116:529–534.

Kumar D, Marshall HJ. Diabetic peripheral neuropathy: amelioration of pain with transcutaneous electrostimulation. *Diabetes Care* 1997; 20:1702–1705.

Lansbury G. Chronic pain management: a qualitative study of elderly people's preferred coping strategies and barriers to management. *Disabil Rehabil* 2000; 22:2–14.

Malmros B, Mortensen L, Jensen MB, Charles P. Positive effects of physiotherapy on chronic pain and performance in osteoporosis. *Osteoporos Int* 1998; 8:215–221.

Mannerkorpi K, Ahlmen M, Ekdahl C. Six- and 24 month follow up of pool exercise therapy and education for patients with fibromyalgia. *Scand J Rheumatol* 2002; 31:306–310.

Marks R, Ghassemi M, Duarte R, Van Nguyen JP. A review of the literature on shortwave diathermy as applied to osteo-arthritis of the knee. *Physiotherapy* 1999; 85:304–316.

Mayer DJ, Price DD. Neural mechanisms in pain. In: Robinson AW, Snyder-Mackler L (Eds). *Clinical Electrophysiology: Electrotherapy and Electrophysiologic Testing,* 2nd ed. Baltimore: Williams & Wilkins, 1995, pp 279–310.

McCarthy CJ, Mills PM, Pullen R, et al. Supplementing a home exercise programme with a class-based programme is more effective than home exercise alone in the treatment of knee osteoarthritis. *Rheumatology* 2004; 43:880–886.

Melzack R, Wall PD. Pain mechanism: a new theory. *Science* 1965; 150:971–979.

Milne S, Welch V, Brosseau L, et al. Transcutaneous electrical nerve stimulation (TENS) for chronic low-back pain. *Cochrane Database Syst Rev* 2000; 4:CD003008.

Moore KC, Hira N, Kumar PS, Jayakumar CS, Oshiro T. A double-blind crossover trial of low-level laser therapy in the treatment of post herpetic neuralgia. *Laser Ther* 1988; 1:7–9.

Oosterveld FG, Rasker JJ, Jacobs JW, Overmars HJ. The effect of local heat and cold therapy on the intraarticular and skin surface temperature of the knee. *Arthritis Rheum* 1992; 35:146–151.

Osiri M, Brosseau L, McGowan J, et al. Transcutaneous electrical nerve stimulation for knee osteoarthritis. *Cochrane Database Syst Rev* 2000; 4:CD002823.

Payne C. Ultrasound for post-herpetic neuralgia: a study to investigate the results of treatment. *Physiotherapy* 1984; 70:96–97.

Petrella RJ, Bartha C. Home based exercise therapy for older patients with knee osteoarthritis: a randomized clinical trial. *J Rheumatol* 2000; 27:2215–2221.

Philadelphia Panel. Philadelphia Panel evidence-based clinical practice guidelines on selected rehabilitation interventions for knee pain. *Phys Ther* 2001; 81:1675–1700.

Sim J, Adams N. Systematic review of randomized controlled trials of nonpharmacological interventions for fibromyalgia. *Clin J Pain* 2002; 18:324–336.

Sluka KA, Walsh D. Transcutaneous electrical nerve stimulation: basic science mechanisms and clinical effectiveness. *J Pain* 2003; 4:109–121.

Sluka KA, Deacon M, Stibal A, Strissel S, Terpstra A. Spinal blockade of opioid receptors prevents the analgesia produced by TENS in arthritic rats. *J Pharmacol Exp Ther* 1999; 289:840–846.

Snyder-Mackler L, Barry AJ, Perkins AI, Soucek MD. Effects of helium-neon laser irradiation on skin resistance and pain in patients with trigger points in the neck or back. *Phys Ther* 1989; 69:336–341.

Templeton MS, Booth DL, O'Kelly WD. Effects of aquatic therapy on joint flexibility and functional ability in subjects with rheumatic disease. *J Orthop Sports Phys Ther* 1996; 23:376–381.

Thorsen SW, Lumsden SG. Trigeminal neuralgia: sudden and long-term remission with transcutaneous electrical nerve stimulation. *J Manipulative Physiol Ther* 1997; 20:415–419.

Thorsen H, Gam AN, Svensson BH, et al. Low level laser therapy for myofascial pain in the neck and shoulder girdle. A double-blind, cross-over study. *Scand J Rheumatol* 1992; 21:139–141.

Thorsteinsson G, Stonnington HH, Stillwell GK, Elveback LR. Transcutaneous electrical stimulation: a double-blind trial of its efficacy for pain. *Arch Phys Med Rehabil* 1977; 58:8–13.

Trudel D, Duley J, Zastrow I, et al. Rehabilitation for patients with lateral epicondylitis: a systematic review. *J Hand Ther* 2004; 17:243–266.

van Tubergen A, Landewe R, van der Heijde D, et al: Combined spa-exercise therapy is effective in patients with ankylosing spondylitis: a randomized controlled trial. *Arthritis Rheum* 2001; 45:430–438.

Wong KY. The effects of a community-based water exercise program on health outcomes for Chinese people with rheumatic disease. Dissertation. Hong Kong Polytechnic University, 2004.

Correspondence to: Rhonda J. Scudds, PhD, PT, Health and Rehabilitation Sciences Research Institute, Faculty of Life and Health Sciences, University of Ulster, Jordanstown Campus, Shore Road, Newtonabbey, Co. Antrim, N. Ireland, BT37 0QB, United Kingdom. Email: rj.scudds@ulster.ac.uk.

Pain in Older Persons, Progress in Pain
Research and Management, Vol. 35, edited
by Stephen J. Gibson and Debra K. Weiner,
IASP Press, Seattle, © 2005.

12

Cognitive-Behavioral Therapy for Pain in Older Adults

Sandra J. Waters, Julia T. Woodward, and Francis J. Keefe

Duke University Medical Center, Durham, North Carolina, USA

Over the past 20 years, recognition has been growing that persistent pain is a major problem for many older adults (Fox et al. 1999; Leveille 2004). The traditional approach to managing persistent pain involves the use of medications (Savage 1999; Fishbain 2000; Freedman 2002; Unutzer et al. 2004). However, it is becoming increasingly clear that the long-term use of pain medications is problematic for older adults because these drugs are likely to cause side effects and interact with other medications (Gloth 2000; Helme 2001; Fick et al. 2003). As a result, there is heightened interest in new approaches to pain management for older adults (Weiner and Hanlon 2001; Wellman et al. 2001; Keefe et al. 2002).

Cognitive-behavioral pain management protocols have shown promise in the treatment of pain caused by a variety of musculoskeletal and disease-related pain conditions (Kroenke and Swindle 2000; Redd et al. 2001; McCracken and Turk 2002), and such approaches are increasingly being used to manage pain in older adults (Keefe et al. 2002). This chapter provides an overview of cognitive-behavioral approaches to managing pain in older adults. It describes the conceptual foundations and basic elements of cognitive-behavioral approaches to pain management and provides a biopsychosocial perspective on some of the special challenges and opportunities that arise when using cognitive-behavioral pain management protocols in older adults. We then review treatment outcome studies that have tested the efficacy of cognitive-behavioral therapy (CBT) for older adults. Specific recommendations for tailoring CBT pain management for older adults are provided, as well as suggestions regarding future directions for research and practice in this important area.

CONCEPTUAL FRAMEWORK

Cognitive-behavioral approaches to pain are guided by a biopsychosocial model (see Fig. 1). This model maintains that pain is a complex phenomenon that is influenced by underlying biological factors (e.g., diseases that cause tissue damage) as well as psychological and social factors. Cognitive-behavioral researchers have identified a number of key psychological factors (e.g., cognitions, emotions, and behaviors) and social factors (e.g., social support, solicitous or critical spousal responses) that can influence pain and disability. A hallmark of the cognitive-behavioral model is that the relationships between biopsychosocial factors and pain are reciprocal. Thus, biopsychosocial factors can directly influence pain and disability, and changes in pain and disability can, in turn, influence important biopsychosocial factors. These reciprocal interrelationships have important implications for treatment. For example, a surgical treatment (e.g., a knee replacement surgery for a patient having osteoarthritic knee pain) can produce substantial reductions in pain and disability and can influence related biological factors (e.g.,

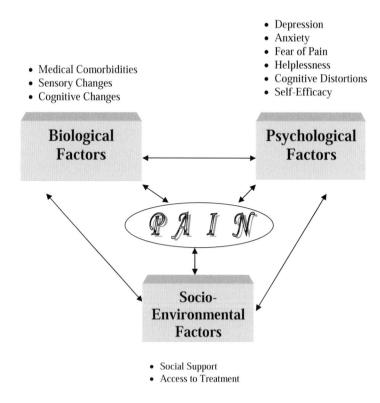

- Depression
- Anxiety
- Fear of Pain
- Helplessness
- Cognitive Distortions
- Self-Efficacy

- Medical Comorbidities
- Sensory Changes
- Cognitive Changes

Biological Factors

Psychological Factors

PAIN

Socio-Environmental Factors

- Social Support
- Access to Treatment

Fig. 1. Recursive cognitive-behavioral model of pain.

by improving joint mechanics and physical conditioning), psychological factors (e.g., by boosting self-efficacy and reducing depression), and social factors (e.g., by reducing caregiver strain). Thus, the impact of one factor on another may be modified with the use of CBT.

Cognitive-behavioral therapy can be characterized by examining both its process-related and content-specific characteristics (Beck 1976; Beck et al. 1979; Dobson and Shaw 1995; see J.S. Beck 1995 for a detailed description of CBT characteristics and techniques). From a process standpoint, CBT is often delivered as a brief intervention (e.g., 8–12 sessions) with an emphasis on current functioning and behaviors. CBT therapists take a directive role in early sessions in order to orient the client to therapy and introduce basic concepts, then transition to a more collaborative stance that involves clients in setting the session's agenda, developing homework assignments, and providing ongoing feedback to the therapist. Within each session, CBT therapists follow a structured sequence in which they: (1) assess the client's current mood; (2) set an agenda; (3) review material covered in the previous session; (4) review the previous homework assignment; (5) introduce a new skill or concept; and finally, (6) establish a homework assignment that will allow for practice and consolidation of the new skill.

Cognitive-behavioral therapy also can be understood by examining its content-specific characteristics (A.T. Beck 1976; Beck et al. 1979; J.S. Beck 1995; Dobson and Shaw 1995). In general, early in treatment patients are provided with a rationale for treatment and informed about the efficacy of CBT in treating their symptoms. Next, the link between cognitions and emotion is established, and patients begin to appreciate the role of distorted cognitions in driving their emotional distress. Throughout the treatment period, patients are taught a variety of specific skills (e.g., identifying automatic thoughts, challenging cognitive distortions) that help them to rationally evaluate and modify thinking (Beck 1995). Challenging the veracity of negative thoughts decreases patients' propensity to accept them as fact and moves patients toward recovery. Finally, the last phase of treatment emphasizes anticipation of potential setbacks and specific steps for relapse prevention.

When patients receive CBT to address their chronic pain, their cognitive experiences become a primary focus of treatment (Thorn 2004). Negative thinking leads chronic pain patients to believe that their life cannot improve and they are victims of pain that will never remit. Thus, the general principles of CBT are particularly effective in this population when the focus is appropriately placed on the pain-related negative cognitions. Further, patient outcome is improved by also providing patients with requisite pain-coping skills training (e.g., relaxation, activity pacing, and pleasant activity scheduling) to enhance self-efficacy for dealing with pain. Such training typically begins with education about the complex nature of pain (e.g., the gate control theory of pain; Melzack and Wall 1965), followed by introduction of specific cognitive and behavioral skills that have demonstrated efficacy in improving patient's ability to cope with their pain. Patients become empowered to actively manage their pain when they are provided with a repertoire of coping skills that can be applied during stressful periods or during pain flares. Table I lists specific skills typically included in pain-coping skills protocols (for a more complete description see Beck 1995; Waters et al. 2004). The final phase of pain-coping skills training focuses on methods of maintaining coping skills practice and dealing with potential setbacks and relapses.

SPECIAL CHALLENGES AND OPPORTUNITIES IN WORKING WITH OLDER ADULTS: A BIOPSYCHOSOCIAL PERSPECTIVE

A number of challenges and opportunities arise when using cognitive-behavioral interventions to manage persistent pain in older adults. These can be grouped into three basic categories: biological, psychological, and social,

Table I
Behavioral and cognitive therapy techniques for pain management

Behavioral Elements	
Activity pacing	Divide each day into periods of limited activity followed by limited rest
Pleasant activity scheduling	Identify and set activity goals that are specific, measurable, and achievable
Social reinforcement	Teach significant others to recognize and reinforce well behaviors and recognize and reduce reinforcement of pain behaviors
Time-contingent medications	Divide pain medication into equal amounts to be delivered at regular intervals over a 24-hour period
Cognitive Elements	
Cognitive restructuring	Identify and modify automatic negative thoughts (e.g., cognitive distortions) associated with increased pain and negative mood
Problem solving	A four-step approach to help patients identify and manage problems associated with their pain experience
Distraction techniques	Techniques that divert attention away from pain (e.g., imagery, progressive muscle relaxation, focal point, and music)
Relapse prevention	Teaches awareness and modification of cognitive factors that can disrupt practice of pain management skills

Source: Adapted from Waters et al. (2004).

which are discussed below (also see Chapter 5 for a discussion of age-related differences in mood, coping, and cognitive beliefs/attitudes that impact on pain perception).

BIOLOGICAL FACTORS

Medical comorbidities. With advances in the management of infectious disease and acute illness, more individuals are living longer and living with chronic diseases (Centers for Disease Control 2003). Many older adults face the challenge of coping with multiple medical conditions that cause persistent and/or episodic pain. Comorbid medical disorders such as diabetes, cardiovascular disorders, cancer, and neurological disorders are common in older populations. In addition to pain, these disorders can produce other symptoms—including fatigue, sleep difficulties, shortness of breath, and nausea—that, in themselves, are challenging. Further complicating the situation is that medications or surgeries designed to manage pain and/or these comorbid medical conditions can have side effects or interactions that limit their effectiveness.

While medical comorbidities can be seen as obstacles to efforts to cope with pain, they also represent an opportunity for intervention (Yonan and Wegener 2003). Cognitive-behavioral skills taught for managing pain due to one condition such as osteoarthritis can also be used to manage pain due to another condition such as diabetic neuropathy. Further, the cognitive-behavioral concepts and coping skills used in managing pain may provide an individual with skills useful in managing symptoms due to comorbidities. Finally, cognitive-behavioral interventions can be easily used in combination with medical and surgical interventions. An effective cognitive-behavioral pain management program can help some older adults decrease their intake of pain medication and delay or enhance the outcome of surgical intervention (Eells 2000; Turk 2003).

Sensory changes. Sensory changes that may occur with increased age can affect pain management efforts. Decreases in sensitivity to touch may prevent older adults from using activity pacing (i.e., shifting positions) as often as they should to alleviate joint pain stiffness. Comprehension of verbal instructions in pain management may be impaired due to hearing losses (auditory presbycusis) that interfere with the ability to hear high-frequency sounds and speech (Bilger and Meyer 1996; Heine and Browning 2002). Older adults with vision problems may experience difficulty reading handouts and written materials commonly used in cognitive-behavioral pain management, unless they are provided in larger type. The low lighting used to facilitate relaxation training in younger adults may be stressful to older adults who are unable to see the therapist due to age-related yellowing of their corneal lenses.

Cognitive changes. It has been suggested that most adults begin to experience declines in cognitive functioning during the second decade of life (Salthouse 2004) and continue to experience age-related cognitive loss as they grow older (Siegler et al. 2002). For example, fluid intelligence, which characterizes the influence of biological factors on intellectual development and represents the ability to reason and solve problems in novel situations, tends to decline with increasing age (McArdle et al. 2002). Research has shown that fluid intelligence has a direct effect on older adults' performance of tasks of daily living (Diehl et al. 1995). Fluid intelligence is also associated with working memory (Beaducel and Kersting 2002; Kane et al. 2005) and with processing speed (Diehl et al. 1995). Both working memory and processing speed are cognitive constructs that exhibit age-related declines (Salthouse 2004). These cognitive declines can hamper pain management in several ways. For example, age-related declines in working memory may reduce the speed of information processing (Salthouse 1996) and the amount of cognitive resources available to simultaneously store and process new information for transference into long-term memory (Baddeley and Hitch 1994; Baddeley 1998). Thus, older adults' ability to learn new information about coping strategies for pain management may be tempered by the amount of information they can process and the speed at which they can perform mental operations on the temporarily stored information before transference into long-term memory (Shifren et al. 1999; Brigman and Cherry 2002; Brown and Park 2003). In addition, age-related declines in inhibitory functioning impair cognitive functioning in older adults (Fisk and Sharp 2004) and make it harder to for them to ignore stimuli irrelevant to their goals and to suppress prepotent behavioral responses (Hasher et al. 1991; Milham et al. 2002; de Beni and Palladino 2004). Consequently, declines in inhibitory functioning may be an impediment to coping skills training if the setting and training format are not structured to minimize distractions. In response to pain episodes, inhibition deficits may diminish older adults' ability to suppress prepotent pain behaviors in favor of more appropriate cognitive and behavioral techniques.

As the number of older adults in the population increases, so does the prevalence of dementias such as Alzheimer's disease (Hebert et al. 2003). Particular challenges for pain management arise because many older adults having Alzheimer's disease also suffer from one or more chronic pain conditions (Sanderson et al. 2002). Various medical conditions, including unrecognized pain, are associated with behavioral disturbances in patients with Alzheimer's disease (Grossberg and Desai 2003). Interestingly, a review of the literature regarding interventions for persons with irreversible dementia suggests that adults in the early, middle, and later stages of dementia can be taught to use modified techniques of CBT to help them cope with various memory, functional, and affective symptoms associated with the dementia (see Burgener and Twigg 2002 for an in-depth review). For example, in the earlier stages of dementia, CBT may be used to reduce cognitive distortions (Teri and Gallagher-Thompson 1991), reduce depression levels (Requena et al. 2004), and improve memory and cognitive performance (Burgener and Twigg 2002). Patients with moderate to severe dementia may benefit from behavioral interventions designed to identify and increase positive activities that may help reduce negative behaviors (Teri and Gallagher-Thompson 1991; Teri and Logsdon 1991; Kasl-Godley and Gatz 2000). The use of cognitive-behavioral interventions has also proven beneficial in reducing anxiety among caregivers of Alzheimer's disease patients (Akkerman and Ostwald 2004).

Fortunately, there are cognitive processes that remain intact across the lifespan that may augment the use of cognitive-behavioral techniques for pain management. Crystallized intelligence, which reflects knowledge and fluency gained through life experiences, acculturation, and education (Beauducel and Kersting 2002) does not begin to show signs of slow decline until around the eighth decade of life (Christensen et al. 1994; McArdle et al. 2002). Crystallized intelligence directly influences older adults' performance of tasks of daily living and mediates the relationship between memory processes and daily task performance (Diehl et al. 1995). Recently, Allain et al. (2005) reported that older adults have more problems formulating a complex strategy to reach a specific goal than in executing a complex, predetermined series of actions to reach a specific goal. Although the authors did not gather direct measures of fluid and crystallized intelligence, the results support the idea that crystallized intelligence may positively contribute to older adults' ability to use CBT techniques for pain management.

In addition, automatic processes (e.g., well-learned skills requiring less cognitive processing of information) are not impaired by increasing age (Hasher and Zacks 1979). Thus, once older adults learn new cognitive and behavioral techniques for coping with their pain, continued practice should make the use of these skills automatic and more likely to be used on a daily basis (Brown et al. 2002; Liu and Park 2004).

In addition to impeding information processing, age-related declines in cognitive functioning are also associated with more self-reported pain, lower self-efficacy, and poorer mental health among older adults (Shifren et al. 1999).

PSYCHOLOGICAL FACTORS

Depression. Depression is prevalent among patients suffering from persistent pain (see, Fishbain et al. 1997; Geerlings et al. 2002; Lepine and Briley 2004). Among older adults, late-life depression is believed to be a primary cause of emotional distress and reduced quality of life (Blazer 2003); it is associated with disability in both instrumental and basic activities of daily living (Ormel et al. 2002). Among older adults with persistent pain, depression exacerbates the impact of pain on physical functioning (Mossey et al. 2000; Mossey and Gallagher 2004) and may complicate the treatment and outcome of chronic medical illnesses (Blazer 2003). Given that depression in later life is often accompanied by chronic medical diseases and disorders, prescribing CBT for older adults may prove beneficial both for managing pain and for reducing depression.

Anxiety. Anxiety is associated with persistent pain (McWilliams et al. 2003; Von Korff et al. 2005) and is often found in patients who report more pain-related functional problems (McCracken et al. 1999) and less acceptance of their pain (McCracken and Eccleston 2003). Among older adults, pain-related anxiety is associated with depression, reduced ability to cope, catastrophizing, and decreases in perceived health status (Bishop et al. 2001).

Because older adults report that they expect to experience increased anxiety as they grow older (Sarkisian et al. 2001), older patients with persistent pain may view increases in anxiety levels as being age-related rather than pain-related. During examinations, health care providers need to address changes in patients' anxiety levels and suggest the use of cognitive-behavioral interventions that have been shown to decrease pain-related anxiety in older patient populations (e.g., guided imagery, Antall and Kresevic 2004).

Fear of pain. Patients who have a heightened fear of pain or are afraid they may cause more injury to themselves if they move about will often eliminate most of their daily activities, including pleasurable activities with friends and family (Heuts et al. 2004). This avoidant coping style increases negative affect and is detrimental to well-being over time (Duke et al. 2002). In persons having chronic musculoskeletal pain, exposure-based CBT interventions can significantly reduce the fear of pain and increase activity levels (Vlaeyen and Linton 2000; Vlaeyen et al. 2002; Boersma et al. 2004; de Jong et al. 2005). In these interventions, patients are encouraged to expose themselves in a graded fashion to activities that they are clearly capable of doing, but which they fear will increase their pain. While exposure-based interventions have shown promise in middle-aged and younger adults, their effectiveness has not been systematically tested in older adults suffering from persistent musculoskeletal or other pain conditions.

Helplessness. Faced with persistent pain, some individuals develop a sense of helplessness in which they feel unable to control their pain (Smith and Wallston 1992). In older adults with osteoarthritis or osteoporosis, feelings of helplessness vary depending on the type of activity being examined and the manner in which the patients adapt to each particular activity (Gignac et al. 2000), suggesting that feelings of helplessness associated with pain management may be modified in older adults.

Cognitive distortions. Cognitive distortions are "errors of logic in interpreting situations," such as focusing solely on the negative aspects of situations, generalizing negative outcomes of a specific event to future similar events, anticipating the worst outcome in any situation, or believing that one is somehow responsible for the occurrence of negative events (Moss-Morris and Petrie 2003). In persons having persistent pain, high levels of cognitive distortions have been linked to increased depression (Smith et al. 1994), fewer positive health practices (Christensen et al. 1999), poorer physical performance (Moseley 2004), and increased disability (Keefe et al. 1989).

In older adults, cognitive distortions may be influenced by aging stereotypes (e.g., beliefs that older adults cannot learn new skills or change acquired behaviors) learned early in life that become self-stereotypes later in life (Levy 2003). For example, older adults who accept age-related stereotypes about the impact of aging on cognitive functioning may feel they are less able to manage their pain. In addition, research has shown that automatic activation of negative age-related (Stein et al. 2002; Hess et al. 2003) and health-related (Auman et al. 2005) stereotypes affects memory performance and physiological responses among older adults. For these reasons, assessing and addressing such stereotypes is an important part of orienting older adults to cognitive-behavioral pain management.

Self-efficacy. Self-efficacy refers to the belief that one has the ability to control various outcomes in one's life (Bandura 1997). For example, functional self-efficacy refers to confidence in one's ability to perform tasks and is associated with pain-related disability among older men with chronic pain (Barry et al. 2003). Individuals having high self-efficacy for pain believe they personally have the capability to control their pain without using medications or other external methods. In older adults having osteoarthritic knee pain, self-efficacy for pain is related to a number of positive outcomes including higher levels of activity, lower levels of physical and psychological disability, lower levels of pain behavior, and higher levels of tolerance for laboratory pain stimuli (Lefebvre et al. 1999; Reid et al. 2003b). Fortunately, studies suggest that self-efficacy beliefs about pain can be modified in older adults (Lorig et al. 1993; Smarr et al. 1997). Further evidence indicates that increases in self-efficacy that occur over the course of spouse-assisted pain-coping skills training are related to short- and long-term treatment outcome (e.g., Keefe et al. 2001, 2003).

SOCIAL FACTORS

Social support. In considering the impact of social support on health, it is important to distinguish between positive and negative social interactions (for a more complete review, see Basford et al. 2003). Social interactions provide informational, instrumental, and emotional support that may foster positive feelings of stability and self-worth for both patients and those with whom they interact. However, long-term social support may cause feelings of resentment in the care provider (Sarason et al. 1990), which may result in negative social interactions. The limited evidence to date suggests that chronic pain is more likely to develop and be maintained if an individual is unmarried, is in a relationship characterized by conflict, or is generally isolated with few supportive relationships (Poleshuck and Dworkin 2004).

Social support in the role of social reinforcement for cognitive-behavioral pain management efforts also may be either negative or positive (Waters et al. 2004). Negative social reinforcement occurs when family members or caregivers are worried that increased activity by patients will increase pain levels. As a result, family members and others become overly solicitous when patients are experiencing pain and tend to suggest behaviors that reinforce a more sedentary lifestyle. Positive social reinforcement occurs when family members or caregivers express interest and confidence in the treatment, reinforce use of skills, and provide instrumental support for home practice assignments and session attendance (see Table I). For older adults who are dependent on family or caregivers, fostering positive social support can be a key component in the successful delivery of cognitive-behavioral pain management (Bortz and O'Brien 1997; Arean et al. 2003; Yonan and Wegener 2003).

Access to treatment. Older adults may experience greater difficulty in accessing clinic-based cognitive-behavioral treatments for pain due to factors such as living on a fixed income and thus having difficulty affording treatment or transportation costs (Kerns et al. 2001). Innovative delivery methods may allow older adults with chronic pain greater access to cognitive-behavioral therapies. For example, in our laboratory, we are currently engaged in research studies using telephone sessions to deliver psychotherapy to patients with lung cancer, prostate cancer, early rheumatoid arthritis, and chronic low back pain. Additionally, researchers have demonstrated the efficacy of therapist-assisted e-mail interventions (Lorig et al.

2002) and mail-delivered, tailored-print self-management interventions (Lorig et al. 2004) in reducing pain, disability, and physician visits among patients with chronic low back pain and arthritis, respectively.

Turning from person-based barriers to program-based barriers, Kee and colleagues (1998) conducted a survey of 96 pain programs in the United States accredited by the Commission on Accreditation of Rehabilitation Facilities. These authors found that although programs did not explicitly turn away patients based on age, they commonly used age-related screening criteria such as the presence of medical comorbidities that effectively exclude a larger proportion of older pain patients. Additionally, the authors found that the same patients were rated as less likely to be admitted to the pain program and less likely to succeed in the program when their true, older age was given than when a false, younger age was given, suggesting age bias. Findings from these studies reinforce the need to examine older adults' ability to access CBT interventions for pain.

EFFICACY OF COGNITIVE-BEHAVIORAL PAIN MANAGEMENT FOR OLDER ADULTS

Despite the prevalence of pain among older adults, only a handful of empirical studies have examined the use of CBT with older pain patients. Possible assumptions contributing to the dearth of studies in this area include: (1) the assumption that pain is a natural part of aging and thus does not merit intervention; (2) the assumption that older adults are difficult to recruit into studies; and (3) the belief that older adults' cognitive deficits would preclude learning pain-coping skills (Arean et al. 2003; Yonan and Wegener 2003). Evidence from both uncontrolled studies and randomized controlled studies, however, suggests that older adults are likely to report the same benefits from CBT pain management protocols as their younger counterparts.

UNCONTROLLED STUDIES

Several uncontrolled studies have examined older adults' response to CBT for chronic pain. Sorkin and colleagues (1990) conducted a single-group outcome study that examined how older and younger patients suffering from chronic pain responded to a cognitive-behavioral pain management group therapy program. Their findings indicated that older adults showed the same levels of attendance, retention, and treatment engagement as younger adults. Further, there were no significant differences in older and younger group members' ratings of pain severity, activity level, interference of pain with activities, or emotional reactions to pain.

Middaugh et al. (1991) conducted a prospective study of the effects of relaxation training in older (55 to 78-year-old) and younger (29 to 48-year-old) patients with persistent pain who were participants in a multidisciplinary pain treatment program. All participants received 8 to 12 sessions of training in progressive muscle relaxation, diaphragmatic breathing, and electromyographic biofeedback. Data analyses revealed that the older patients learned to relax just ask quickly as younger patients and achieved levels of relaxation (as measured by increases in skin temperature and decreases in respiration rate) and reductions in pain that were equivalent to those of younger patients.

Reid et al. (2003a) delivered a group CBT protocol to a group of cognitively intact chronic low back pain patients aged 65 and older who were living in a senior housing center. The treatment consisted of 10 50-minute sessions led by a psychologist. The only modifications to the authors' standard treatment protocol were that age-appropriate examples were used and handouts were printed in a larger font. The authors reported impressive attendance and retention figures, with 93% of participants completing all 10 treatment sessions. After completing treatment, participants reported significant reductions in pain intensity and pain-related disability. These improvements in pain and disability levels had lessened somewhat by 24 weeks follow-up, yet levels still remained below the pretreatment baseline.

RANDOMIZED CONTROLLED STUDIES

Six randomized, controlled studies have tested the efficacy of cognitive-behavioral pain management protocols for older adults. Puder (1988) conducted one of the few controlled studies that directly examined the effect of age on treatment outcome. In this study, 69 outpatients (mean age = 53 years old, range = 27–80 years old) having persistent pain were randomly assigned either to a 10-session CBT group (Stress Inoculation Training) or to a waiting-list control group. Patients who received cognitive-behavioral treatment showed a significant reduction in the degree to which pain interfered with their activities and medication intake and an increase in their ability to cope with pain. These gains were maintained at a 6-month follow-up. Interestingly, age was unrelated to treatment outcome; younger and older participants benefited equally from treatment.

Results from a randomized, controlled trial of CBT in patients between the ages of 18 and 80 with recent-onset rheumatoid arthritis provided even stronger evidence for the ability of older adults to commit to and participate in psychological treatment (Sharpe et al. 2001). Older participants in this study were more likely to complete the CBT intervention trial than were the younger participants. One reason for the higher attendance and retention seen in this study may be the structure of older adults' lives, often involving fewer commitments and responsibilities that interfere with self-care and skills practice.

In our own laboratory, we conducted a controlled study testing the efficacy of a cognitive-behavioral pain-coping skills training protocol for managing osteoarthritic knee pain (Keefe et al. 1990a). Older adults (mean age = 64 years) with osteoarthritic knee pain were randomly assigned to one of three conditions: pain-coping skills training, an arthritis education comparison condition, or standard medical care. Patients in both the coping skills and arthritis education conditions met in 10 weekly group sessions that each lasted 90 minutes. At the end of treatment, participants who received pain-coping skills training reported significant reductions in pain and psychological disability when compared to those who received arthritis education or standard medical care. At a 6-month follow-up, participants who received pain-coping skills maintained their reductions in psychological disability and began to show a trend towards improvements in physical disability as compared to participants in the arthritis education group (Keefe et al. 1990b). Taken together, these findings support the notion that pain-coping skills training may be useful in the management of individuals who have persistent pain due to osteoarthritis.

Cook (1998) conducted a controlled study testing the efficacy of cognitive-behavioral pain management in older adults living in a nursing home. Participants included 22 residents between the ages of 61 and 98 years (mean age = 77 years) who had persistent pain of varied etiologies and no more than mild cognitive impairment. Participants were randomly assigned to either a cognitive-behavioral pain management group or an attention/support control group. Group sessions were conducted at the nursing home and involved 10 weekly sessions lasting 60 to 75 minutes. Although no significant effects on depression were found in either group, participants who received the CBT intervention reported significantly less pain and pain-related disability than those in the attention control condition. Effects were maintained at a 4-month follow-up. These results are particularly noteworthy given the study's small sample size and the heterogeneity of pain diagnoses represented in the groups.

In a study conducted on-site in three retirement communities, Ersek and colleagues (2003) randomized 45 older persons with persistent pain (mean age = 82) to either a pain self-management group or an educational booklet control condition. The group met for seven 90-minute sessions facilitated by a doctoral-level health professional. Sessions emphasized discussion of chronic pain topics as well as development of individual pain management goals. At a 3-month follow-up, the pain self-management group showed significantly greater improvement in physical role functioning and pain intensity. No significant group differences emerged for pain-related activity interference, pain-related beliefs, or depression. The authors concluded that a brief, community-based self-management intervention may be beneficial for older adults coping with persistent pain.

Finally, Fry and Wong (1991) investigated the effects of matching the type of CBT intervention provided with participants' preferred style of coping with their pain. Sixty-nine homebound older adults between the ages of 63 and 82 years were given the *Ways of Coping Checklist* and were classified as either predominantly problem-focused or emotion-focused copers. Participants were then assigned either to a matched intervention group or a control group. The problem-focused intervention emphasized problem-solving approaches for coping with pain, including relaxation, cognitive restructuring regarding pain intensity and pain sensations, and physiotherapy. The emotion-focused intervention emphasized expressions of hope and faith, seeking social support, and talking with others who had experienced similar pain. The control group received a mixed intervention composed of randomly selected problem- and emotion-focused pain management strategies. Participants completed 3 weeks of daily practice with the assigned intervention strategies and 12 weeks of continued monitoring.

Participants in all three groups (including the control group) showed significant pre- to post-treatment reductions in pain and anxiety and significant increases in satisfaction and adjustment. These gains were maintained at a 24-week follow-up (Fry and Wong 1991). Although the groups did not differ overall in outcome, there were differences based on participants' preferred coping styles. Specifically, participants who received the CBT intervention that matched their dispositional problem-focused coping style showed significantly better outcomes in terms of pain, anxiety, satisfaction, and adjustment as compared to participants in the control group. Participants who received the CBT intervention that matched their dispositional emotion-focused coping style showed significantly better outcomes only in terms of pain and anxiety as compared to participants in the control group. These data suggest that understanding the ways in which older adults cope with pain and tailoring CBT interventions to match dispositional coping efforts may be particularly beneficial.

TAILORING COGNITIVE-BEHAVIORAL PAIN MANAGEMENT FOR OLDER ADULTS

As the use of cognitive-behavioral interventions in older adults has grown, there has been increasing recognition of the need to tailor these interventions so as to best meet the needs of older adults (Arean et al. 2003; see also Gibson et al. 1996). In this section, we describe some of specific recommendations for tailoring treatment that have been advanced and discuss their relevance to CBT approaches to pain management. These modifications are summarized in Table II.

As Arean et al. (2003) note, older adults may be less familiar with the nature and process of therapy or skills training and therefore may need an introduction to its fundamental components. This orientation might include a review of the training and orientation of the therapist, the collaborative nature of treatment, the autonomy of the client, and a clear description of the treatment rationale and methods. It is helpful to ask clients to verbalize the rationale for treatment to ensure they understand it (Yonan and Wegener 2003). It is also important to give the patient a chance to ask questions in order to gain accurate information and dispel preconceptions or myths about treatment (Arean et al. 2003). This is especially important in pain management, where the patient might consider a referral to a psychologist for CBT as a sign that the pain is not considered "real" (Keefe et al. 1996). It is also very important to normalize feelings of anxiety about seeking treatment and to clearly communicate the message that pursuing treatment does not mean that one is weak, but rather that one is simply interested in learning new skills for coping (Bortz and O'Brien 1997).

Table II
Modifying cognitive-behavioral therapy protocols for use with older adults

Screen for cognitive impairment
Regularly assess for factors that can hinder cognitive-behavioral therapy (e.g., changes in pain, health status, medication compliance, or life circumstances)
Assess for auditory impairment: use a lower-pitched voice, inquire about hearing aids
Assess for visual impairment: use large font and high contrast colors in written materials
Provide socialization to cognitive-behavioral therapy
Involve spouses or caregivers, particularly in the socialization process
Thoroughly assess client's developmental history
Present material at a slower pace by conducting shorter, more numerous sessions
Allow additional time for repetition and slower processing of material
Ask older adults to summarize the topics addressed and the home practice assignment to ensure comprehension
Use multimodal presentation of material (e.g., written summary, session audiotape)
Provide repeated reinforcement of treatment gains or skills use
Make age-appropriate behavioral recommendations

A particularly useful way of decreasing the stigma associated with seeking treatment is to conduct treatment or training sessions in community settings, rather than in traditional mental health settings (Arean et al. 2003). In our own clinical research we have conducted partner-guided coping skills training for cancer patients who were near the end of life in patients' homes (Keefe et al. 2004). Many of our current projects use a telephone-based approach to delivering coping-skills training, which minimizes the burden of travel and thus appeals to older clients.

Another strategy for enhancing older adults' level of engagement in cognitive-behavioral treatment is to include a review of important life milestones early in the treatment protocol (Bortz and O'Brien 1997). In a pain-coping skills training protocol, having patients review key milestones in their life provides valuable information about significant life experiences, self-beliefs, typical coping strategies, and strengths and weaknesses that may influence their ability to cope with persistent pain.

Involving a family member or caregiver in cognitive-behavioral treatment can be especially beneficial for older adults (Keefe et al. 1996). Caregivers who are involved in treatment are more likely to encourage or help older adults to attend sessions and prompt them or work with them to complete home practice assignments. Along these lines, we carried out a controlled study to test the effects of a spouse-assisted pain coping skills training protocol for older adults having pain due to osteoarthritis of the knee. Eighty-eight osteoarthritis patients and their spouses were randomly assigned to one of three conditions: (1) spouse-assisted pain-coping skills training, (2) a conventional coping-skills training intervention with no spouse involvement, or (3) an arthritis education intervention that involved spousal support. Patients and spouses in the spouse-assisted coping-skills training condition attended group sessions together, where they were trained in pain-coping skills and couples skills to enhance pain management. Patients in the conventional coping-skills training condition attended group sessions without their spouses and were trained in pain-coping skills only. Patients and spouses in the arthritis education and spousal support condition attended group sessions together, where with they received detailed educational information about pain. Data analyses revealed a consistent pattern of improvement across a variety of outcomes (e.g., pain, psychological disability, pain behavior, coping, and self-efficacy), in which patients in the spouse-assisted coping-skills training condition had the best outcomes, those in the conventional coping-skills training condition the next best outcomes, and those in the arthritis education and spousal support condition the worst outcomes. These findings indicate that involving spouses in cognitive-behavioral training in pain coping can be quite beneficial in reducing pain and disability.

Research on the effect of aging on information-processing speed and inferential reasoning suggests that older adults are likely to experience declines in these areas (Bortz and O'Brien 1997; Arean et al. 2003). The pace of psychotherapy may need to be adjusted to accommodate these changes (Arean et al. 2003). Specifically, each therapy session might be shortened slightly to ensure sustained attention and to prevent client fatigue. For example, a protocol that is delivered in 10 sessions with younger adults might be extended to 12 or 14 sessions when delivered to older adults. Information may need to be reviewed regularly during sessions. Arena et al. (1988) found that despite providing what they viewed as clear instructions about the importance of home skills practice and the frequency of recommended practice during the upcoming week, their older participants were initially unable to accurately describe home practice assignments. The authors began allowing additional time at the end of sessions to review home practice recommendations and asking clients to verbalize their understanding of recommendations before leaving the session. Providing clients with written summaries of session content and allowing them to review the material in written or audiotaped format is likely to improve comprehension and retention of information.

Patients who have very significant cognitive impairment are poor candidates for cognitive-behavioral approaches to pain management (Keefe et al. 1996). Treatment approaches, however, can be modified to meet the needs of patients with less severe cognitive deficits. For example, therapists can use concrete examples and avoid abstractions, use audiovisual aids, repeat key content material, and conduct shorter, more frequent therapy sessions (Solomon and Szwabo 1992; Bonder 1994; Bortz and O'Brien 1997).

FUTURE DIRECTIONS

Evidence of the efficacy of CBT in treating older adults' persistent pain is supported by the research described in this chapter. The next step is to determine how we can increase the use of CBT in the older adult population. In addition to modifying protocols as discussed in the previous section, providing alternative settings may increase the likelihood that older adults will engage in, and benefit from, cognitive-behavioral interventions. For instance, support for the efficacy of self-management and clinician-assisted group interventions has been demonstrated in a variety of studies (e.g., Rybarczyk et al. 2001; Ersek et al. 2003). In addition, the Internet is increasingly being viewed as a viable alternative to face-to-face therapy sessions (e.g., Riley and Veale 1999; Taylor and Luce 2003) and has been used in studies for data collection (e.g., Chang 2004) and for delivery of CBT (Christensen et al. 2002).

Finally, how responsive are physicians to the growing evidence that older adults with pain can actively engage in and benefit from cognitive-behavioral interventions? How can we increase CBT referral rates for this population? There is some evidence suggesting that many older adults prefer to be treated by their primary care physician for both physical and psychological problems (Klausner and Alexopoulos 1999). Perhaps having mental health professionals available at primary care settings might increase physicians' awareness of nonpharmacological intervention options and may increase older adult patients' willingness to participate in CBT. These and many other questions regarding the potential of CBT for pain in older adults await exploration.

REFERENCES

Akkerman RL, Ostwald SK. Reducing anxiety in Alzheimer's disease family caregivers: the effectiveness of a nine-week cognitive-behavioral intervention. *Am J Alzheimers Dis Other Demen* 2004; 19(2):117–123.

Allain P, Nicoleau S, Pinon K, et al. Executive functioning in normal aging: a study of action planning using the Zoo Map Test. *Brain Cogn* 2005; 57:4–7.

Antall GF, Kresevic D. The use of guided imagery to manage pain in an elderly orthopaedic population. *Orthop Nurs* 2004; 23(5):335–340.

Arean PA, Cook BL, Gallagher-Thompson D, et al. Guidelines for conducting geropsychotherapy research. *Am J Geriatr Psychol* 2003; 11(1):9–16.

Arena JG, Hightower NE, Chong GC. Relaxation therapy for tension headache in the elderly: a prospective study. *Psychol Aging* 1988; 3(1):96–98.

Auman LC, Bosworth HB, Hess TM. Effect of health-related stereotypes on physiological responses of hypertensive middle-aged and older men. *J Gerontol Soc Am* 2005; 60:P3–P10.

Baddeley A. The central executive: a concept and some misconceptions. *J Int Neuropsychol Soc* 1998; 4:523–526.

Baddeley AD, Hitch GJ. Developments in the concept of working memory. *Neuropsychology* 1994; 8(4):485–493.

Bandura A. *Self-Efficacy: The Exercise of Control*. New York: W.H. Freeman, 1997.

Barry LC, Guo Z, Kerns RD, Duong BD, Reid MC. Functional self-efficacy and pain-related disability among older veterans with chronic pain in a primary care setting. *Pain* 2003; 104:131–137.

Basford L, Poon LW, Dowzer C, Booth A. Coping with specific chronic health conditions. In: Poon LW, Gueldner SH, Sprouse BM. (Eds). *Successful Aging and Adaptation with Chronic Diseases*. New York: Springer, 2003, pp 151–180.

Beauducel A, Kersting M. Fluid and crystallized intelligence and the Berlin model of intelligence structure (BIS). *Eur J Psychol Assess* 2002; 18(2):97–112.

Beck AT. *Cognitive Therapy and the Emotional Disorders*. New York: International Universities Press, 1976.

Beck AT, Rush AJ, Shaw BF, Emery G. *Cognitive Therapy of Depression*. New York: Guilford Press, 1979.

Beck JS. *Cognitive Therapy: Basics and Beyond.* New York: Guilford Press, 1995.

Bilger RC, Meyer TA. Localization and speech perception in noise by aging listeners. *J Acoustical Soc Am* 1996; 99(4):2516–2529.

Bishop KL, Ferraro FR, Borowiak DM. Pain management in older adults: role of fear and avoidance. *Clin Gerontol* 2001; 23(1–2):33–42.

Blazer DG. Depression in late life: review and commentary. *J Gerontol A Biol Sci Med Sci* 2003; 58:M249–M265.

Boersma K, Linton S, Overmeer T, et al. Lowering fear-avoidance and enhancing function through exposure in vivo. A multiple baseline study across six patients with back pain. *Pain* 2004; 108(1–2):8–16.

Bonder BR. Psychotherapy for individuals with Alzheimer's disease. *Alzheimer Dis Assoc Disord* 1994; 8(Suppl 3):75–81.

Bortz JJ, O'Brien KP. Psychotherapy with older adults: theoretical issues, empirical findings, and clinical applications. In: Nussbaum PD (Ed). *Handbook of Neuropsychology and Aging: Critical Issues with Neuropsychology.* New York: Plenum, 1997, pp 431–451.

Brigman S, Cherry KE. Age and skilled performance: contributions of working memory and processing speed. *Brain Cogn* 2002; 50(2):242–256.

Brown SC, Park DC. Theoretical models of cognitive aging and implications for translational research in medicine. *Gerontologist* 2003; 43 (Special Issue 1):57–67.

Brown SC, Glass JM, Park DC. The relationship of pain and depression to cognitive function in rheumatoid arthritis patients. *Pain* 2002; 96:279–284.

Burgener SC, Twigg P. Interventions for persons with irreversible dementia. *Annu Rev Nurs Res* 2002; 20:89–124.

Centers for Disease Control. Public health and aging: projected prevalence of self-reported arthritis or chronic joint symptoms among persons aged ≥65 years: United States, 2005–2030. *Morb Mortal Wkly Rep* 2003; 52(21):489–491.

Chang BL. Internet intervention for community elders. *West J Nurs Res* 2004; 26(4):461–466.

Christensen H, Mackinnon A, Jorm AF, et al. Age differences and interindividual variation in cognition in community-dwelling elderly. *Psychol Aging* 1994; 9(3):381–329.

Christensen AJ, Moran PJ, Wiebe JS. Assessment of irrational health beliefs: relation to health practices and medical regimen adherence. *Health Psychol* 1999; 18(2):169–176.

Christensen H, Griffiths KM, Korten A. Web-based cognitive behavior therapy: analysis of site usage and changes in depression and anxiety. *J Med Internet Res* 2002; 4(1):e3. Available at: www.jmir.org/2002/1/e3.

Cook AJ. Cognitive-behavioral pain management for elderly nursing home residents. *J Gerontol B Psychol Sci Soc Sci* 1998; 53B(1):P51–P59.

de Beni R, Palladino P. Declines in working memory updating through ageing: intrusion error analyses. *Memory* 2004; 12(1):75–89.

de Jong JR, Vlaeyen JW, Onghena P, et al. Fear of movement/(re)injury in chronic low back pain: education or exposure in vivo as mediator to fear reduction? *Clin J Pain* 2005; 21(1):9–17.

Diehl M, Willis SL, Schaie KW. Everyday problem solving in older adults: observational assessment and cognitive correlates. *Psychol Aging* 1995; 20(3):478–491.

Dobson KS, Shaw BF. Cognitive therapies in practice. In: Bongar B, Beutler LE (Eds). *Comprehensive Textbook of Psychotherapy: Theory and Practice.* New York: Oxford University Press, 1995, pp 159–172.

Duke J, Leventhal H, Brownlee S, Leventhal EA. Giving up and replacing activities in response to illness. *J Gerontol B Psychol Sci Soc Sci* 2002; 57B(4):P367–P376.

Eells TD. Can therapy affect physical health? *J Psychother Pract Res* 2000; 9(2):100–104.

Ersek M, Turner JA, McCurry SM, Gibbons L, Kraybill BM. Efficacy of a self-management group intervention for elderly persons with chronic pain. *Clin J Pain* 2003; 19:156–167.

Fick DM, Cooper JW, Wade WE, et al. Updating the Beers criteria for potentially inappropriate medication use in older adults. *Arch Intern Med* 2003; 163:2716–2724.

Fishbain D. Evidence-based data on pain relief with antidepressants. *Ann Med* 2000; 32(5):305–316.

Fishbain DA, Cutler R, Rosomoff HL, Rosomoff RS. Chronic pain-associated depression: antecedent or consequence of chronic pain? A review. *Clin J Pain* 1997; 13(2):116–137.

Fisk JE, Sharp CA. Age-related impairment in executive functioning: updating, inhibition, shifting, and access. *J Clin Exp Neuropsychol* 2004; 26(7):874–890.

Fox PO, Raina P, Jadad AR. Prevalence and treatment of pain in older adults in nursing homes and other long-term care institutions: a systematic review. *CMAJ* 1999; 160(3):329–333.

Freedman GM. Chronic pain. Clinical management of common causes of geriatric pain. *Geriatrics* 2002; 57(5):36–41.

Fry PS, Wong PTP. Pain management training in the elderly: matching interventions with subjects' coping styles. *Stress Med* 1991; 7:93–98.

Geerlings SW, Twisk JWR, Beekman ATF, Deeg DJH, van Tilburg W. Longitudinal relationship between pain and depression in older adults: sex, age and physical disability. *Soc Psychiatry Psychiatr Epidemiol* 2002; 37(1):23–30.

Gibson SJ, Farrell MJ, Katz B, Helme RD. Multidisciplinary management of chronic nonmalignant pain in older adults. In: Ferrell BR, Ferrell BA (Eds). *Pain in the Elderly*. Seattle: IASP Press, 1996, pp 91–99.

Gignac MAM, Cott C, Baley EM. Adaptation to chronic illness and disability and its relationship to perceptions of independence and dependence. *J Gerontol B Psychol Sci Soc Sci* 2000; 55B(6):P362–P372.

Gloth FM. Geriatric pain. Factors that limit pain relief and increase complications. *Geriatrics* 2000; 55(10):46–48:51–54.

Grossberg GT, Desai AK. Management of Alzheimer's disease. *J Gerontol A Biol Sci Med Sci* 2003; 58A(4):331–353.

Hasher L, Zacks RT. Automatic and effortful processes in memory. *J Exp Psychol Gen* 1979; 108:356–388.

Hasher L, Stoltzfus ER, Zacks RT, Rypma B. Age and inhibition. *J Exp Psychol Learn Mem Cogn* 1991; 17(1):163–169.

Hebert LE, Scherr PA, Bienias JL, Bennett DA, Evans DA. Alzheimer disease in the US population: prevalence estimates using the 2000 census. *Arch Neurol* 2003; 60(8):1119–1122.

Heine C, Browning CJ. Communication and psychosocial consequences of sensory loss in older adults: overview and rehabilitation directions. *Disabil Rehabil* 2002; 24(15):763–773.

Helme RD. Chronic pain management in older people. *Eur J Pain* 2001; Suppl A:31–36.

Hess TM, Auman C, Colcombe SJ, Rahhal TA. The impact of stereotype threat on age differences in memory performance. *J Gerontol B Psychol Sci Soc Sci* 2003; 5:P3–P11.

Heuts PHTG, Vlaeyen JWS, Roelofs J, et al. Pain-related fear and daily functioning in patients with osteoarthritis. *Pain* 2004; 110:228–235.

Kane MJ, Hambrick DZ, Conway ARA. Working memory capacity and fluid intelligence are strongly related constructs: Comment on Ackerman, Beier, and Boyle (2005). *Psychol Bull* 2005; 131(1):66–71.

Kasl-Godley J, Gatz M. Psychosocial interventions for individuals with dementia: an integration of theory, therapy, and a clinical understanding of dementia. *Clin Psychol Rev* 2000; 20(6):755–782.

Kee WG, Middaugh SJ, Redpath S, Hargadon R. Age as a factor in admission to chronic pain rehabilitation. *Clin J Pain* 1998; 14(2):121–128.

Keefe FJ, Brown GK, Wallston KA, Caldwell DS. Coping with rheumatoid arthritis pain: catastrophizing as a maladaptive strategy. *Pain* 1989; 37:51–56.

Keefe FJ, Caldwell DS, Williams DA, et al. Pain coping skills training in the management of osteoarthritic knee pain: a comparative study. *Behav Ther* 1990a; 21:49–62.

Keefe FJ, Caldwell DS, Williams DA, et al. Pain coping skills training in the management of osteoarthritic knee pain. II: Follow-up results. *Behav Ther* 1990b; 21:435–447.

Keefe FJ, Caldwell DS, Baucom D, et al. Spouse-assisted coping skills training in the management of osteoarthritic knee pain. *Arthritis Care Res* 1996; 9(4):279–291.

Keefe FJ, Caldwell DS, Baucom D, et al. M. Spouse-assisted coping skills training in the management of knee pain in osteoarthritis: long-term follow-up results. *Arthritis Care Res* 2001; 12(2):101–111.

Keefe FJ, Smith SJ, Buffington ALH, et al. Recent advances and future directions in the biopsychosocial assessment and treatment of arthritis. *J Consult Clin Psychol* 2002; 70:640–655.

Keefe FJ, Ahles TA, Porter LS, et al. The self-efficacy of family caregivers for helping cancer patients manage pain at the end of life. *Pain* 2003; 103(1–2):157–162.

Keefe FJ, Rumble ME, Scipio CD, Giordano LA, Perri LM. Psychological aspects of persistent pain: current state of the science. *J Pain* 2004; 5(4):195–211.

Kerns RD, Otis JD, Marcus KS. Pain management in the elderly: cognitive-behavioral therapy for chronic pain in the elderly. *Clin Geriatr Med* 2001; 17(3):1–18.

Klausner EJ, Alexopoulos GS. The future of psychosocial treatments for elderly patients. *Psychiatr Serv* 1999; 50(9):1198–1204.

Kroenke K, Swindle R. Cognitive-behavioral therapy for somatization and symptom syndromes: a critical review of controlled clinical trials. *Psychother Psychosom* 2000; 69(4):205–215.

Lefebvre JC, Keefe FJ, Affleck G, et al. The relationship of arthritis self-efficacy to daily pain, daily mood, and daily pain coping in rheumatoid arthritis patients. *Pain* 1999; 80:425–435.

Lepine JP, Briley M. The epidemiology of pain in depression. *Hum Psychopharmacol* 2004; 19(Suppl 1):S3–S7.

Leveille SG. Musculoskeletal aging. *Curr Opin Rheumatol* 2004; 16(2):114–118.

Levy BR. Mind matters: cognitive and physical effects of aging self-stereotypes. *J Gerontol B Psychol Sci Soc Sci* 2003; 58B(4):P203–P211.

Liu LL, Park DC. Aging and medical adherence: the use of automatic processes to achieve effortful things. *Psychol Aging* 2004; 19(2):318–325.

Lorig K, Mazonson P, Holman H. Evidence suggesting that health education for self-management in patients with chronic arthritis has sustained health benefits which reducing health care costs. *Arthritis Rheum* 1993; 36:439–446.

Lorig KR, Laurent DD, Deyo RA, et al. Can a back pain e-mail discussion group improve health status and lower health care costs? A randomized study. *Arch Intern Med* 2002; 162(7):792–796.

Lorig KR, Ritter PL, Laurent DD, Fries JF. Long-term randomized controlled trials of tailored-print and small-group arthritis self-management interventions. *Med Care* 2004; 42(4):346–354.

McArdle JJ, Ferrer-Caja E, Hamagami F, Woodcock RW. Comparative longitudinal structural analyses of the growth and decline of multiple intellectual abilities over the life span. *Dev Psychol* 2002; 38(1):115–142.

McCracken LM, Eccleston C. Coping or acceptance? What to do about chronic pain? *Pain* 2003; 105:197–204.

McCracken LM, Turk DC. Behavioral and cognitive-behavioral treatment for chronic pain: outcome, predictors of outcome, and treatment process. *Spine* 2002; 27(22):2564–2573.

McCracken LM, Spertus IL, Janeck AS, Sinclair D, Wetzel FT. Behavioral dimensions of adjustment in persons with chronic pain: pain-related anxiety and acceptance. *Pain* 1999; 80:283–289.

McWilliams LA, Cox BJ, Enns MW. Mood and anxiety disorders associated with chronic pain: an examination in a nationally representative sample. *Pain* 2003; 106:127–133.

Melzack R, Wall PD. Pain mechanisms: a new theory. *Science* 1965; 150:971–979.

Middaugh SJ, Woods SE, Kee WG, Harden RN, Peters JR. Biofeedback-assisted relaxation training for the aging chronic pain patient. *Biofeedback Self-Regul* 1991; 16(4):361–377.

Milham MP, Erickson KI, Banich MT, et al. Attentional control in the aging brain: Insights from an fMRI study of the Stroop task. *Brain Cogn* 2002; 49:277–296.

Moseley GL. Evidence for a direct relationship between cognitive and physical change during an education intervention in people with chronic low back pain. *Eur J Pain* 2004; 8:39–45.

Moss-Morris R, Petrie KJ. Cognitive distortions of somatic experiences: Revision and validation of a measure. *J Psychosom Res* 2003; 43(3):293–306.

Mossey JM, Gallagher RM. The longitudinal occurrence and impact of comorbid chronic pain and chronic depression over two years in continuing care retirement community residents. *Pain Med* 2004; 5(4): 335–348.

Mossey JM, Gallagher RM, Tirumalasett F. The effects of pain and depression on physical functioning in elderly residents of a continuing care retirement community. *Pain Med* 2000; 1(4):340–350.

Ormel J, Rijsdijk FV, Sullivan M, von Sonderen E, Kempen GIJM. Temporal and reciprocal relationship between IADL/ADL disability and depressive symptoms in late life. *J Gerontol B Psychol Sci Soc Sci* 2002; 57:P338–P347.

Poleshuck EL, Dworkin RH. Risk factors for chronic pain in patients with acute pain and their implications for prevention. In: Dworkin RH, Breitbart WS (Eds). *Psychosocial Aspects of Pain: A Handbook for Health Care Providers*, Progress in Pain Research and Management, Vol. 27. Seattle: IASP Press, 2004, pp 589–606.

Puder RS. Age analysis of cognitive-behavioral group therapy for chronic pain outpatients. *Psychol Aging* 1988; 3(2):204–207.

Redd WH, Montgomery GH, DuHamel KN. Behavioral intervention for cancer treatment side effects. *J Natl Cancer Inst* 2001; 93(11):810–823.

Reid MC, Otis J, Barry LC, Kerns RD. Cognitive-behavioral therapy for chronic low back pain in older persons: a preliminary study. *Pain Med* 2003a; 4(3):223–232.

Reid MC, Williams CS, Gill TM. The relationship between psychological factors and disabling musculoskeletal pain in community-dwelling older persons. *J Am Geriatr Soc* 2003b; 51:1092–1098.

Requena C, Lopez Ibor MI, Maestu F, et al. Effects of cholinergic drugs and cognitive training on dementia. *Dement Geriatr Cogn Disord* 2004; 18:50–54.

Riley S, Veale D. The internet and its relevance to cognitive behavioural psychotherapists. *Behav Cogn Psychother* 1999; 27:37–46.

Rybarczyk B, DeMarco G, DeLaCruz M, Lapidos S, Fortner B. A classroom mind/body wellness intervention for older adults with chronic illness: comparing immediate and 1-year benefits. *Behav Med* 2001; 27(1):15–27.

Salthouse TA. The processing speed theory of adult age differences in cognition. *Psychol Rev* 1996; 103:403–428.

Salthouse TA. What and when of cognitive aging. *Curr Direct Psychol Sci* 2004; 13(4):140–144.

Sanderson M, Wang J, Davis DR, et al. Co-morbidity associated with dementia. *Am J Alzheimers Dis Other Demen* 2002; 17(2):73–78.

Sarason IG, Sarason BR, Pierce GR. Anxiety, cognitive interference, and performance. *J Soc Behav Personal* 1990; 5:1–18.

Sarkisian CA, Hays RD, Berry SH, Mangione CM. Expectations regarding aging among older adults and physicians who care for older adults. *Med Care* 2001; 39(9):1025–1036.

Savage SR. Opioid use in the management of chronic pain. *Med Clin N Am* 1999; 83(3):761–786.

Sharpe L, Senskl T, Timberlake N, et al. A blind, randomized, controlled trial of cognitive-behavioral intervention for patients with recent onset rheumatoid arthritis: preventing psychological and physical morbidity. *Pain* 2001; 89:275–283.

Shifren K, Park DC, Bennett JM, Morrell RW. Do cognitive processes predict mental health in individuals with rheumatoid arthritis? *J Behav Med* 1999; 22(6):529–547.

Siegler IC, Bastian LA, Steffens DC, Bosworth HB, Costa PT. Behavioral medicine and aging. *J Consult Clin Psychol* 2002; 70(3):843–851.

Smarr KL, Parker JC, Wright GE, et al. The importance of enhancing self-efficacy in rheumatoid arthritis. *Arthritis Care Res* 1997; 10:18–26.

Smith CA, Wallston KA. Adaptation in patients with chronic rheumatoid arthritis: application of a general model. *Health Psychol* 1992; 11:151–162.

Smith TW, Christensen AJ, Peck JR, Ward JR. Cognitive distortion, helplessness, and depressed mood in rheumatoid arthritis: a four-year longitudinal analysis. *Health Psychol* 1994; 13(3): 213–217.

Solomon K, Szwabo P. Psychotherapy for patients with dementia. In: Morley JE, Coe RM, Strong R, Grossberg GT (Eds). *Memory Function and Aging-Related Disorders.* New York: Springer, 1992, pp 295–319.

Sorkin BA, Rudy TE, Hanlon RB, Turk DC, Stieg RL. Chronic pain in old and young patients: differences appear less important than similarities. *J Gerontol* 1990; 45:P64–P68.

Stein R, Blanchard-Fields F, Hertzog C. The effects of age-stereotype priming on the memory performance of older adults. *Exp Ageing Res* 2002; *28*(2):169–181.

Taylor CB, Luce KH. Computer- and internet-based psychotherapy interventions. *Curr Direct Psychol Sci* 2003; 12(1):18–22.

Teri L, Gallagher-Thompson D. Cognitive-behavioral interventions for treatment of depression in Alzheimer's patients. *Gerontologist* 1991; 31(3):413–416.

Teri L, Logsdon RG. Identifying pleasant activities for Alzheimer's disease patients: the pleasant events schedule-AD. *Gerontologist* 1991; 31(3):124–127.

Thorn BE. *Cognitive Therapy for Chronic Pain: A Step-by-Step Approach.* New York: Guilford Press, 2004.

Turk DC. Cognitive-behavioral approach to the treatment of chronic pain patients. *Reg Anesth Pain Med* 2003; 28(6):573–579.

Unutzer J, Ferrell B, Lin EH, Marmon T. Pharmacotherapy of pain in depressed older adults. *J Am Geriatr Soc* 2004; 52(11):1916–1922.

Vlaeyen JW, Linton SJ. Fear-avoidance and its consequences in chronic musculoskeletal pain: a state of the art. *Pain* 2000; 85(3):317–332.

Vlaeyen JW, de Jong JR, Onghena P, Kerckhoffs-Hanssen M, Kole-Snijders AM. Can pain-related fear be reduced? The application of cognitive-behavioural exposure in vivo. *Pain Res Manage* 2002; 7(3):144–153.

Von Korff M, Crane P, Lane M, et al. Chronic spinal pain and physical-mental comorbidity in the United States: results from the national comorbidity survey replication. *Pain* 2005; 113:331–339.

Waters SJ, Campbell LC, Keefe FJ, Carson JW. The essence of cognitive-behavioral pain management. In: Dworkin RH, Breitbart WS (Eds.) *Psychosocial Aspects of Pain: A Handbook for Health Care Providers,* Progress in Pain Research and Management, Vol. 27. Seattle: IASP Press, 2004, pp 261–284.

Wellman B, Kelner M, Wigdor BT. Older adults' use of medical and alternative care. *J Appl Gerontol* 2001; 20(1):3–23.

Weiner DK, Hanlon JT. Pain in nursing home residents: management strategies. *Drugs Aging* 2001; 18(1):13–29.

Yonan CA, Wegener ST. Assessment and management of pain in the older adult. *Rehabil Psychol* 2003; 48(1):4–13.

Correspondence to: Sandra J. Waters, PhD, Duke University Medical Center, Department of Psychiatry and Behavioral Medicine, Box 90399, Durham, NC 27708, USA. Email: water017@mc.duke.edu.

Pain in Older Persons, Progress in Pain
Research and Management, Vol. 35, edited
by Stephen J. Gibson and Debra K. Weiner,
IASP Press, Seattle, © 2005.

13

Interventional Pain Management Procedures in Older Patients

Cheryl Bernstein,[a] Bud Lateef,[b] and Perry Fine[c]

Departments of [a]Anesthesiology and [b]Pain Medicine, University of Pittsburgh School of Medicine, Pittsburgh, Pennsylvania, USA; [c]University of Utah Pain Management Center, Salt Lake City, Utah, USA

Interventional procedures have become an important option in pain management for older adults. In these patients, in whom polypharmacy is common, well-selected interventional techniques may reduce or eliminate the need for systemic oral analgesics. Notwithstanding the value of opioid analgesics in the treatment of moderate to severe pain in appropriately selected cases, many patients are unable to tolerate these medications due to adverse side effects such as constipation, sedation, cognitive impairment ("mental clouding," confusion), and respiratory depression.

Interventional pain procedures can serve both diagnostic and therapeutic functions. With the addition of high-resolution fluoroscopy, interventional procedures have become safer and more exact, facilitating delivery of medications directly and more precisely to target sites. These procedures are ideally performed in specialized clinic settings, outpatient surgery centers, or hospital operating rooms, where aseptic technique and conditions can be maintained. Appropriate monitoring equipment and emergency resuscitation supplies are necessary, particularly in fragile older adults. Consideration should always be given to coagulation status in these patients, since they are often prescribed anti-platelet and anti-thrombotic drugs. Despite these precautions, most injection procedures can be done safely in the outpatient setting. This chapter will discuss a variety of procedures used in the treatment of chronic pain including those for neuroaxial, myofascial, and diskogenic pain, implantable technologies including intrathecal opioid pumps and spinal cord stimulators, and sympathetic blockade. A summary of the indications and complications associated with the procedures reviewed in this chapter is provided in Table I.

Table I
Interventional pain management procedures: indications and complications

Procedure	Indications	Complications
Epidural steroids	Radiculopathy Symptoms referable to spinal stenosis HNP Flare of chronic low back or neck pain Tumor invasion of nerve roots	Back pain Dural-puncture headache Epidural hematoma Epidural abscess Meningitis Neurological dysfunction
Sacroiliac joint injections	LBP with SIJ dysfunction	Infection Bleeding Back pain flare
Trigger point injections	Myofascial pain syndrome	Infection Pneumothorax Intravascular injection of local anesthetic Neural blockade from inadvertent perineural, epidural, subarachnoid injection
Facet injections	Nonradicular neck and back pain Degenerative arthritis of facet joints Pain with facet joint loading	Infection Radicular pain Subarachnoid injection Somatic nerve block or injury
Vertebroplasty/ kyphoplasty	Vertebral body compression fractures	Infection Needle trauma Cement leakage Neurological dysfunction Intravascular injection/pulmonary embolism
Intradiskal electrothermal therapy	Diskogenic low back pain Failure of conservative therapy	Infection/diskitis Catheter breakage Nerve root injury Vertebral body osteonecrosis Cauda equina syndrome
Percutaneous nucleoplasty	Diskogenic low back pain with positive diskogram HNP or disk bulge on MRI	Infection/diskitis Catheter breakage Nerve root injury
Intrathecal opioid pumps	Malignant and nonmalignant opioid-responsive pain	Infection Hematoma Catheter breakage/failure Catheter granuloma Spinal cord injury Neurological injury CSF leakage Pump complications

Table I *(Cont.)*

Procedure	Indications	Complications
Spinal cord stimulators	Neuropathy/CRPS/SMP Radicular pain with failed back surgery syndrome Postherpetic neuralgia Peripheral neuropathy Vascular insufficiency	Bleeding Injection Lead migration Lead failure/breakage
Lumbar sympathetic block	CRPS/SMP of the lower extremity Vascular insufficiency Postherpetic neuralgia Peripheral neuropathy	Back pain Hematoma Intravascular or subarachnoid injection Renal or ureteral trauma Genitofemoral neuralgia
Stellate ganglion block	CRPS/SMP of the head and neck or upper extremity Postherpetic neuralgia Vascular insufficiency Raynaud's disease	Pneumothorax Horner's syndrome Intravascular/subarachnoid injection Recurrent laryngeal nerve block Cervical root block
Celiac plexus block	Pancreatic cancer pain Acute and chronic pancreatitis Abdominal visceral pain syndrome Abdominal angina	Pneumothorax Intrathecal/intravascular injection Hypotension Diarrhea Paraplegia (artery of Ademkiewicz) spasm

Abbreviations: CSF = cerebrospinal fluid; CRPS = complex regional pain syndrome; HNP = herniated nucleus pulposus; LBP = low back pain; MRI = magnetic resonance imaging; SIJ = sacroiliac joint; SMP = sympathetically maintained pain.

EPIDURAL CORTICOSTEROID INJECTIONS

First introduced in 1953 for the treatment of radiculopathy, lumbar epidural steroid injections are one of the most common procedures pain physicians perform. These injections are most effective for patients with symptoms of nerve root irritation, including radicular pain, numbness, weakness, and hypesthesia.

Epidural corticosteroid administration has the advantage of direct application of steroids to inflamed nerve roots. The potential causes of nerve root inflammation include pressure changes from herniated disks, chemical irritation from disk substances, structural abnormalities, and postsurgical fibrosis. Epidural steroids reduce inflammation by inhibiting phospholipase A2, a chemical constituent in disk material, blocking the rate-limiting step in the synthesis of prostaglandins and leukotrienes. There may be other antinociceptive mechanisms, but these have not been clearly elucidated.

Indications for epidural steroid injections include symptomatic treatment of herniated disks, postural back pain, intermittent flare-ups of chronic back pain, painful spinal stenosis, and cancer pain (Raj 2000). Various techniques are described in the literature, including selective epidural needle placement for more localized placement of lower doses of injectate. Comparative studies of efficacy, risks, and long-term outcomes are lacking. Cervical epidural steroid injections are used to treat neck pain of similar etiologies, although very few controlled studies support this practice, and it may be fraught with hazards. Depot steroids, methylprednisolone acetate, and triamcinolone diacetate are commonly used for epidural injections. Steroid formulations containing polyethylene glycol have been associated with arachnoiditis, sterile meningitis, and pachymeningitis.

Contraindications include coagulopathy and systemic or overlying skin infections. Postlumbar laminectomy/fusion patients are treated with additional caution given previous disruption of the epidural space. In these patients, the practitioner may use fluoroscopic guidance and inject via the caudal epidural space. Complications are rare, and the most common side effects are transient increase in back pain and radicular symptoms. Potentially adverse steroid effects should be monitored, including elevated blood glucose, hypertension, and fluid retention. Patients at risk for volume overload (e.g., patients with heart failure) and "brittle" diabetes require close follow-up. Serious complications including adhesive arachnoiditis, meningitis, epidural abscess, and hematoma formation are rare but require prompt attention.

The success rate for epidural steroid injections is not convincingly established in the literature, despite their widespread use to treat radiculopathy. Since the 1950s, only 14 double blind, placebo-controlled trials have been reported. In 1995, Koes et al. reviewed the 12 randomized trials that were available and concluded that six of the studies demonstrated effectiveness versus the control treatment, while the other six showed no benefit. The authors also rated the quality of these studies and found no difference between the half that showed effectiveness versus the half that did not (Koes et al. 1995). Since that review, two additional randomized placebo-controlled trials of lumbar epidural steroids have appeared. One studied a total of 158 patients treated with either epidural steroid injection or epidural isotonic saline. The authors demonstrated short-term benefit of epidural steroids in decreasing leg pain and sensory deficits, but showed no significant functional benefit or reduction in need for surgery (Carette et al. 1997). The most recent study evaluated 85 patients treated with either epidural steroids or epidural isotonic saline and showed no improvement with epidural steroids (Valat et al. 2003).

Kraemer et al. (1997) introduced selective epidural injections that access the epidural space via a transforaminal approach. The procedure's advantage is the use of lower steroid doses applied directly to the affected nerve root. There are only two controlled prospective studies of this approach, but both demonstrate success. Lutz et al. (1998) published a study of 69 patients treated with transforaminal epidural steroids for herniated nucleus pulposus and severe radicular back pain. Approximately three-quarters of subjects had greater than 50% pain reduction and reported improved functioning. Eighty percent of subjects reported satisfaction with the procedure.

While the popularity of lumbar epidural steroids appears to be a continuing trend in the treatment of low back pain, the long-term consequences of these injections remain unclear. The overall success of this intervention in terms of functional improvement, return to work, and prevention of surgery has yet to be determined. Currently, the main benefit from epidural steroid injection procedures in older patients appears to be purely palliative. By reducing pain, improving mobility, reducing the risk of falls, and enhancing overall quality of life, this procedure may be of great value, and so these end-outcomes should warrant further study.

SACROILIAC JOINT INJECTIONS

Sacroiliac (SI) joint pain is complex, thus its designation as SI joint syndrome, described in detail in Chapter 16 of this text. Studies of diagnostic, fluoroscopically guided SI injections identify the SI joint as the cause of 15% of chronic low back pain (Dreyfuss et al. 2004). Among the many causes of SI joint syndrome are trauma, osteoarthritis, ligamentous strain, and hypermobility. The practitioner may have difficulty recognizing SI joint etiology from other common causes of chronic low back pain, including disk disease, lumbar radiculopathy, facet joint pain, and myofascial pain. This difficulty in diagnosis is largely due to the fact that SI joint pain radiates to a variety of locations, most commonly to the thigh, but also to the lower leg, foot, groin, and abdomen. Physical examination that elicits sacral sulcus tenderness is highly sensitive for SI pain, but has poor specificity (Dreyfuss et al. 1996). Provocative testing may also be helpful for diagnosis (i.e., stressing the joint), and leg length measurement may identify a discrepancy that often accompanies SI joint dysfunction.

Local anesthetic SI joint injections are considered the diagnostic "gold standard" for SI joint pain (Chou et al. 2004). Most published studies use over 75% pain relief as diagnostic of SI-joint-mediated pain. Less than 50% pain relief is considered nondiagnostic. Low volumes of local anesthetic should be used to enhance specificity, since high volumes may spread out of the joint space, block nearby structures, and lead to false-positive results.

Sacroiliac joint injections are optimally done under either fluoroscopic or computed tomography (CT) guidance. Blind techniques are generally unsatisfactory secondary to poor needle placement (Rosenberg et al. 2000). A variety of observational studies of patients with spondyloarthropathy have shown the therapeutic benefit of injecting lidocaine and corticosteroid into the SI joint (Dreyfuss et al. 2004). There are no prospective, placebo-controlled studies evaluating therapeutic injections for idiopathic sacroiliitis. One retrospective study of 20 patients with idiopathic sacroiliitis reported modest relief after injection of steroid (Slipman et al. 2001).

Prolotherapy consists of injecting a mixture of dextrose/glycerol/phenol and lidocaine within the ligaments surrounding the SI joint, to create an inflammatory response that putatively strengthens the joint. Two randomized trials have shown superiority of this technique over sham injections (Ongley et al. 1987; Klein et al. 1993). Viscosupplementation has been reported to provide partial pain relief in a few case reports, although no controlled studies are available.

Some pain practitioners utilize radiofrequency denervation of the L5 dorsal ramus and the lateral branches of the S1–S3 roots to treat persistent SI joint pain. Once pain has been confirmed as originating from the SI joint with diagnostic blockade and other causes of low back pain have been excluded, radiofrequency ablation may be considered (Ferrante et al. 2001). One retrospective study of 14 patients treated with radiofrequency neurotomy of the SI joint demonstrated 50% pain reduction in 64% of study subjects. Prior to enrollment in this study, patients not only had clinical findings consistent with SI joint dysfunction, but responded to two diagnostic SI joint blocks and failed to respond to facet joint blocks (Yin et al. 2003). Further prospective studies are needed to determine the effectiveness of therapeutic injections for SI dysfunction compared with other more conservative treatments for SI joint pain.

TRIGGER POINT INJECTIONS

Trigger point (TP) injections are commonly used procedures for the treatment of myofascial pain syndromes (MPS). Both latent and active TPs are identified by palpating taut muscle bands, with pain often referred to distal sites. Trigger point injections are rarely effective as the sole therapy for myofascial pain (Criscuolo 2001), but they may improve response to physical therapy. Several potential mechanisms by which TP therapy reduces pain are postulated, including the release of potassium through depolarization, "washout" of sensitizing substances, inhibition of pain centralization, and focal necrosis (Esenyel et al. 2000).

Prior to injection, the TP is identified and stabilized by applying pressure on either side of the site. A twitch may be noted with dry needling and injection of a local anesthetic. Use of steroids in TP injections is controversial, and may potentially lead to muscle wasting, hypopigmentation, and dimpling with prolonged use (Criscuolo 2001). Dry needling alone, with redirection of the needle though various planes, may also be performed and is reported to be as beneficial as injection with local anesthetic (Esenyel et al. 2000). Focal pain and bruising are the most common side effects of TP therapy. Syncopal episodes, as a result of the vasovagal response, also may occur. Serious complications including infection, inadvertent spinal anesthesia, and pneumothorax are rare, but added caution is indicated when injecting in the thoracic region or in highly neurovascular areas such as the head and neck.

Some experts deny scientific evidence supporting the use of TP injections, while others recognize their benefit (Melzack and Wall 1999). The literature reports several controlled studies, including one by Fine et al. (1988) that showed significant results. The value of TP injections for the treatment of the more generalized muscular pain that occurs in patients with fibromyalgia syndrome is not clear. Studies show mixed results (Borg-Stein and Stein 1996; Hong and Hsueh 1996). Additional research is needed to clarify the indications for and long-term benefits of this commonly performed procedure.

FACET JOINT INJECTIONS

Lumbar zygapophyseal (facet joint) syndrome is estimated to account for 15–52% of patients with chronic low back pain (Slipman et al. 2003). The zygapophyseal joints are true synovial joints innervated by the medial branches of the dorsal rami. Almost 100 years ago, Goldthwait (1911) was the first to recognize the lumbar facet joints as sources of low back pain. Many years later, Mooney and Robertson (1976) reported local anesthetic block of the lumbar facet joint. There are several possible causes of zygapophyseal joint pain including inflammatory arthritis, microtrauma, and osteoarthritis. While physical examination and radiological data may suggest facet joint dysfunction, local anesthetic blockade of the joint or its nerve supply helps to confirm the diagnosis (Dreyfuss and Dreyer 2003). Therapeutic facet joint injections with corticosteroid and local anesthetic may reduce inflammation and provide longer pain relief than local anesthetic alone. Radiofrequency ablation of the medial branch nerve is used for long-term pain relief in patients responding to diagnostic blockade. Contraindications include coagulopathy, systemic infection, malignancy, and acute neurological impairment. Injections performed under fluoroscopic guidance can show spread of radio-opaque contrast in the joint or in the vicinity of the medial branch nerve. Success rates with fluoroscopically guided injections are superior to blind injections (Purcell-Jones et al. 1989).

Lumbar facet joint steroid injections are reportedly successful in 18–63% of cases (Dreyfuss and Dreyer 2003). Both intra-articular and medial branch blocks provide pain relief. Marks and Houston (1992) compared intra-articular injection versus medial branch nerve block. Their study of 86 patients with chronic low back pain demonstrated no statistical difference between the two groups immediately following the block or at 3 months. At one month, however, there was statistically superior pain relief in the intra-articular group. Not all studies support the utility of facet joint injections for low back pain. Nash (1990) studied 67 patients receiving articular injection or medial branch blocks. One month after the injection there was no significant benefit in terms of pain relief, work status, or drug intake.

Although it is clear from the available literature that diagnostic facet blocks may be helpful in elucidating the etiology of low back pain, controversy is ongoing over the therapeutic benefits of these injections. A recent systematic review of available data found only "sparse evidence" supporting facet injections for the treatment of low back pain, with moderate (level II) to limited (level IV) evidence in the literature. Similarly, the evidence for the success of radiofrequency medial nerve ablation also was determined to be between moderate and limited (level III) in quality (Slipman et al. 2003). In light of these data, these procedures need to be justified on the basis of degree of debility, lack of response to other treatments, and a thoughtful "cost-benefit-risk" assessment in each specific case.

VERTEBROPLASTY AND KYPHOPLASTY

Osteoporotic vertebral compression fractures are a significant source of back pain in older adults, affecting about 70,000 individuals per year. About one-third of these fractures cause chronic pain (Riggs and Melton 1995) that results from incomplete vertebral healing and progressive bony collapse, spinal deformity, and pseudoarthrosis (Amar et al. 2001; Aebli et al. 2002).

Conservative treatment is limited and includes analgesic medications, activity modification, and bracing. Opioid medications, commonly used for treatment of acute and chronic pain from compression fractures, are oftentimes poorly tolerated and may lead to confusion, falls, and constipation (see Chapter 10). Purely palliative treatments do not address the kyphosis, adverse effects (e.g., atelectasis, reduced vital capacity, and ventilation/perfusion mismatch), and gastrointestinal dysfunction that can result from spinal deformity. Surgical intervention and spinal cord decompression are typically reserved for patients with neurological compromise (Rao and Singrakhia 2003).

Vertebroplasty and kyphoplasty represent new and rapidly evolving procedures used to treat the refractory pain of compression fractures. Vertebroplasty, the injection of polymethylmethacrylate (PMMA) directly into the vertebral body, was first used in 1987 to treat vertebral body hemangiomas (Galbert et al. 1987). Kyphoplasty involves insertion of a balloon tamp into the collapsed vertebral body prior to the injection of PMMA (Lieberman et al. 2001). Indications for vertebroplasty include stabilization of painful osteoporotic compression fractures, as well as treatment of painful vertebrae because of metastases, multiple myeloma, Kümmell's disease (avascular necrosis), and vertebral hemangiomas (Phillips 2003). Kyphoplasty has similar indications, but is not currently recommended for nonosteolytic infiltrative spinal metastases.

Prior to considering these treatments, physicians need to establish that compression fractures are the source of the patient's pain. Patients should have symptoms refractory to conservative treatment. Both procedures are done under general anesthesia or monitored sedation and utilize either CT or fluoroscopic guidance. While both may relieve pain, kyphoplasty provides greater restoration of vertebral height.

Retrospective studies of percutaneous vertebroplasty from the United States, Europe, and Asia report success rates between 70% and 95%. The largest retrospective study of vertebroplasty included 245 patients who were questioned 7 months after the procedure. Mean pain scores decreased from 8.9 pre-procedure to 3.4 post-procedure, with 50% of the patients improving their ability to ambulate. The failure rate in this study was 4.9% (Evans et al. 2003). Barr et al. (2000) retrospectively evaluated 38 patients with symptomatic compression fractures, reporting complete pain relief in 63% and moderate pain relief in 32%. A retrospective look at 37 patients 11 months post-procedure found complete relief in nearly half of the patients and partial relief in the remaining half (Peh et al. 2002).

Only a handful of prospective studies of vertebroplasty are available. The success rates in these studies are similar to those that examined retrospective data. The largest study evaluated 100 patients treated for compression fractures. At final follow-up 21 months after the procedure, 97% of patients reported significant reductions in pain, with a mean decrease in visual analogue scale (VAS) scores from 8.9 to 2.0 (McGraw et al. 2002). Another study of 16 vertebroplasty patients showed statistically significant improvement immediately post-procedure, with pain relief lasting up to 180 days. General health status, mobility, emotional status, involvement in social activities, and energy improved as well (Cortet et al. 1999).

For kyphoplasty, success rates are similar (Heini et al. 2000; Garfin et al. 2001). A study of over 2000 kyphoplasties found both significant pain relief and decreased medication use (Garfin et al. 2001). Kyphoplasty and vertebroplasty also improve vertebral body strength and structure. Results of ex-vivo studies report vertebral height restoration to 97% of original with kyphoplasty and to 30% with vertebroplasty (Belkoff et al. 2001). Clinically, however, a study of 70 consecutive kyphoplasties showed that 30% of patients had no height restoration (Lieberman et al. 2001).

While short-term pain relief from vertebroplasty and kyphoplasty has been demonstrated, the long-term success rates vary. In their study of 13 patients, Perez-Higueras et al. (2002) reported pain relief as long as 5 years post-procedure, and nearly all participants reported that they would have the procedure done again under similar circumstances. Grados et al. (2000) reported sustained relief for up to 5 years post-procedure. Other data are less satisfactory, with 11 of 38 patients having moderate to severe recurrent pain 2 years post-procedure (Yoem et al. 2003).

Serious complications occur in 4–6% of vertebroplasty patients (Mehbod et al. 2003). These include rib fractures, neuritis, pedicle fracture, and infection. Researchers report leakage of cement (PMMA) into the spinal canal, causing neurological complications including transient neuropathy or paraplegia (Jensen et al. 1997; Lee et al. 2002). Other reports have shown no neurological sequelae from cement leakage (Cotten et al. 1996; Weill et al. 1996; Nakano et al. 2002; Perez-Higueras et al. 2002). Pulmonary embolism may also result from cement leakage into the venous system, and paradoxical cerebral artery embolization was reported in one patient with a patent foramen ovale (Padovani et al. 1999; Jang et al. 2002; Scroop et al. 2002). Kyphoplasty appears to be associated with less leakage as compared with vertebroplasty, with only one report of pulmonary embolus following kyphoplasty (Mehbod et al. 2003). One recently recognized complication is the development of new compression fractures adjacent to previously treated fracture sites (Grados et al. 2000).

In summary, both retrospective and prospective studies have shown relative effectiveness and safety of vertebroplasty and kyphoplasty for patients not responding to conservative therapies. Further prospective studies evaluating long-term effectiveness and complications are needed. Both procedures have their own particular advantages; vertebroplasty is less costly, but kyphoplasty offers greater restoration of vertebral height while using more viscous cement with less risk of leakage (Phillips 2003). Prospective randomized trials are needed to demonstrate the cost-effectiveness of both procedures and to identify their impact on morbidity and mortality (Rao and Singrakhia 2003).

INTRADISKAL ELECTROTHERMAL ANNULOPLASTY

Diskogenic pain may account for up to 40% of pain complaints in patients with chronic low back pain. The pathophysiology of diskogenic pain is thought to be from internal disk disruption that results in central ingrowth of nociceptive nerve fibers. High-intensity signals visualized on magnetic resonance imaging (MRI) of the intervertebral disk, especially in the posterior annulus fibrosis, may correlate with symptomatic diskogenic pain associated with annular fissuring (Aprill and Bogduk 1992). Although MRI and CT scans can diagnose degenerative disk disease, only provocative diskography can diagnose diskogenic pain. Injection of these degenerated disks through diskography has shown 86% concordance when suspected as a cause of low back pain (Schellhas et al. 1996).

The treatment of diskogenic low back pain after failure of conservative therapy is challenging. Intradiskal electrothermal therapy (IDET) appears to be a safe and effective alternative to surgical fusion in patients with one- or two-level disk disease based upon the results of uncontrolled studies. This minimally invasive outpatient procedure uses a fluoroscopically guided catheter to deliver thermal energy in a controlled fashion directly to the annular wall and disk nucleus, thereby altering the biomechanics of the disk. Evidence for efficacy is mixed, however, most likely because of variance among patients being studied (Saal and Saal 2002; Davis 2004).

PERCUTANEOUS NUCLEOPLASTY

Disk decompression for herniated disks has traditionally been accomplished via surgical means. Percutaneous methods have emerged more recently, with early techniques using chemical, mechanical, and laser technology. Excessive risks, complications, and lack of significant benefits have, however, prevented their ongoing use.

Disk nucleoplasty is an emerging percutaneous procedure that utilizes coblation technology, allowing for a controlled method of tissue ablation with low bipolar radiofrequency energy that causes molecular dissociation.

Singh and colleagues (2003) reported clinical outcomes data from a case series of 80 patients with contained lumbar disk herniations who underwent disk nucleoplasty. Although there was no control group, 75% of the patients reported a decrease in their pain 12 months after the procedure.

Similarly, Sharps and Isaac (2002), in a single-site prospective outcome study of the disk nucleoplasty procedure, observed success rates as high as 82% for patients with no prior surgical intervention that sustained greater than 50% VAS pain reduction at 1-year follow-up. Ruano (2003) presented a study in which 25 consecutive patients who underwent disk nucleoplasty returned to work in about 1.5 weeks, with overall cost being less than half the cost of a diskectomy.

These minimally invasive outpatient procedures may be appropriate for symptomatic patients with contained herniated disks. They require minimal recovery and, in older patients, minimize the greater risks associated with spinal surgery. Although there are no controlled trials to date, the literature suggests that this may be a promising interventional pain procedure.

INTRATHECAL OPIOID PUMPS

Growing understanding of the neurophysiology, neurochemistry, and neuroanatomy of pain transmission and modulation, along with technological developments and applied pharmaceutics, provides new options for patients with refractory pain syndromes. Percutaneous spinal delivery systems and programmable implantable infusion devices represent a major advance in this field. This option is especially important in cancer pain treatment, since severe pain occurs in up to 80% of patients with advanced cancer, is frequently difficult to control, and may result in significant impairments in quality of life and physical function (Gilmer-Hill et al. 1999). Advances in opioid delivery systems into either the epidural or subarachnoid space have emerged as an option for many types of patients with refractory pain. These implantable drug delivery systems provide neuroaxial delivery of opioids, which may be combined with alpha-2 adrenergic agonists. When delivered through this mechanism, these agents are believed to exert their primary effects in the substantia gelatinosa (lamina II) of the dorsal horn of the spinal cord. Combined with local anesthetics, spinal opioid analgesia may be enhanced through additional spinal and nerve root blockade.

Traditionally, selection criteria have allowed for placement of intrathecal opioid pumps in patients with chronic intractable pain for whom systemic opioids and adjunctive agents have failed to provide adequate analgesia or have caused intolerable side-effects. The ability of the older adult or his or her caregiver to operate and maintain the system is also an important consideration, in addition to a successful trial demonstrating pain relief with epidural or intrathecally administered medications. Patients must also undergo careful psychological screening prior to implantation to help predict the potential effectiveness of this rather costly intervention (Oakley and Staats 2000).

Numerous studies have now shown cost-effective outcomes from implantable drug delivery systems in patient with cancer and certain noncancer pain-producing conditions (Hassenbusch et al. 2004; Sloan 2004). Smith and colleagues (2002) demonstrated reduced pain scores and drug-related adverse effects, and improved survival from early use of spinal opioid analgesia compared with systemic drug therapy in cancer patients. These findings require corroboration and cannot be generalized to other populations of patients, but they provoke considerable thought about the value of targeted drug delivery versus systemic delivery, especially in older patients with lowered therapeutic indices.

Although implantable pumps were initially reserved for patients with intractable cancer pain, studies have shown the pump to be a viable alternative in the management of failed back surgery syndrome (FBSS) and other nonmalignant pain conditions (Angel et al. 1998). Paice et al. (1996) showed positive outcomes in his study of patients with FBSS that had a mean 14.6 month follow-up. Ninety-five percent had good to excellent pain relief and 81% had improvement in activities in daily living. Coyne et al. demonstrated 27% reduction in pain scores and 50% reduction of opioid toxicities (P.J. Coyne et al., unpublished manuscript). Intrathecal delivery of morphine and bupivacaine has also been successful in treating other atypical pain such as refractory restless leg syndrome (Jakobsson and Ruuth 2002).

Studies on the cost-effectiveness of long-term intrathecal morphine therapy for pain associated with FBSS have suggested that a pump implant is less costly than alternative methods providing comparable analgesia for treatment exceeding 12–18 months, even when the cost of complications or pump replacements is included (de Lissovoy et al. 1997). Side effects of intrathecal morphine are similar to those seen with oral morphine. They may occur less frequently with intrathecal morphine, however, because of lower medication doses. Common side effects still include nausea and vomiting, urinary retention, and pruritis (Paice et al. 1996).

Post-implantation complications from implantable pumps include catheter disconnection, kinks or breakage, cerebrospinal fluid leaks, infected seromas, and component failure that may result in loss of therapeutic effect or clinically significant drug withdrawal or overdose signs and symptoms. In rare instances, an inflammatory mass may develop at the tip of an implanted spinal catheter that can lead to progressive neurological effects. Care must be taken during magnetic resonance imaging (MRI) because the infusion system will temporarily shut down for the duration of MRI exposure. The pump should resume its normal operation upon completion of the test, but its operation should be reconfirmed.

In select patients with chronic intractable pain, intrathecal administration of opioids and other agents via an implanted pump can reduce pain with minimal long-term adverse effects or complications when properly monitored. All published data regarding the utility of this technology must be extrapolated to older adults, because no studies have specifically addressed these individuals.

SPINAL CORD STIMULATORS

Until recently, few treatment options were available for patients suffering from chronic intractable neuropathic pain. Along with newer pharmacotherapies and spinal delivery systems, implantable spinal cord stimulators are another possibility when more conservative treatments have provided unsatisfactory pain relief for certain conditions. Spinal cord stimulators induce neurostimulation by delivering electrical impulses to the dorsal columns of the spinal cord via the placement of epidural electrodes. Neurostimulation activates the body's pain inhibitory systems and blocks incoming pain-generating signals, according to a theory that derives from the landmark "gate control theory of pain" by Melzack and Wall (1965), who hypothesized that peripheral nociceptive information is transmitted to the dorsal horn of the spinal cord via nerve fibers. All nerve fibers, including small-diameter unmyelinated C fibers and myelinated Aδ fibers, which carry afferent nociceptive information, in addition to larger myelinated Aβ fibers, which carry touch and vibration sensory information, terminate in the substantia gelatinosa (and deeper layers) of the dorsal horn of the spinal cord. The theory proposed that stimulation of these large myelinated Aβ fibers would inhibit reception of afferent small fibers at the respective spinal levels (Shealy et al. 1967). Although the original theory has undergone much refinement over the last 40 years, the basic tenets still hold.

Spinal cord stimulators can be used to treat a variety of chronic intractable types of pain, especially neuropathic or radicular conditions of the extremities. Specific conditions that have been shown to respond to spinal cord stimulation include complex regional pain syndrome (CRPS) types I and II (previously termed reflex sympathetic dystrophy and causalgia, respectively) and FBSS. Kemler et al. (2000) demonstrated a reduction in the intensity of pain and an improvement in the health-related quality of life in their cohort of subjects. Likewise, Turner et al. (1995) demonstrated that an average of 59% of FBSS patients had greater than 50% pain relief in their analysis of 39 studies. Minor complications were frequent, with an average of 42%. Moreover, North et al. (1991) demonstrated similar findings in a series of FBSS patients, with at least 50% reduction in pain in 53% of patients at 2.2 years and 47% at 5 years after implantation. North and colleagues also found that spinal cord stimulation reduced hospitalizations, surgical procedures, and related health care costs, while promoting greater independence and improvement in quality of life. De La Porte et al. (1993) reported that neurostimulation in FBSS patients produced more than 50% reduction of pain in 55% of those studied, while improving functional capacity by 61% and reducing pain medication use by 90% during a mean 4-year follow-up.

Other types of treatment-refractory pain conditions have been found to respond to neurostimulation, including phantom limb or post-amputation stump pain, ischemic pain, and painful peripheral neuropathies from diabetes mellitus, AIDS, chemotherapy, and chronic heavy alcohol use (Ceballos et al. 2000; Cata et al. 2004). Hautvast et al. (1998) demonstrated the effectiveness of spinal cord stimulation in patients with chronic intractable angina pectoris, demonstrated by reduced anginal pain, decreased sublingual nitrate requirements, and improved quality of life indicators.

Screening protocols and selection guidelines have been put in place to optimize outcomes and minimize deleterious effects (Scalzitti 1997). Some models of stimulators are contraindicated in patients with an implantable cardiac pacemaker or defibrillator, and in those who are likely to require MRI on a regular basis. Furthermore, diathermy is contraindicated because of possible transfer of energy through the implanted system, which could result in tissue injury and damage to the neurostimulation system. Patients need to be forewarned of these situations, and a "medical alert" identifier (e.g., a bracelet or necklace) is advised for those with a spinal cord stimulator.

Serious adverse events are rare, but some undesirable effects include uncomfortable jolting or shocking sensations, requiring adjustment of the stimulus or lead placement. According to current evidence, spinal cord stimulation may represent a valuable treatment option, particularly for patients with chronic pain of predominately neuropathic origin and topographical distribution involving the extremities. As with other interventional pain therapies, benefits and risks must be extrapolated to older adults because of a paucity of data emerging specifically from this demographic group.

SYMPATHETIC NERVE BLOCKS

Sympathetically mediated pain may be treated with either temporary or permanent blockade at a number of sites along the sympathetic nervous system. Pain practitioners utilize stellate ganglion blockade in the treatment of face or arm pain, thoracic or intrapleural injections for arm and thoracic visceral pain, and lumbar sympathetic blocks for lower extremity pain. Sympathetic blocks are also effective for the treatment of visceral pain, especially in cancer patients. Celiac plexus and hypogastric plexus blockade treat upper abdominal and lower abdominal/pelvic pain respectively. Blockade of the sacrococcygeal ganglion (the ganglion of Walther), the termination of the sympathetic chain, is effective for the treatment of sympathetically mediated perineal pain.

The stellate ganglion provides most of the sympathetic innervation to the face and upper extremity. Stellate ganglion block is used to treat a variety of sympathetically mediated pain syndromes including herpes zoster, CRPS, and phantom limb pain. It is typically achieved with an anterior paratracheal approach at the level of C6–C7, although a variety of techniques are described and advocated. Both "blind" and fluoroscopically guided techniques are considered to be within the standard of care because of the safe track record and objective measures of success (e.g., Horner's syndrome) in experienced hands. After blockade, arm temperature increases, and the resultant pain relief may last longer than local anesthesia. A similar but slightly modified technique is used to block the superior cervical sympathetic ganglion. This technique has been beneficial in the treatment of certain ocular pain syndromes such as photo-oculodynia and blepharospasm (McCann et al. 1999).

For treatment of sympathetically mediated pain in the lower extremities, the sympathetic block is performed at the second and third lumbar levels. A needle is placed along the superior, anterior, lateral border of the L2 or L3 vertebral body via a posterior approach. Fluoroscopy verifies needle placement. As with stellate ganglion blockade, limb temperature increases following the block.

Serious complications from stellate ganglion blockade and lumbar sympathetic blockade are rare. Pneumothorax, intraspinal or intravascular injection, laryngeal nerve block, brachial plexus block, and persistent Horner's syndrome are potential complications of stellate ganglion blockade. The major life-threatening complication is intravascular (vertebral artery or intravenous) injection, necessitating immediately available resuscitation equipment and skill in airway management. The most common side effect of lumbar sympathetic block is lower back pain, and hypotension may also be seen. Monitoring is essential during both of these procedures to recognize possible hemodynamic changes. Careful aspiration prior to injection may prevent inadvertent vascular or subarachnoid injection. Other rare complications of lumbar sympathetic blockade include renal trauma and genitofemoral neuralgia. Patients who are medically anticoagulated or have coagulopathies are at risk for hematoma formation.

There are mixed reports of the efficacy of sympathetic blocks for the treatment of CRPS. Cepeda et al. (2002) reviewed 29 available studies and found overall poor study quality, with most reports being case series lacking long-term follow-up. Clear benefit over placebo has not been demonstrated. Better methodology is required to specifically define the potential benefits of sympathetic blocks in patients thought to have sympathetically maintained pain. Sympathetic blockade has been shown to be effective in predicting a positive response to spinal cord stimulation (Hord et al. 2003).

Celiac plexus blocks are performed at the lower thoracic and first lumbar vertebral levels and have been used mainly for the treatment of pancreatic cancer pain, as well as other gastrointestinal malignancies that cause pain. The recently published randomized controlled trial by Wong et al. (2004) demonstrated superiority of celiac plexus block in the treatment of pancreatic cancer pain compared with standard analgesic medications. Their study did not demonstrate any difference in survival or quality of life between those treated with celiac plexus blockade versus analgesic therapy. The usefulness of this technique for nonmalignant pain is debatable (Eisenberg et al. 1995). Generally, self-limited back pain is the most common side effect following celiac plexus blockade. Post-procedure hypotension is expected and can be treated and avoided with adequate volume replacement. Diarrhea, occurring in less than 1% of patients, is a predictable result of lost sympathetic tone. Lower-extremity paralysis secondary to spasm of the artery of Adamkiewicz is an extremely rare complication (Raj 2000).

CONCLUSIONS

Interventional pain-relieving procedures can offer substantial benefit to older patients with pain syndromes that do not improve with less invasive measures. Proper procedure selection and ongoing monitoring, coupled with a context-appropriate rehabilitative program, leads to optimal outcomes. Most importantly, awareness of this rapidly evolving field by primary care clinicians is essential, both to safeguard vulnerable patients from needless (excessively risky or costly) interventions, and for timely referral to capable specialists when indications support the use of such therapies.

REFERENCES

Aebli N, Krebs J, Davis G, Theis JC. Fat embolism and acute hypotension during vertebroplasty: an experimental study in sheep. *Spine* 2002; 27:460–466.

Amar AP, Larsen DW, Esnaahari N, et al. Percutaneous transpedicular polymethylmethacrylate vertebroplasty for the treatment of spinal compression fractures. *Neurosurgery* 2001; 49:1105–1114.

Angel IF, Gould HJ, Carey ME. Intrathecal morphine pump as a treatment option in chronic pain of nonmalignant origin. *Surg Neurol* 1998; 49(1):92–99.

Aprill CN, Bogduk N. High-Intensity zone: a diagnostic sign of painful lumbar disc on magnetic resonance imaging. *Br J Radiol* 1992; 65:361–369.

Barr JD, Barr MS, Lemley TJ, McCann RM. Percutaneous vertebroplasty for pain relief and spinal stabilization. *Spine* 2000; 25:923–928.

Belkoff SM, Mathis JM, Fenton DC, et al. An ex vivo biomechanical evaluation of an inflatable bone tamp used in the treatment of compression fracture. *Spine* 2001; 26:151–156.

Borg-Stein J, Stein J. Controversies in fibromyalgia and related conditions. *Rheum Dis Clin North Am* 1996; 22(2):305–322.

Carette S, Leclaire R, Marcoux, S, et al. Epidural corticosteroid injection for sciatica due to herniated nucleus pulposus. *New Engl J Med* 1997; 336(23):1634–1640.

Cata JP, Cordella JV, Burton AW, et al. Spinal cord stimulation relieves chemotherapy-induced pain: a clinical case report. *J Pain Symptom Manage* 2004; 27(1):72–78.

Ceballos A, Cabezudo L, Bovaira M, Fenollosa P, Moro B. Spinal cord stimulation: a possible therapeutic alternative for chronic mesenteric ischemia. *Pain* 2000; 87(1):99–101.

Cepeda MS, Lau J, Carr DB. Defining the therapeutic role of local anesthetic sympathetic blockade in complex regional pain syndrome: a narrative and systematic review. *Clin J Pain* 2002; 18:216–233.

Chou LH, Slipman CW, Bhagia SM, et al. Inciting events initiating injection-proven sacroiliac joint syndrome. *Pain Med* 2004; 5:26–32.

Cortet B, Cotten A, Boutry N, et al. Percutaneous vertebroplasty in the treatment of osteoporotic vertebral compression fractures: an open prospective study. *J Rheumatol* 1999; 26:2222–2228.

Cotten A, Dewatre F, Cortet B, et al. Percutaneous vertebroplasty for osteolytic metastases and myeloma: effects of the percentage of the lesion filling and the leakage of methylmethacrylate at clinical follow-up. *Radiology* 1996; 200:525–530.

Criscuolo CM. Interventional approaches to the management of myofascial pain syndrome. *Curr Pain Headache Rep* 2001; 5:407–411.

Davis TT. The IDET procedure for chronic discogenic low back pain. *Spine* 2004; 29(7):752–756.

de Lissovoy G, Brown R, Halpern M, et al. Cost-effectiveness of long-term intrathecal morphine therapy for pain associated with failed back surgery syndrome. *Clin Ther* 1997; 19(1)96–112.

De La Porte C, Van de Kelft E. Spinal cord stimulation in failed back surgery syndrome. *Pain* 1993; 52(1):55–61.

Dreyfuss PH, Dreyer SJ. Lumbar zygapophysial (facet) joint injections. *Spine J* 2003; 3(3 Suppl):50S–59S.

Dreyfuss P, Michaelsen M, Pauza K, McLarty J, Bogduk N. The value of medical history and physical examination in diagnosing sacroiliac joint pain. *Spine* 1996; 21:2594–2602.

Dreyfuss P, Dreyer SJ, Cole A, Mayo, K. Sacroiliac joint pain. *J Am Acad Orthop Surg* 2004; 12:255–265.

Eisenberg E, Carr DB, Chalmers TC. Neurolytic celiac plexus block for the treatment of chronic pain: a meta-analysis. *Anesth Analg* 1995; 80(2):290–295.

Esenyel M, Caglar N, Aldemir T. Treatment of myofascial pain. *Am J Phys Med Rehabil* 2000; 79(1):48–52.

Evans AJ, Jensen ME, Kip KE, et al. Vertebral compression fractures: pain reduction and improvement in functional mobility after percutaneous polymethylmethacrylate vertebroplasty: retrospective report of 245 cases. *Radiology* 2003; 226:366–372.

Ferrante FM, King LF, Roche EA, et al. Radiofrequency sacroiliac joint denervation for sacroiliac syndrome. *Reg Anesth Pain Med* 2001; 26(2):137–142.

Fine PG, Milano R, Hare BD. The effects of myofascial trigger point injections are naloxone reversible. *Pain* 1988; 32(1):15–20.

Galbert P, Deramond H, Rosat P, Le Gars D. Preliminary note on the treatment of vertebral angioma by percutaneous acrylic vertebroplasty. *Neurochirurgie* 1987; 33:166–168.

Garfin SR, Hansen AY, Reiley MA. Kyphoplasty and vertebroplasty for the treatment of painful osteoporotic compression fractures. *Spine* 2001; 26:1511–1515.

Gilmer-Hill HS, Bobban JE, Smith KA, Wagner FC. Intrathecal morphine delivered via subcutaneous pump for intractable cancer pain. *Surg Neurol* 1999; 51(1):12–15.

Goldthwait JE. The lumbosacral articulation: an explanation of many cases of lumbago, sciatica and paraplegia. *Boston Med Sci J* 1911; 164:365–372.

Grados F, Depriester C, Cayrolle G, et al. Long-term observations of vertebral osteoporotic fractures treated by percutaneous vertebroplasty. *Rheumatology* 2000; 39:1410–1414.

Hassenbusch SJ, Portenoy RK, Cousin M, et al. Polyanalgesic Consensus Conference 2003: an update on the management of pain by intraspinal drug delivery—report of an expert panel. *J Pain Symptom Manage* 2004; 27(6):540–563.

Hautvast RW, DeJongste MJ, Staal MJ, van Gilst WH, Lie KI. Spinal cord stimulation in chronic intractable angina pectoris: a randomized, controlled efficacy study. *Am Heart J* 1998; 136(6):1114–1120.

Heini PF, Walchi B, Berlemann U. Percutaneous transpedicular vertebroplasty with PMAA: operative technique and early results. *Eur Spine J* 2000; 9:445–450.

Hong C-Z, Hsueh T-C. Difference in pain relief after trigger point injections in myofascial pain patients with and without fibromyalgia. *Arch Phys Med Rehabil* 1996; 77:1161–1166.

Hord ED, Cohen SP, Cosgrove GR, et al. The predictive value of sympathetic block for the success of spinal cord stimulation. *Neurosurgery* 2003; 53(3):626–631.

Jakobsson B, Ruuth K. Successful treatment of restless legs syndrome in an implanted pump for intrathecal drug delivery. *Acta Anaesthesiol Scand* 2002; 46(1):114–117.

Jang JS, Lee SH, Jung SK. Pulmonary embolism of polymethylmethacrylate after percutaneous vertebroplasty: a report of three cases. *Spine* 2002; 27:E416–418.

Jensen ME, Evans AJ, Mathis JM, et al. Percutaneous polymethylmethacrylate vertebroplasty in the treatment of osteoporotic vertebral body compression fractures: technical aspects. *Am J Neuroradiol* 1997; 18:1897–1904.

Koes BW, Scholten R, Mens J, et al. Efficacy of epidural steroid injections for low-back pain and sciatica: a systematic review of randomized clinical trials. *Pain* 1995; 63:279–288.

Kemler MA, Barendse GA, van Kleef M, et al. Spinal cord stimulation in patients with chronic reflex sympathetic dystrophy. *N Engl J Med* 2000; 343(9):618–624.

Klein RG, Eek BC, DeLong WB, Mooney V. A randomized double-blind trial of dextrose-glycerine-phenol injections for chronic, low back pain. *J Spinal Disord* 1993; 6:23–33.

Kraemer J. Ludwig J, Bicker U, et al. Lumbar epidural perineural injection: a new technique. *Eur Spine J* 1997; 6:357–361.

Lee BJ, Lee SR, Yoo TY. Paraplegia as a complication of percutaneous vertebroplasty with polymethylmethacrylate: a case report. *Spine* 2002; 27:E419–422.

Lieberman IH, Dudeney S, Reinhardt MK, et al. Initial outcome and efficacy of "kyphoplasty" in the treatment of painful osteoporotic vertebral compression fractures. *Spine* 2001; 26:1631–1638.

Lutz GE, Vad VB, Wisneski RJ. Fluoroscopic transforaminal lumbar epidural steroids: an outcome study. *Arch Phys Med Rehabil* 1998; 79: 1362–1366.

Marks RC, Houston T. Facet joint injection and facet nerve block—a randomized comparison in 86 patients. *Pain* 1992; 49:325–328.

McCann JD, Gauthier M, Morschbacher R, et al. A novel mechanism for benign essential blepharospasm. *Ophthal Plastic Reconstr Surg* 1999; 15(6):384–389.

McGraw JK, Lippert JA, Minkus KD, et al. Prospective evaluation of pain relief in 100 patients undergoing percutaneous vertebroplasty: results and follow-up. *J Vasc Interv Radiol* 2002; 13:883–886.

Mehbod A, Aunoble S, Le Huec JC. Vertebroplasty for osteoporotic spine fracture: prevention and treatment. *Eur Spine J* 2003; 12(Suppl 2):S155–S162.

Melzack R, Wall PD. Pain mechanisms: a new theory. *Science* 1965; 150(699):971–979.

Melzack R, Wall PD (Eds). *Textbook of Pain*, 4th ed. Philadelphia: Churchill Livingstone, 1999.

Mooney V, Robertson J. Facet joint syndrome. *Clin Orthop* 1976; 115:149–156.

Nakano M, Hirano N, Matsuura K, et al. Percutaneous transpedicular vertebroplasty with calcium phosphate cement in the treatment of osteoporotic vertebral compression and burst fractures. *J Neurosurg* 2002; 97:287–293.

Nash TP. Facet joints. Intraarticular steroids or nerve blocks? *Pain Clinic* 1990; 3:77–82.

North RB, Ewend MG, Lawton MT, et al. Failed back surgery syndrome: 5-year follow-up after spinal cord stimulator implantation. *Neurosurgery* 1991; 28(5):692–699.

Oakley J, Staats P. The use of implanted drug delivery systems. In: Raj PP (Ed). *Practical Management of Pain*, 3rd ed. St. Louis: Mosby, 2000.

Ongley MJ, Klein RG, Dorman TA, Eek BC, Hubert LJ. A new approach to the treatment of chronic low back pain. *Lancet* 1987; 2:143–146.

Padovani B, Kasriel O, Brunner P, et al. Pulmonary embolism caused by acrylic cement: a rare complication of percutaneous vertebroplasty. *Am J Neuroradiol* 1999; 20:375–377.

Paice JA, Penn RD, Shott S. Intraspinal morphine for chronic pain: a retrospective multicenter study. *J Pain Symptom Manage* 1996; 11(2):71–80.

Peh W, Gilula L, Peck D. Percutaneous vertebroplasty for severe osteoporotic vertebral body compression fractures. *Radiology* 2002; 223:121–126.

Perez-Higueras A, Alvarez L, Rossi RE, Quinones D, Al-Assor I. Percutaneous vertebroplasty: long term clinical and radiolgical outcome. *Neuroradiology* 2002; 44:950–954.

Phillips FM. Minimally invasive treatments of osteoporotic vertebral compression fractures. *Spine* 2003; 28(15S):S45–S53.

Purcell-Jones G, Pither CE, Justins DM. Paravertebral somatic nerve block: A clinical, radiographic and computed tomographic study in chronic pain patients. *Anesth Analg* 1989; 68:32–39.

Raj PP (Ed). *Practical Management of Pain*, 3rd ed. St. Louis: Mosby, 2000.

Rao RD, Singrakhia MD. Painful osteoporotic vertebral fracture: pathogenesis, evaluation, and roles of vertebroplasty and kyphoplasty in its management. *J Bone Joint Surg* 2003; 85(10):2010–2022.

Riggs BL, Melton LJ. The worldwide problem of osteoporosis: insights afforded by epidemiology. *Bone* 1995; 5:S505–S511.

Rosenberg JM, Quint DJ, deRosayro AM. Computerized tomographic localization of clinically-guided sacroiliac joint injections. *Clin J Pain* 2000; 16:18–21.

Ruano A. Nucleoplasty treatment of symptomatic disc herniation. Paper presented at: 6th Congress of the European Federation of Orthopaedics and Traumatology, 2003, Helsinki.

Saal JA, Saal JS. Intradiscal electrothermal treatment for chronic discogenic low back pain: prospective outcome study with a minimum 2 year follow up. *Spine* 2002; 27(9):966–973.

Scalzitti DA. Screening for psychological factors in patients with low back pain: Waddell's nonorganic signs. *Phys Ther* 1997; 77(3):306–312.

Schellhas KP, Pollei SR, Gundry CR, Heithoff K. Lumbar disc high-intensity zone: correlation of magnetic resonance imaging and discography. *Spine* 1996; 21(1):79–86.

Scroop R, Eskridge J, Britz GW. Paradoxical cerebral arterial embolization of cement during intraoperative vertebroplasty: case report. *Am J Neuroradiol* 2002; 23:868–870.

Sharps L, Isaac Z. Percutaneous disc decompression using nucleoplasty. *Pain Physician* 2002; 5(2):121–126.

Shealy CN, Mortimer JT, Reswick JB. Electrical inhibition of pain by stimulation of the dorsal columns: Preliminary clinical report. *Anesth Analg* 1967; 46(4):489–491.

Singh V, Piryani C, Liao K. Evaluation of percutaneous disc decompression using coblation in chronic back pain with or without leg pain. *Pain Physician* 2003; 6:273–280.

Slipman CW, Lipetz JS, Plastaras CT, et al. Fluoroscopically guided therapeutic sacroiliac joint injections for sacroiliac joint syndrome. *Am J Phys Med Rehabil* 2001; 80:425–432.

Slipman CW, Bhat AL, Gilchrist RV, et al. A critical review of the evidence for the use of zygapophysial injections and radiofrequency denervation in the treatment of low back pain. *Spine J* 2003; 3:310–316.

Sloan PA. The evolving role of interventional pain management in oncology. *J Support Oncol* 2004; 2(6):491–500, 503; discussion 503–506.

Smith TJ, Staats PS, Deer T, et al. Randomize clinical trial of an implantable drug delivery system compared with comprehensive medical management for refractory cancer pain: impact on pain, drug-related toxicity, and survival. *J Clin Oncol* 2002; 20(19):4040–4049.

Turner JA, Loeser JD, Bell KG. Spinal cord stimulation for chronic low back pain: a systematic literature synthesis. *Neurosurgery* 1995; 37(6):1088–1096.

Valat J-P, Giraudeau B, Rozenberg S, et al. Epidural corticosteroid injects for sciatica: a randomised, double blind, controlled clinical trial. *Ann Rheum Dis* 2003; 62: 639–643.

Weill A, Chiras J, Simon JM, Sola-Martinez T, Enkaoua E. Spinal metastases: indications for and results of percutaneous injection of acrylic cement. *Radiology* 1996; 199:241–247.

Wong GY, Schroeder DR, Carns PE et al. Effect of neurolytic celiac plexus block on pain relief, quality of life, and survival in patients with unresectable pancreatic cancer. *JAMA* 2004; 291(9):1092–1099.

Yin W, Willard F, Carreiro J, Dreyfuss P. Sensory stimulation-guided sacroiliac join radiofrequency neurotomy: technique based on neuroanatomy of the dorsal sacral plexus. *Spine* 2003; 28:2419–9425.

Yoem JS, Kim WJ, Choy WS, et al. Percutaneous transpedicular vertebroplasty: two-year follow-up results of 38 cases. Presented at: Annual Meeting of the American Academy of Orthopaedic Surgeons, February 5–9, 2003, New Orleans.

Correspondence to: Prof. Cheryl D. Bernstein, MD, Department of Anesthesiology, University of Pittsburgh School of Medicine, UPMC Pain Medicine at Centre Commons, 5750 Centre Avenue, Suite 400, Pittsburgh, PA 15206, USA. Email: berncd@anes.upmc.edu.

Pain in Older Persons, Progress in Pain
Research and Management, Vol. 35, edited
by Stephen J. Gibson and Debra K. Weiner,
IASP Press, Seattle, © 2005.

14

Complementary and Alternative Medicine for the Treatment of Pain in Older Adults

Karen Prestwood

*Center on Aging, University of Connecticut Health Center,
Farmington, Connecticut, USA*

Complementary and alternative medicine (CAM), as defined by the National Center for Complementary and Alternative Medicine (NCCAM), is a group of diverse medical and health care systems, practices, and products that are not considered to be part of conventional medicine, defined as medicine practiced by medical doctors (which in the United States includes doctors of osteopathy) and other allied health professionals. Complementary medicine involves the use of modalities *in conjunction with* conventional medicine, while alternative medicine implies that a modality is used *in place of* conventional medicine. Integrative medicine, another relevant term, combines conventional medical therapies and CAM therapies for which there is high-quality scientific evidence of safety and effectiveness. This chapter will discuss CAM pain management for older adults according to NCCAM's categorization system, shown in Fig. 1.

CAM use in the United States is increasing (Eisenberg et al. 1993, 1998). Seventy percent of 31,000 U.S. adults recently surveyed by the National Health Interview Survey and Centers for Disease Control and Prevention had ever used CAM, and 60% had done so during the past year (Barnes et al. 2004). Excluding prayer, 49% of respondents had ever used CAM, and 36% had done so within the last year. The largest category given as a reason for CAM use was the belief that CAM plus conventional medicine would be more beneficial than either alone. The most popular category in the survey was mind-body medicine, which includes prayer, meditation, and deep breathing; 6 of the 10 most commonly used therapies used are in mind-body medicine.

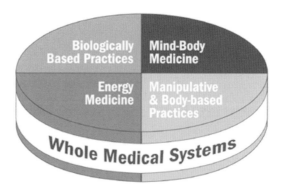

Fig. 1. Domains of complementary and alternative medicine (CAM) as recognized by the U.S. National Center for Complementary and Alternative Medicine (2005). NCCAM groups CAM practices into four domains, recognizing there can be some overlap. In addition, NCCAM studies CAM medical systems, which cut across all domains.

The use of CAM, excluding prayer and megavitamins, decreases with age. The most common CAM modalities used by older adults are mind-body medicine, biologically based therapies, and manipulative/body-based therapies. Six of the 10 most common conditions reported by persons using CAM are related to pain. Thus, the use of CAM for pain is quite common in U.S. adults, particularly in older adults.

BIOLOGICALLY BASED THERAPIES

This category includes botanicals, animal-derived extracts, vitamins, minerals, fatty acids, amino acids, proteins, prebiotics and probiotics, whole-food diets, and functional foods. Dietary supplements, a subset of this category, contains vitamins, minerals, herbs, amino acids, and substances such as enzymes, organ tissues, glandular extracts, and metabolites. The U.S. Food and Drug Administration (FDA) regulates dietary supplements differently than drugs: manufacturers of drugs are required to follow defined good manufacturing practices, while manufacturers of dietary supplements must follow existing manufacturing requirements for foods. Drugs also must be approved by the FDA prior to marketing, while manufacturers of dietary supplements are responsible for ensuring product safety, and new dietary supplements are not subject to pre-market approval. Manufacturers of dietary supplements may cite existing literature to validate claims. The Federal Trade Commission has primary responsibility for monitoring dietary supplements for truth in advertising (Dietary Supplement Health and Education

Act; see U.S. Food and Drug Administration 1994). An Institute of Medicine report (2002) on the safety of dietary supplements recommended developing a system for cost-effective and science-based evaluation by the FDA.

Use of vitamin and mineral supplements by the U.S. population has been increasing since the 1970s. National surveys indicate that 40–46% of U.S. residents reported taking at least one vitamin or mineral supplement at some time within the month surveyed. In 2002, sales of dietary supplements increased to an estimated U.S.$18,700 million per year, with botanical supplements accounting for an estimated U.S.$4,300 million (Ervin et al. 1999; Radimer et al. 2004).

Many clinical studies of dietary supplements are flawed because of poor study design, including inadequate sample size, limited preliminary dosing data, lack of masking, and failure to incorporate rigorous outcome measures. In addition, the lack of reliable data on absorption, disposition, metabolism, and excretion in humans has complicated the selection of products to be used in clinical trials. The lack of consistent and reliable botanical products represents a challenge both in clinical trials and in basic research. NCCAM now has strict requirements regarding standardization of botanical and dietary products for research to address some of these concerns. Additionally, NCCAM has funded major centers to specifically complete research related to dietary supplements for use in human conditions.

SPECIFIC COMPOUNDS

Glucosamine sulfate and chondroitin sulfate. Glucosamine sulfate and chondroitin sulfate, popular supplements for osteoarthritis (OA), have been available for many years and are frequently combined, although there is little evidence for synergistic or additive effects. Glucosamine is an essential component of cell membranes, cell surface proteins, and interstitial structural proteins and plays a role in the formation of articular cartilage, tendons, ligaments, and synovial fluid. The primary biological role for glucosamine in arthritis is its action as a substrate for the synthesis of the glycoaminoglycans and of hyaluronic acid, which are essential for the formation of proteoglycans found in the structural matrix of joints. Chondroitin provides additional substrates for the formation of healthy joints. Glucosamine may also have anti-inflammatory effects (Alvarez-Soria et al. 2002).

Several systemic reviews and meta-analyses have evaluated the efficacy of glucosamine for arthritis (McAlindon et al. 2000; Towheed et al. 2001; Richy et al. 2003). The Cochrane review (Towheed et al. 2001) found 16 high-quality randomized controlled trials. Glucosamine improved pain and function in 12 of 13 placebo-controlled studies. Of four randomized controlled trials that compared glucosamine to nonsteroidal anti-inflammatory drugs (NSAIDs), two studies found that glucosamine was superior and the other two determined that it was equivalent in reducing pain and improving function. A meta-analysis (McAlindon et al. 2000) that included six studies of glucosamine and nine of chondroitin for knee and hip OA found that overall, glucosamine and chondroitin were effective in improving pain and function. Glucosamine had a moderate effect (0.42) while chondroitin had a substantial effect (0.78). The data suggested publication bias in that more positive studies were published than negative, which is true of most clinical trials. Another meta-analysis demonstrated that glucosamine was effective in improving pain, function, and joint space, and its overall safety was excellent (Richy et al. 2003).

More recently, in a 3-year randomized, placebo-controlled study in 212 patients (mean age 65 years) with mild to moderate OA, Reginster et al. (2001) found that glucosamine reduced pain and improved function. Side effects were similar between groups, with GI complaints being the most common. The correlation between joint space outcomes and pain was poor, and most persons in the glucosamine group had decreased pain regardless of the severity of the joint space measurements. A smaller randomized, placebo-controlled study examined the effect of 6 months of glucosamine supplementation in 80 patients (mean age 62 years) with OA, of whom 60% had moderate to severe disease. The glucosamine subjects had significant improvement in knee flexion, but not in pain, which suggests that glucosamine may not be effective in more severe OA (Hughes and Carr 2002). Another long-term placebo-controlled study ($N = 202$; mean age 62 years), which allowed acetaminophen for rescue analgesia, found that glucosamine was effective in decreasing pain, increasing function, and preserving joint space. The improvement in pain in the glucosamine group was 20–25% over the course of 3 years according to a per protocol analysis and 15–20% by an intent-to-treat analysis (Pavelka et al. 2002).

A large ongoing multicenter trial comparing the effects of glucosamine, chondroitin, combined glucosamine and chondroitin, or placebo on knee OA plans to enroll over 1500 subjects, who will be treated for 2 years. With anticipated completion in late 2005, this study, at the University of Utah, will determine whether the combination of glucosamine and chondroitin is additive or synergistic.

In addition to knee and hip OA, studies have evaluated the effect of glucosamine on OA in other joints. One small study ($N = 52$) examined the effect of glucosamine on the temporomandibular joint; participants received either glucosamine (500 mg t.i.d.) or ibuprofen (400 mg t.i.d.) for 3 months (Thie et al. 2001). Both groups showed significant symptomatic improvement, with a greater decrease ($P < 0.05$) in pain and acetaminophen use between days 90 and 120 in the glucosamine group.

Overall, the relative quality of studies evaluating chondroitin has been lower than those of glucosamine. However, chondroitin also appears to decrease pain and improve function in patients with mild to moderate OA. Chondroitin treatment for 2–4 months is typically required for symptomatic improvement, and the addition of chondroitin to NSAIDs can significantly reduce pain to a greater degree that NSAIDs alone. Intermittent dosing with chondroitin is also possible, e.g., 800 mg/d for 3 months and then off for 3 months (Verbruggen et al. 2002; McAlindon et al. 2000). See Table I for recommended doses of glucosamine and chondroitin.

The most common adverse effects of glucosamine are mild GI symptoms such as nausea, heartburn, diarrhea, and constipation. In clinical trials the incidence of these adverse effects are comparable to placebo. Glucosamine is at least as well tolerated as ibuprofen and better than piroxicam (Lopes-Vaz 1982; Forster et al. 1996). Since glucosamine is derived from the exoskeletons of shrimp, lobster, and crabs, some may be concerned that persons with shellfish allergies may also be allergic to glucosamine. However, shellfish allergy is due to IgE antibodies in the meat of shellfish, not in the shells, and there have been no reported cases of glucosamine allergy in those with shellfish allergy (Gray et al. 2004).

Chondroitin sulfate is generally well tolerated, with the most commonly reported adverse effects being epigastric pain and nausea. Preliminary data suggest that versican, a proteoglycan of chondroitin sulfate, may facilitate the invasion of cancer cells into the prostrate stroma (Sakko et al. 2003), but this effect has not been shown with supplemental chondroitin. Nevertheless, men with prostate cancer should avoid chondroitin until further studies are available.

Table I
Recommended doses for dietary supplements and herbs used for pain

Supplement/Herb	Daily Dose
Glucosamine sulfate	1500 mg in divided doses (500 mg t.i.d.)
Chondroitin sulfate	200–400 mg BID to t.i.d. or 1000–1200 mg in single dose
S-adenosyl L-methionine (SAMe)	200 mg t.i.d.*
Avocado-soybean unsaponifiables (1/3 avocado and 2/3 soybean oil)	300 mg daily
Devil's claw	2.6 g/d (Harpadol)
Capsicum	0.025–0.075%

* Most trials that showed benefit used 600–800 mg/d; several used up to 1200 mg/d.

Potential glucosamine-chondroitin drug interactions either have negative clinical trial evidence or have not been evaluated in clinical trials (Table II). In the United States, patients should look for products containing the USP (U.S. Pharmacopeia) seal, the best assurance of quality at this time.

S-adenosyl L-methionine (SAMe). SAMe is a naturally occurring molecule in most body tissues and fluids; it is synthesized from L-methionine and adenosine triphosphate (ATP). SAMe plays a role in transmethylation, transsulfuration, and aminopropylation and is important for the synthesis, activation, and metabolism of hormones, neurotransmitters, and nucleic acids. SAMe may be beneficial for OA through its analgesic and anti-inflammatory effects; it also may stimulate articular cartilage growth and repair (Hardy et al. 2002).

Several clinical trials support the use of SAMe to reduce pain and improve function in patients with OA. SAMe appears to be as effective as NSAIDs, including celecoxib, with fewer side effects. However, the onset of significant symptom relief may take longer with SAMe (30 days) than with NSAIDs (15 days) (Najm et al. 2004; Soeken 2004). Side effects of SAMe are more common with higher doses (such as those used for depression) and include GI symptoms (flatulence, nausea, vomiting, diarrhea, constipation), dry mouth, headache, dizziness, and nervousness. SAMe may interact with drugs and supplements that have serotonergic properties (e.g., dextromethorphan, meperidine, monoamine oxidase inhibitors, selective serotonin reuptake inhibitors, pentazocine, and tramadol) since it is associated with increased serotonin turnover and with higher epinephrine and norepinephrine levels. SAMe has been shown to cause Parkinson's-like symptoms in rats that may be due to interference with the effectiveness of levodopa (Soeken 2004).

Table II
Potential drug interactions with glucosamine sulfate and chondroitin sulfate

Medication	Theoretical Interaction	Clinical Evidence
Acetaminophen	Reduces serum sulfur concentrations and may decrease effectiveness	Not supported in clinical trials
Antidiabetic medications	May increase insulin resistance or decrease insulin production	Not supported in clinical trials
Antimitotic medications	May induce resistance to etoposide, doxorubicin, and teniposide by reducing drugs inhibition of topoisomerase II (enzyme required for DNA replication in tumor cells)	Not tested in clinical trials
Warfarin	High-dose glucosamine (>3000 mg/d) combined with high-dose chondroitin (>2400 mg/d) may increase the international normalized ratio	No reports at recommended doses

Avocado-soybean unsaponifiables. Avocado-soybean unsaponifiables (ASU) are the fraction of avocado and soybean oils that do not produce soap after hydrolysis. A systematic review of four randomized, double-blind, placebo-controlled studies evaluated the effects of ASU on OA (Ernst 2003) as evidenced by pain relief, NSAID intake reduction, and functional improvement. Two short-term studies (3 and 6 months; $N = 424$) demonstrated that the ASU groups improved in all outcomes (Maheu et al. 1998; Appelboom et al. 2001). Another short-term study (3 months; $N = 163$) demonstrated a reduction in NSAID intake but no difference in pain reduction (Blotman et al. 1997). In a 2-year study ($N = 163$) of patients with hip OA, pain was not decreased, but progression of joint space narrowing was slowed (Lequesne et al. 2002).

The combination of avocado and soybean oils may inhibit cartilage degradation and promote cartilage repair in osteoarthritic chondrocytes (Henrotin et al. 2003). Clinical trials have not reported adverse effects, but there may be cross-sensitivity in patients who are sensitive to latex. Interactions with drugs and supplements are minimal; there has been one case report of an interaction with ASU and warfarin (Ernst 2003).

Devil's claw. Devil's claw (*Harpagophytum procumbens*) is a traditional African herb that has been used for pain due to OA and a number of other conditions, with preliminary data suggesting that it may have anti-inflammatory effects (Gagnier et al. 2004). While numerous studies have suggested that aqueous or alcoholic extracts or powdered devil's claw material may reduce pain, standardized outcome measures were not used. In a placebo-controlled study, devil's claw appeared to decrease low back pain as measured with a visual analogue scale (Chrubasik et al. 1999). A later study demonstrated that devil's claw was comparable to rofecoxib after 6 weeks of treatment (Chrubasik et al. 2003). A recent uncontrolled, open-label study of devil's claw in 75 elderly patients with hip and knee OA (800 mg t.i.d. for 12 weeks) showed significant improvement in pain and function (Chrubasik et al. 2002). These and other preliminary data (Wegener and Lupke 2003) suggest that devil's claw is worthy of further study and may be useful in reducing NSAID dose in patients with low back pain and hip or knee OA.

Devil's claw is generally well tolerated when given orally. Diarrhea is the most common adverse effect, and other GI side effects are possible. There are no known interactions with other herbs and supplements. A number of theoretical interactions may occur with devil's claw but have not been reported in humans. These include a reduction of blood glucose and blood pressure that may add to the therapeutic effect of antidiabetic and antihypertensive medications; an increase of stomach acid that may blunt the effects of H_2 blockers and proton pump inhibitors; and an inhibition of CYP2C9, CYP2C19, and CYP3A4 that may alter the metabolism of drugs by the liver.

Capsicum. Capsicum, also known as cayenne or chili pepper, has been shown to decrease pain due to OA, rheumatoid arthritis, and postherpetic neuralgia when used topically. A short-term, double-blind, placebo-controlled trial that examined the effect of capsicum plaster on nonspecific low back pain in 320 subjects aged 18–75 years resulted in 42% pain reduction in the active treatment group compared to 31% in the placebo group ($P = 0.0001$). Sixty-seven percent of subjects in the capsicum group had >30% pain reduction compared to 49% in the placebo group ($P = 0.002$). Local skin reactions were more common in the capsicum group (7.5% vs. 3.1%), but there were no systemic adverse effects. The number needed to treat to see 30% reduction in pain was 5.8 (Frerick et al. 2003). Capsaicin binds to skin nociceptors, which initially increases and then later reduces sensitivity. Repeated application results in persistent desensitization, possibly through substance P depletion. One major issue in conducting clinical trials with capsicum is that it is quite difficult to completely mask subjects to treatment since the capsicum group may initially feel a burning or tingling sensation with application and thus are likely to suspect that they are receiving the active treatment.

ALTERNATIVE MEDICAL SYSTEMS

Alternative medical systems are complete systems of theory and practice that have evolved independently from conventional Western medicine. Major Eastern systems include traditional Chinese medicine (TCM) and Ayurvedic medicine from India. Major Western systems include homeopathy and naturopathy. Other systems have been developed by Native American, African, Middle Eastern, Tibetan, and Central and South American cultures.

TRADITIONAL CHINESE MEDICINE

TCM is a complete system of healing that dates back to 200 B.C. in written form. One of the major tenets of TCM is that health is achieved by maintaining the body in a balanced state, based on the belief that disease is caused by an internal imbalance of yin and yang. This imbalance leads to blockage in the flow of qi or vital energy along pathways known as meridians. TCM practitioners typically use herbs, acupuncture, and massage to rebalance the flow of qi to bring the body back into harmony and wellness. Other TCM practices are tai chi, qi gong, and various forms of meditation.

Two excellent books that provide information on TCM are *The Web That Has No Weaver* (Kaptchuk 2000) and *Between Heaven and Earth* (Beinfield and Korngold 1992).

AYURVEDIC MEDICINE

Ayurveda is a comprehensive medical system that places equal emphasis on the body, mind, and spirit and strives to restore the innate harmony of the individual. Some of the primary treatments include diet, exercise, meditation, herbs, massage, sunlight exposure, and controlled breathing. In India, Ayurvedic treatments have been developed for various diseases such as diabetes, cardiovascular conditions, and neurological disorders, but the quality of published clinical trials generally falls short of contemporary methodological standards with regard to randomization criteria, sample size, and control group design. An excellent overview of Ayurveda is *The Science of Self-Healing* (Lad 1985).

NATUROPATHY

Naturopathy, literally translated as "nature disease," emphasizes health restoration as well as disease treatment. Six principles form the basis of naturopathic practice in North America: recognition of the healing power of nature, identification and treatment of the cause of disease, the concept of "first do no harm," the concept of the doctor as teacher, treatment of the whole person, and prevention. The core modalities supporting these principles include diet modification and nutritional supplements, herbal medicine, acupuncture and Chinese medicine, hydrotherapy, massage and joint manipulation, and lifestyle counseling. Practitioners design individualized treatment protocols according to each patient's needs. The *Textbook of Natural Medicine* (Pizzorno and Murray 1999) is an excellent reference for naturopathy.

HOMEOPATHY

Samuel Hahnemann founded homeopathy in the late 1700s on the "principle of similars." He hypothesized that therapies can be selected on the basis of how closely symptoms produced by a remedy match the symptoms of the patient's disease. Hahnemann gave repeated doses of many common substances to healthy volunteers and carefully recorded the symptoms produced. As a result of this experience, Hahnemann developed treatments (called remedies) for sick patients by matching the symptoms produced by a substance in healthy persons to symptoms in sick patients. The remedies used in homeopathy are greatly diluted from the original substance. Homeopathy emphasizes the careful examination of all aspects of a person's health status, including emotional and mental states, and idiosyncratic characteristics (Vithoulkas 1980).

PRACTICES FROM ALTERNATIVE MEDICAL SYSTEMS FOR PAIN

ACUPUNCTURE

Acupuncture involves the placing of fine needles at specific points (acupoints) along the channels through which qi flows, called meridians. Needles placed along meridians may not necessarily correspond to the area of pain but to the system that is related to the pain. Acupuncture needles may also be placed locally in the area of pain or in and around trigger points.

Prior to 1995, only seven randomized controlled trials of acupuncture for knee OA had been published in English (Ernst 1997), although many were published in Chinese. Overall, these studies had three methodological drawbacks: lack of credible control groups for the placebo effect, inadequate assessment of long-term treatment benefits, and insufficient sample sizes. A meta-analysis examining the effectiveness of acupuncture in OA was inconclusive (Ezzo et al. 2001). However, better designed and longer term studies suggest that acupuncture is useful in OA.

Over the past several years, higher quality acupuncture studies have been published, including studies on electroacupuncture and percutaneous electrical nerve stimulation (PENS). Contemporary studies of the effectiveness of acupuncture and related modalities for pain in older adults are summarized in Table III. One of the largest studies, in outpatients with knee OA, demonstrated a significant decrease in pain and function with acupuncture compared to sham acupuncture. However, true acupuncture was not significantly different from sham until 14 weeks into the 26-week study; both sham and true acupuncture had significant benefit compared to the education control group, indicating a significant nonspecific effect of needling, even when sham points were utilized. One limitation of the study was the large dropout rate, especially in the education control (45%) compared to 25% in each acupuncture group (Berman et al. 2004).

A single-blind, randomized, placebo-controlled study in patients with chronic mechanical neck pain also demonstrated nonspecific effects. Subjects received eight treatments over 4 weeks with either acupuncture or mock transcutaneous electrical stimulation delivered to acupoints. Both groups improved considerably, and adverse effects were minimal. The decrease in pain was still present in both groups at 1-year follow-up, suggesting a powerful nonspecific effect of acupoint manipulation (White et al. 2004). Another large study conducted in primary care found acupuncture to be useful for chronic tension and migraine headaches (Vickers et al. 2004). This study also found that acupuncture improved health-related quality of life at low cost (Wonderling et al. 2004).

Acupuncture given by placing needles in the ear is known as auricular acupuncture. One study randomized patients with chronic pain (at least 30 mm on a 100-mm visual analogue scale) after cancer treatment to auricular acupuncture, placebo acupuncture, or auricular seeds fixed at placebo points. The study found that acupuncture reduced pain by 36%, compared to 2% in the placebo groups (Alimi et al. 2003).

Electroacupuncture uses acupuncture needles connected to electrical stimulation of variable frequency. Most studies that have evaluated electroacupuncture for a variety of pain conditions have been small and short-term. Several studies that included middle-aged and older adults with chronic low back pain demonstrated that electroacupuncture had a greater effect on disability, pain, and function than did control conditions, including an exercise control group (Meng et al. 2003; Ng et al. 2003, Yeung et al. 2003; Tsui and Cheing 2004). Another study found that electroacupuncture decreased pain in patients with knee OA to the same degree as transcutaneous electrical nerve stimulation and to a greater extent than an education control group. An ongoing trial will examine the effectiveness of periosteal electroacupuncture for the treatment of chronic knee pain in older adults with knee OA.

Percutaneous electrical nerve stimulation (PENS) is a neuroanatomical form of acupuncture that also combines acupuncture needles with electrical stimulation. Instead of being placed along meridians, needles are placed directly at the site of pain along corresponding dermatomes, myotomes, and sclerotomes (Ghoname et al. 1999a). Although the exact mechanism of analgesia is not known, PENS may act by neural modulation and by increasing endogenous opioid-like substances (Hamza et al. 2000). Several studies in various age groups have demonstrated the efficacy of PENS in reducing chronic low back pain compared to various control groups (Ghoname et al. 1999a,b; Weiner et al. 2003). In addition to reducing pain intensity, PENS has been shown to decrease use of oral nonopioid analgesics and to improve physical activity, quality of sleep, and sense of well-being. In one small study performed in older adults with chronic low back pain, PENS plus physical therapy significantly improved psychosocial function, timed chair rise, and isoinertial lifting endurance. Also, although none of the subjects

Table III

Contemporary studies of the effectiveness of acupuncture and related modalities for pain in older adults

Study	Pain Condition	Acupuncture Technique	Duration of Treatment	Study Design	No. Subjects (Mean Age)	Comments and Conclusions
Berman et al. 2004	Knee OA	Traditional	26 wk	RCT (true vs. sham vs. education)	570 (66 y)	Pain and function improved in true acupuncture at 14 and 26 wk; true and sham improved pain and function compared to education at all time points
White et al. 2004	Neck pain	Traditional	4 wk	RCT (true vs. sham)	135 (53 y)	Pain improved in both groups with a significant difference between groups at weeks 5 and 12; not considered clinically significant
Vickers et al. 2004	Headache	Traditional	3 months	RT (true vs. usual care)	401 (46 y)	Lower headache scores and fewer days of headache in acupuncture group
Tsui et al. 2004	Chronic low back pain	EA	4 wk	RCT (EA vs. electrical heat acupuncture vs. control)	42 (39 y)	Electroacupuncture had a greater effect on disability (by straight-leg raise), while electrical heat acupuncture had a greater effect on pain
Meng et al. 2003	Chronic low back pain	EA	5 wk	RCT (EA vs. usual care)	55 (72 y)	Function significantly improved with acupuncture at 6 and 9 wk
Yeung et al. 2003	Chronic low back pain	EA	4 wk	RCT (EA + exercise vs. exercise alone)	52 (56 y)	Electroacupuncture resulted in improvement in pain and disability, but not in ROM and strength
Ng et al. 2003	Knee OA	EA	2 wk	RCT (EA vs. TENS vs. usual care)	24 (85 y)	Both treatments reduced pain with prolonged effects
Alimi et al. 2003	Chronic pain after cancer treatment	Ear acupuncture	2 treatments 1 month apart	RCT (auricular vs. placebo acupuncture vs. auricular seeds fixed at placebo points)	90 (56 y)	Significant pain reduction in the acupuncture group compared to both placebo groups

Study	Condition	Intervention	Duration	Design	N (mean age)	Results
Ghoname et al. 1999a	Chronic low back pain	PENS	3 wk	RCT/cross-over (PENS, sham PENS, TENS, or exercise)	64 (43 y)	PENS decreased pain and use of oral nonopioid analgesics; 91% of patients felt that PENS was most effective for pain. PENS also improved physical activity, quality of sleep, and sense of well-being.
Ghoname et al. 1999b	Sciatica, L2 disk herniation	PENS	3 wk	RCT/cross-over (PENS, TENS, or sham PENS)	64 (43 y)	PENS and TENS were more effective than sham PENS in decreasing pain and oral analgesic use. PENS was more effective than TENS in improving physical activity and quality of sleep
Weiner et al. 2003	Low back pain	PENS	6 wk	RCT (PENS + PT vs. sham PENS + PT)	34 (65 y)	PENS plus PT decreased pain and pain-related disability, and improved psychosocial function, timed chair rise, and isoinertial lifting endurance
Ahmed et al. 2000	Headache	PENS	2 wk	RCT, crossover, single blind	30 (36 y)	PENS decreased pain, increased physical activity, and improved quality of sleep; also decreased oral analgesic requirements by 50%
Hamza et al. 2000	Diabetic neuropathy	PENS	3 wk	RCT/ crossover (PENS, sham PENS)	50 (55 y)	PENS decreased extremity pain and need for oral analgesics; improved sense of well-being and quality of sleep

Abbreviations: EA = electroacupuncture; OA = osteoarthritis; PENS = percutaneous electrical nerve stimulation; PT = physical therapy; RCT = randomized control trial; ROM = range of motion; TENS = transcutaneous electrical nerve stimulation.

were clinically depressed, Geriatric Depression Scale scores decreased immediately after treatment and remained lower than baseline at a 3-month follow-up (Weiner et al. 2003). An ongoing larger clinical trial at the University of Pittsburgh will disentangle the effectiveness of PENS and physical therapy for the treatment of chronic low back pain in older adults (D. Weiner et al., unpublished data).

PENS has been studied for a variety of other pain conditions, including headaches and diabetic neuropathy. PENS may be helpful in headache management by reducing pain, permitting increased physical activity, improving quality of sleep, and reducing oral analgesic requirements (Ahmed et al. 2000). A single-blind, randomized crossover study in 50 patients with diabetic neuropathy found that PENS significantly decreased lower-extremity pain and oral analgesic requirements, while improving patients' sense of well-being and quality of sleep (Hamza et al. 2000).

Acupuncture and related modalities are quite safe when administered by a trained practitioner (Weiner and Ernst 2004). For patients with bleeding disorders (including those taking systemic anticoagulants), practitioners should discuss the increased risk of bruising and bleeding (generally minor). Infection is rare when pre-packaged, sterilized needles are used. The most common serious adverse consequence associated with acupuncture is pneumothorax, although the risk is extremely low (Rampes and James 1995; Ernst and White 1997). Caution should be exercised when administering electroacupuncture with leads that cross the thorax in patients with a pacemaker or other implanted cardiac device.

ENERGY THERAPIES

Energy medicine, practiced in many cultures, is based on the concept that human beings are infused with a subtle form of energy that flows in and around the body. Practitioners of energy medicine believe that illness results from disturbances or blocks in this energetic biofield and work with this subtle energy to effect changes in the physical body and influence health. Energy can be transferred to the body either by another human or by a machine. Energy can be measured as mechanical vibration (such as sound) and as electromagnetic forces including visible light, magnetism, monochromatic radiation (such as laser), and rays from other parts of the electromagnetic spectrum. Treatment uses specific, measurable wavelengths and frequencies. Putative energy fields or biofields have been more difficult to reproducibly measure, although energy emanating from the hands of treating healers has been documented. Common examples of this subtle energy work include Reiki, qigong, Healing Touch, and Therapeutic Touch. Energy medicine is gaining popularity and has become the subject of investigation at academic medical centers. A recent National Center for Health Statistics survey indicated that approximately 1% of participants had used Reiki, 0.5% had used qigong, 4.6% had used some kind of healing ritual, and approximately 30% had had others pray for their health.

Most of the published studies in energy medicine are small and focus on Therapeutic Touch (TT). The effectiveness of TT has been demonstrated in wound healing, osteoarthritis, migraine headaches, and pain and anxiety in burn patients (Keller and Bzdek 1986; Wirth 1990; Gordon et al. 1998; Turner et al. 1998). Two meta-analyses reported overall positive results of TT without adverse effects (Winstead-Fry and Kijek 1999; Astin et al. 2000). In the most recent meta-analysis (Astin et al. 2000), 7 of 11 controlled studies had positive outcomes, 3 showed no effect, and in one the controls healed faster than the TT group. One controlled study demonstrated the effectiveness of short-term TT in decreasing pain and improving function in knee OA (Gordon et al. 1998).

Another form of energy medicine is external qigong. In one small study, 10 patients with chronic orofacial pain who received one 5–10-minute treatment of qi transmission demonstrated widely variable responses. Eight of 10 subjects experienced up to 21% pain reduction (Chen and Marbach 2002). Lee et al. (2003) specifically examined qi therapy as compared with placebo for 104 older adults with chronic pain. Subjects who received qi reported a decrease in both pain intensity and number of pain points.

MANIPULATIVE AND BODY-BASED METHODS

This category includes chiropractic and osteopathic manipulation and massage therapy, as well as other methods listed in Table IV. Surveys of the U.S. population suggest that between 3% and 16% of adults receive chiropractic manipulation, which primarily involves adjustments of the spine and other joints, while between 2% and 14% receive massage therapy, which involves manipulation of the soft tissues of the body through pressure and movement. In 1997, U.S. adults made an estimated 192 million visits to chiropractors and 114 million visits to massage therapists, which combined represented 50% of all visits to CAM practitioners. Fewer data exist regarding the use of the remaining manipulative and body-based practices, and it is estimated that collectively they are used by less than 7% of the U.S. population.

Manipulative and body-based practices focus primarily on the structures and systems of the body, including the bones and joints, soft tissues, and circulatory and lymphatic systems. Most of these practices share the philosophy that the human body is self-regulating and has the ability to heal itself, and that its parts are interdependent. There have been several reviews of the effectiveness of manipulation for pain (Koes et al. 1995; Bronfort 1999; Assendelft et al. 2003; Cherkin et al. 2003) and two notable clinical trials (Cherkin et al. 1998; Hurwitz et al. 2002). Overall, chiropractic manipulation seems to be effective for acute uncomplicated low back pain and for chronic low back pain compared to sham or treatments considered to be ineffective. However, chiropractic does not seem to be superior to usual medical management including physical therapy for low back pain. Neck pain also may benefit from spinal manipulation; a study that compared spinal mobilization techniques to physical therapy and usual care found manual therapy to be superior to both control groups (Hoving et al. 2002; Gross et al. 2004). There may be a dose-response relationship of the number of spinal manipulations regarding improvements in pain and disability (Haas et al. 2004). There are also data to suggest that mobilization (lower velocity treatment) is as effective as manipulation (which includes higher velocity treatments) and may result in fewer symptoms after treatment. Childs et al. (2004), in a randomized controlled study, demonstrated that it is possible to select patients who are more likely to respond to chiropractic manipulation using clinical prediction rule criteria: symptom duration, symptom location, fear-avoidance beliefs, lumbar mobility, and hip range of motion. Treatment with spinal manipulation was more effective if four out of the criteria were met. Chiropractic treatment is quite safe; there are reports of minor symptoms including dizziness and headache, but more serious adverse effects such as vertebrobasilar artery dissection and cauda equine syndrome are rare (Assendelft et al. 1996, 2003).

MIND-BODY MEDICINE

Mind-body medicine focuses on interactions between the brain, mind, body, and behavior and on the powerful ways in which emotional, mental, social, spiritual, and behavioral factors can directly affect health. It respects and enhances each person's capacity for self-knowledge and self-care and emphasizes techniques that are grounded in this approach.

Mind-body medicine includes interventions that are thought to promote health such as relaxation, hypnosis, visual imagery, meditation, cognitive-behavioral therapies, group support, autogenic training, spirituality, and prayer. The field views illness as an opportunity for personal growth and transformation, seeing health care providers as catalysts and guides in this process. Mind-body interventions constitute a major portion of the overall use of CAM by the public. In 2002, five relaxation techniques and imagery, biofeedback, and hypnosis, taken together, were used by more than 30% of the adult U.S. population, and prayer was used by more than 50%.

The concept that the mind is important in the treatment of illness is integral to the healing approaches of Eastern cultures. Hippocrates recognized the moral and spiritual aspects of healing and believed that treatment included consideration of attitude, environmental influences, and natural remedies. While this integrated approach was maintained in traditional healing systems in the East, developments in the Western world by the 16th and 17th centuries had separated human spiritual or emotional dimensions from the physical body. During the Renaissance and Enlightenment eras, science was redirected to the purpose of enhancing humankind's control over nature. Technological advances (e.g., microscopy, the stethoscope, the blood pressure cuff, and refined surgical techniques) demonstrated a cellular world that seemed distant from the world of belief and emotion. The discovery of bacteria and later antibiotics further dispelled the notion of beliefs influencing health. Fixing or curing an illness became a matter of science and took precedence over healing of the soul.

In the 1920s, the work of physiologist Walter Cannon revealed the direct relationship between stress and neuroendocrine responses in animals. Coining the phrase "fight or flight," Cannon described the primitive reflexes of sympathetic and adrenal activation in response to perceived danger and other environmental pressures. In the mid-20th century, endocrinologist Hans Selye further defined the deleterious effects of stress and distress on health. At the same time, technological advances in medicine that could identify specific pathological changes and new discoveries in pharmaceuticals were occurring at a very rapid pace. The disease-based model, the search for a specific pathology, and the identification of external cures were dominant in all fields of medicine.

During World War II, the importance of belief re-entered health care, when morphine for the wounded soldiers was in short supply and anesthetist Henry Knowles Beecher discovered that much of the pain could be controlled by saline injections. He coined the term "placebo effect," claiming that one-third of patients improve on placebo (Beecher 1955), and his subsequent research showed that up to 35% of a therapeutic response to any medical treatment could be the result of belief. Investigation into the placebo effect is ongoing at several academic centers. Since the 1960s, mind-body interactions have been extensively researched. The evidence for benefits from biofeedback, cognitive-behavioral interventions, and hypnosis is quite extensive, and evidence is emerging regarding their physiological effects.

Music therapy is fairly common in conventional medical settings and may be effective in various situations. It is considered by many to be part of mind-body medicine. One unmasked study evaluated the effects of music on OA pain in 66 older adults randomized to either listening to music or sitting quietly for 20 minutes per day over 14 days. The music group had significantly less pain after each session. The weaknesses of the study were that it was not masked and that the music group appeared to have greater pain at baseline than the control group. However, given the lack of adverse events and the low cost, this intervention may well be worth instituting (McCaffrey and Freeman 2003).

Mind-body techniques are potentially effective for fibromyalgia, a common condition in older women (Wolfe et al. 1995). In one study, 128 patients with fibromyalgia were randomly assigned to an 8-week mind-body training program (mindfulness meditation plus qigong movement therapy) or to an education support group. Pain, disability, and depression all decreased in both groups by the eighth week and were maintained at a 6-month follow-up (Astin et al. 2003b). An earlier systematic review reported strong evidence that mind-body therapies improved self-efficacy compared to a waiting list or usual care, but there was less evidence for improvement in pain and other outcomes. There is limited evidence that mind-body therapies reduce pain, but fairly strong evidence that, when combined with moderate-to high-intensity exercise, they improve pain and function (Hadhazy et al. 2000).

A recent excellent review summarized mind-body techniques for multiple clinical conditions, including seven pain conditions (Astin et al. 2003a). Moderate to large effects were demonstrated for chronic pain including migraines, OA, low back pain, chronic benign headaches, and cancer pain. The evidence was strongest for cancer symptoms, headache, OA, and chronic low back pain. Mind-body therapies have few side effects. Most are related to reduced medication needs, for example in patients with hypertension and diabetes mellitus.

CLINICAL USE AND PRECAUTIONS IN OLDER ADULTS

Most clinical trials support excellent safety of the modalities discussed in this chapter. In older adults, however, adverse interactions of medication with herbs and supplements are potentially problematic. The medication most likely to interact with an herb or supplement is warfarin. Most other interactions are theoretical and have little clinical evidence-based support. To assure patient safety, however, it is important to check for interactions between drugs and herbal or supplements in the Natural Medicines Comprehensive Database (www.naturaldatabase.com). This database is available as an online resource (updated daily) or in book form. The online resource allows one to search by product name, common name, or disease and has specific sections on interactions and efficacy, with direct reference links.

Practitioners should also be mindful of potential adverse interactions between medication and alternative modalities in older adults, particularly when modalities that result in significant relaxation, such as mind-body techniques, energy medicine, or acupuncture are used. In these situations, patient monitoring is important because a decrease in or discontinuation of medication may be indicated. Specific information about various CAM modalities is available in English and Spanish for practitioners and patients on the NCCAM Web site (www.nccam.nih.gov).

There are several practical guidelines for use of CAM in older adults. Clinicians should consider the following questions before advising CAM: (1) Is the conventional medical evaluation complete? (2) What is the diagnosis? (3) What are the conventional treatment options for this diagnosis? (4) Have conventional treatments been tried? Refused? Exhausted? It is important to identify the chief symptom for which CAM will be used and to follow that symptom using a diary completed by the patient. A discussion of patient and doctor preferences is important in selecting a CAM modality because these preferences will affect compliance and safety. It is important to review safety and efficacy data using the available resources and to pay special attention to real or potential toxicity. Finally, one must acknowledge incomplete information and important studies in progress. Eisenberg (1997) has provided an excellent review to help clinicians choose and prescribe CAM. The reality is that research on CAM is rapidly expanding to address critical issues related to patient care and safety. Over the next 5–10 years we will have a much clearer perspective on what constitutes good medicine, rather than simply what differentiates conventional medicine from CAM.

REFERENCES

Ahmed HE, White PF, Craig WF, et al. Use of percutaneous electrical nerve stimulation (PENS) in the short-term management of headache. *Headache* 2000; 40:311–315.

Alimi D, Rubino C, Pichard-Leandri E, et al. Analgesic effect of auricular acupuncture for cancer pain: a randomized, blinded, controlled trial. *J Clin Oncol* 2003; 21:4120–4126.

Alvarez-Soria MA, Largo R, Diez-Ortego E, et al. Glucosamine inhibits IL-1β-induced NF-κB activation in human osteoarthritic chondrocytes. Presented at: American College of Rheumatology meeting, October 25–29, 2002.

Appelboom T, Schuermans J, Verbruggen G, Henrotin G, Reginster JY. Symptoms modifying effect of avocado/soybean unsaponifiables (ASU) in knee osteoarthritis. *Scand J Rheumatol* 2001; 30:242–247.

Assendelft WJ, Bouter LM, Knipschild PG. Complications of spinal manipulation: a comprehensive review of the literature. *J Fam Pract* 1996; 42:475–480.

Assendelft WJ, Morton SC, Yu EI, Suttorp MJ, Shekelle PG. Spinal manipulative therapy for low back pain. Meta-analysis of effectiveness relative to other therapies. *Ann Intern Med* 2003; 138:871–881.

Astin JA, Harkness E, Ernst E. The efficacy of "distant healing": a systematic review of randomized trials. *Ann Intern Med* 2000; 132:903–910.

Astin JA, Shapiro SL, Eisenberg DM, Forys K. Mind-body medicine: state of the science, implications for practice. *J Am Board Fam Pract* 2003a; 16:131–147.

Astin JA, Berman B, Bausell B, et al. The efficacy of mindfulness meditation plus Qigong movement therapy in the treatment of fibromyalgia: a randomized controlled trial. *J Rheumatol* 2003b; 30:2257–2262.

Barnes P, Powell-Griner E, McFann K, Nahin R. *Complementary and Alternative Medicine Use among Adults: United States, 2002.* CDC Advance Data Report No. 343. May 27, 2004. Available at: www.nccam.nih.gov.

Beecher HK. The powerful placebo. *JAMA* 1955;159(17):1602–1606.

Beinfield H, Korngold E. *Between Heaven and Earth.* New York: Ballantine Books, 1992.

Berman BM, Lao L, Langenberg P, et al. Effectiveness of acupuncture as adjunctive therapy in osteoarthritis of the knee. *Ann Inter Med* 2004; 141:901–910.

Blotman F, Maheu E, Wulwik A, Caspard H, Lopez A. Efficacy and safety of avocado/soybean unsaponifiables in the treatment of symptomatic osteoarthritis of the knee and hip. A prospective, multicenter, three-month, randomized, double-blind, placebo-controlled trial. *Rev Rhum Engl Ed* 1997; 64:825–834.

Bronfort G. Spinal manipulation: current state of research and its indication. *Neurol Clin* 1999; 17:91–111.

Chen KW, Marbach J. External qigong therapy for chronic orofacial pain. *J Altern Complement Med* 2002; 8:532–534.

Cherkin DC, Deyo, RA, Battie M, Street J, Barlow W. A comparison of physical therapy, chiropractic manipulation and provision of an educational booklet for the treatment of patients with low back pain. *N Engl J Med* 1998; 339:1021–1029.

Cherkin DC, Sherman KJ, Deyo RA, Shekelle PG. A review of the evidence for the effectiveness, safety and cost of acupuncture, massage therapy and spinal manipulation for back pain. *Ann Int Med* 2003; 138:898–906.

Childs JD, Fritz JM, Flynn TW, et al. A clinical prediction rules to identify patients with low back pain most likely to benefit from spinal manipulation: a validation study. *Ann Int Med* 2004; 141:920–928.

Chrubasik S, Junck H, Breitschwerdt H, Conradt C, Zappe H. Effectiveness of *Harpagophytum* extract WS 1531 in the treatment of exacerbation of low back pain: a randomized, placebo-controlled, double-blind study. *Eur J Anaesthesiol* 1999; 16(2):118–129.

Chrubasik S, Thanner J, Kunzel O, et al. Comparison of outcome measures during treatment with the proprietary *Harpagophytum* extract Doloteffin in patients with pain in the lower back, knee or hip. *Phytomedicine* 2002; 9(3):181–194.

Chrubasik S, Model A, Black A, Pollak S. A randomized double-blind pilot study comparing Doloteffin and Vioxx in the treatment of low back pain. *Rheumatology (Oxford)* 2003; 42(1):141–148.

Eisenberg DM. Advising patients who seek alternative medical therapies. *Ann Intern Med* 1997; 27:61–69.

Eisenberg DM, Kessler RC, Foster C, et al. Unconventional medicine in the United States: prevalence, costs and patterns of use. *N Engl J Med* 1993; 328:246–252.

Eisenberg DM, Davis RB, Ettner SL, et al. Trends in alternative medicine use in the United States, 1990–1997: results of a follow-up national survey. *JAMA* 1998; 280:1569–1575.

Ernst E. Acupuncture as a symptomatic treatment of osteoarthritis. A systematic review. *Scand J Rheumatol* 1997; 26(6):444–4447.

Ernst E. Avocado-soybean unsaponifiables (ASU) for osteoarthritis: a systemic review. *Clin Rheumatol* 2003; 22:285–288.

Ernst E, White A. Life-threatening adverse reactions after acupuncture? A systematic review. *Pain* 1997; 71:123–126.

Ervin RB, Wright JD, Kennedy-Stephenson J. Use of dietary supplements in the United States, 1988–94. *Vital Health Stat* 1999; 244:1–14.

Ezzo J, Hadhazy V, Birch S, et al. Acupuncture for osteoarthritis of the knee: a systemic review. *Arthritis Rheum* 2001; 44:819–825.

Forster K, Schmid K, Rovati L, et al. Longer-term treatment of mild-to-moderate osteoarthritis of the knee with glucosamine sulfate- a randomized controlled, double-blind clinical study. *Eur J Clin Pharmacol* 1996; 50:542.

Frerick H, Keitel W, Kuhn U, et al. Topical treatment of chronic low back pain with a capsicum plaster. *Pain* 2003; 106:59–64.

Gagnier JJ, Chrubasik S, Manheimer E. *Harpagophytum procumbens* for osteoarthritis and low back pain: a systemic review. *BMC Complement Altern Med* 2004; 4:4–13.

Ghoname EA, Craig WF, White PF, et al. Percutaneous electrical nerve stimulation for low back pain: a randomized crossover study. *JAMA* 1999a; 281:818–823.

Ghoname EA, White PF, Ahmed HE, et al. Percutaneous electrical nerve stimulation: an alternative to TENS in the management of sciatica. *Pain* 1999b; 83:193–199.

Gordon A, Merenstein JH, D'Amico F, Hudgens D. The effects of therapeutic touch on patients with osteoarthritis of the knee. *J Fam Pract* 1998; 47:271–277.

Gray HC, Hutcheson PS, Slavin RG. Is glucosamine safe in patients with seafood allergy? (letter) *J Allergy Clin Immunol* 2004; 114:459–460.

Gross AR, Hoving JL, Haines TA, et al. Cervical Overview Group. A Cochrane review of manipulation and mobilization for mechanical neck disorders. *Spine* 2004; 29:1541–1548.

Haas M, Groupp E, Kraemer DF. Dose-response for chiropractic care of chronic low back pain. *Spine* 2004; 4:574–583.

Hadhazy VA, Ezzo J, Creamer P, Berman B. Mind-body therapies for the treatment of fibromyalgia: a systemic review. *J Rheumatol* 2000; 27:2911–2918.

Hamza MA, White PF, Craig WF, et al. Percutaneous electrical nerve stimulation: a novel analgesic therapy for diabetic neuropathic pain. *Diabetes Care* 2000; 23(3):365–370.

Hardy M, Coulter I, Morton SC, et al. *S-Adenosyl-L-Methionine for Treatment of Depression, Osteoarthritis, and Liver Disease.* Evidence Report/Technology Assessment No. 64, AHRQ Publication 02-E033. Rockville, MD: Agency for Healthcare Research and Quality, U.S. Department of Health and Human Services, 2002. Available at: www.ahrq.gov/clinic/tp/sametp.htm.

Henrotin YE, Sanchez C, Deberg MA, et al. Avocado/soybean unsaponifiables increase aggrecan synthesis and reduce catabolic and proinflammatory mediator production by human osteoarthritic chondrocytes. *J Rheumatol* 2003; 30:1825–1834.

Hoving JL, Koes BW, de Vet HCW, et al. Manual therapy, physical therapy or continued care by a general practitioner for patients with neck pain. *Ann Int Med* 2002; 136:713–722.

Hughes R, Carr A. A randomized, double-blind, placebo-controlled trial of glucosamine sulphate as an analgesic in osteoarthritis of the knee. *Rheumatology* 2002; 41:279–284.

Hurwitz EL, Morgenstern H, Harber P, et al. A randomized trial of medical care with and without physical therapy and chiropractic care with and without physical modalities for patients with low back pain: 6-month follow-up outcomes from the UCLA low back pain study. *Spine* 2002; 27:2193–2204.

Institute of Medicine. *Dietary Supplements: Framework for Evaluating Safety.* Institute of Medicine, July 24, 2002. Available at: www.iom.edu.

Kaptchuk TJ. *The Web That Has No Weaver: Understanding Chinese Medicine,* 2nd ed. Chicago: Contemporary Books, 2000.

Keller E, Bzdek VM. Effects of therapeutic touch on tension headache pain. *Nurs Res* 1986; 35:101–106.

Koes BW, Assendelft WJ, van der Heijden GJ, Bouter LM, Knopschild PG. Spinal manipulation for low back pain: an updated systemic review. *Spine* 1995; 21:2860–2871.

Lad V. *The Science of Self-Healing: A Practical Guide.* Santa Fe, NM: Lotus Press, 1985.

Lee MS, Jang JW, Jang HS, Moon SR. Effects of qi-therapy on blood pressure, pain and psychological symptoms in the elderly: a randomized controlled pilot trial. *Complement Ther Med* 2003; 11:159–164.

Lequesne M, Maheu E, Cadet C, Dreiser RL. Structural effect of avocado/soybean unsaponifiables on joint space loss in osteoarthritis of the hip. *Arthritis Care Res* 2002; 47:50–58.

Lopes-Vaz A. Double-blind clinical evaluation of the relative efficacy of ibuprofen and glucosamine sulphate in the management of osteoarthrosis of the knee in out-patients. *Curr Med Res Opin* 1982; 8(3):145–149.

Maheu E, Mazieres B, Valat JP, et al. Symptomatic efficacy of avocado/soybean unsaponifiables in the treatment of osteoarthritis of the knee and hip: a prospective, randomized, double-blind, placebo-controlled, multicenter clinical trial with a six-month treatment period and a two-month followup demonstrating a persistent effect. *Arthritis Rheum* 1998; 41:81–91.

McAlindon TE, LaValley MP, Gulin JP, Felson DT. Glucosamine and chondroitin for treatment of osteoarthritis. *JAMA* 2000; 283:1469–1475.

McCaffrey R, Freeman E. Effect of music on chronic osteoarthritis pain in older people. *J Adv Nurs* 2003; 44:517–524.

Meng CF, Wang D, Ngeow J, et al. Acupuncture for chronic low back pain in older patients: a randomized, controlled trial. *Rheumatology (Oxford)* 2003; 42(12):1508–1517.

Najm WI, Reinsch S, Hoehler F, et al. S-adenosyl methionine (SAMe) versus celecoxib for the treatment of osteoarthritis symptoms: a double-blind crossover trial. *BMC Musculoskelet Disord* 2004; 5:6.

National Center for Complementary and Alternative Medicine. Available at: nccam.nih.gov/ news/images/campractice.htm. Accessed August 3, 2005.

Ng MML, Leung MCP, Poon DMY. The effects of electro-acupuncture and transcutaneous electrical nerve stimulation on patients with painful osteoarthritic knees: a randomized controlled trial with follow-up evaluation. *J Altern Complement Med* 2003; 9:641–649.

Pavelka K, Gatterova J, Olejarova M, et al. Glucosamine sulfate use and delay of progression of knee osteoarthritis. *Arch Intern Med* 2002; 162:2113–2123.

Pizzorno JE Jr, Murray MT. *Textbook of Natural Medicine.* Edinburgh: Churchill Livingstone, 1999,

Radimer K, Bindewald B, Hughes J, et al. Dietary supplement use by US adults: data from the National Health and Nutrition Examination Survey, 1999–2000. *Am J Epidemiol* 2004; 160(4):339–349.

Rampes H, James R. Complications of acupuncture. *Acupuncture Med* 1995; 8:26–33.

Reginster JY, Deroisy R, Rovati LC, et al. Long-term effects of glucosamine sulphate on osteoarthritis progression: a randomized, placebo-controlled clinical trial. *Lancet* 2001; 357:251–256.

Richy F, Bruyere O, Ethgren O, et al. Structural and symptomatic efficacy of glucosamine and chondroitin in knee osteoarthritis. *Arch Intern Med* 2003; 163:1514–1522.

Sakko AJ, Ricciardelli C, Mayne K, et al. Modulation of prostate cancer cell attachment to matrix by versican. *Cancer Res* 2003; 63:4786–4791.

Soeken KL. Selected CAM therapies for arthritis-related pain: the evidence from systematic reviews. *Clin J Pain* 2004; 20:13–18.

Thie NM, Prasad NG, Major PW. Evaluation of glucosamine sulfate compared to ibuprofen for the treatment of temporomandibular joint osteoarthritis: a randomized double blind controlled 3 month clinical trial. *J Rheumatol* 2001; 28:1347–1355.

Towheed TE, Anastassiades TP, Shea B, et al. Glucosamine therapy for treating osteoarthritis. *Cochrane Database Syst Rev* 2001 (1).

Tsui MLK, Cheing GLY. The effectiveness of electroacupuncture versus electrical heat acupuncture in the management of chronic low back pain. *J Altern Complement Med* 2004; 10:803–809.

Turner J, Clark A, Gauthier D, Williams M. The effect of therapeutic touch on pain and anxiety in burn patients. *J Adv Nurs* 1998; 28:10–20.

U.S. Food and Drug Administration. *Dietary Supplement Health and Education Act of 1994.* U.S. Food and Drug Administration Center for Food Safety and Applied Nutrition. Available at www.cfsan.fda.gov/~dms/supplmnt.html; accessed October 1, 2004.

Verbruggen G, Goemaere S, Veys EM. Systems to assess the progression of finger joint osteoarthritis and the effects of disease modifying osteoarthritis drugs. *Clin Rheumatol* 2002; 21:231–243.

Vickers AJ, Rees RW, Zollman CE, et al. Acupuncture for chronic headache in primary care: large, pragmatic, randomised trial. *BMJ* 2004; 328:744.

Vithoulkas G. *The Science of Homeopathy.* New York: Grove Press, 1980.

Wegener T, Lupke NP. Treatment of patients with arthrosis of hip or knee with an aqueous extract of devil's claw (*Harpagophytum procumbens*). *Phytother Res* 2003; 17:1165–1172.

Weiner DK, Ernst E. Complementary and alternative approaches to the treatment of persistent musculoskeletal pain. *Clin J Pain* 2004; 20:244–255.

Weiner DK, Rudy TE, Glick RM, et al. Efficacy of percutaneous electrical nerve stimulation for the treatment of chronic low back pain in older adults. *J Am Geriatr Soc* 2003; 51:599–608.

White P, Lewith G, Prescott P, Conway J. Acupuncture versus placebo for the treatment of chronic mechanical neck pain. *Ann Int Med* 2004; 141:911–919.

Winstead-Fry P, Kijek J. An integrated review and meta-analysis of therapeutic touch research. *Altern Ther Health Med* 1999; 5:58–67.

Wirth DP. The effect of non-contact therapeutic touch intervention on the healing rate of full thickness dermal wounds. *Subtle Energies* 1990; 1:1–20.

Wolfe F, Ross K, Anderson J, Russell IJ, Hebert L. The prevalence and characteristics of fibromyalgia in the general population. *Arthritis Rheum* 1995; 38:19–28.

Wonderling D, Vickers AJ, Grieve R, McCarney R. Cost effectiveness analysis of a randomised trial of acupuncture for chronic headache in primary care. *BMJ* 2004; 328:747.

Yeung CKN, Leung MCP, Chow DHK. The use of electro-acupuncture in conjunction with exercise for the treatment of chronic low-back pain. *J Altern Complement Med* 2003; 9:479–490.

Correspondence to: Karen Prestwood, MD, Center on Aging, University of Connecticut Health Center, Farmington, CT 06030-5215, USA. Email: karenprestwood7722@sbcglobal.net.

Pain in Older Persons, Progress in Pain
Research and Management, Vol. 35, edited
by Stephen J. Gibson and Debra K. Weiner,
IASP Press, Seattle, © 2005.

15

Multidisciplinary Pain Management Clinics for Older Adults

Benny Katz,[a] Sam Scherer,[b] and Stephen J. Gibson[c,d,e]

*[a]Austin Health, Heidelberg, Victoria; [b]Pain Management Clinic for the Elderly,
Melbourne Health, Parkville, Victoria; [c]National Ageing Research Institute,
Parkville, Victoria; [d]Department of Medicine, University of Melbourne,
Melbourne, Victoria; [e]Caulfield Pain Management and Research Centre,
Caulfield, Victoria, Australia*

John Bonica's experiences in treating patients with chronic pain during World War II led to the establishment of a multidisciplinary pain program at the University of Washington in the 1960s. Bonica's pioneering work was pivotal in the establishment of the International Association for the Study of Pain (IASP) and in the proliferation of multidisciplinary pain clinics around the world. By the time of Bonica's death in 1994, some 2,000 pain centers had been established in 36 countries.

Where medical interventions have failed, a multidisciplinary biopsychosocial approach has become established as the preferred method of dealing with the complexity of persistent pain. Modern technology and pharmacological advances over recent decades have had a more profound impact on the management of acute and cancer pain than on persistent pain. The need for a multidisciplinary approach to the management of persistent pain is therefore likely to continue in the foreseeable future.

Despite the growth in the number of older people in our population and a higher prevalence of persistent pain with advancing age, older patients are often underrepresented in pain management clinics (Harkins and Price 1992; Kee et al. 1998). Older patients attending pain treatment centres are offered less treatment and fewer treatment options than younger counterparts, particularly behavioral and nonpharmacological therapies (Kee et al. 1998). The underrepresentation may be due to reluctance by physicians to refer older adults to pain management clinics, to the difficulties older individuals have traveling to clinics, or to restrictive admission criteria. Kee and colleagues reported that none of 96 multidisciplinary pain treatment programs surveyed excluded patients on the basis of age, although no patient over 70 years old had been admitted to 28% of the programs surveyed. Patients were excluded from 6% of programs if they did not have plans to return to work, and 34% of the programs surveyed excluded patients with concurrent medical illnesses. Both criteria represent indirect age-related barriers to admission and are likely to result in the exclusion of older patients. Kee et al. also found a significant age bias among pain program personnel when faced with identical clinical vignettes for patients of different ages. Older patients were perceived to be 14.8% less suitable for admission to the program and were considered 12.5% less likely to succeed if admitted. Few clinics specifically focus on pain management in older people, while others may lack the experience or expertise to deal with the special needs of this group, particularly those who are frail. This chapter describes two decades of experience in a pain management clinic focusing exclusively on older adults.

MULTIDISCIPLINARY PAIN CLINICS

Persistent pain is a significant problem for many people and is often associated with adverse effects on function, mood, and social interaction. There is no single way to treat these patients because no current treatment can eliminate pain in all circumstances. In the majority of patients with persistent pain, medications will fail to totally eradicate the pain. The average pain reduction with long-term opioid therapy is approximately 32% (Turk 2002). A multidisciplinary approach is the preferred method of delivering health care to patients with persistent pain that is accompanied by functional disability and adverse psychosocial consequences, regardless of etiology. Multidisciplinary pain management aspires to achieve more than diminution in pain intensity: it also targets restoration of physical and psychosocial function. A distinguishing characteristic of the multidisciplinary approach is that it addresses physical disabilities and patients' beliefs about their pain, as well as resultant behavior changes, in an integrated manner (Bogduk 2004). The primary goal is to provide those who suffer persistent pain with effective, humane care. Not every person with chronic pain needs a multidisciplinary clinic to receive appropriate care.

There is no universal definition of what constitutes multidisciplinary therapy, nor is there agreement about how it should be delivered. The operation of a pain management service will depend on the patient mix and on the resources available. The IASP has developed guidelines for the desirable characteristics for pain treatment facilities (Loeser 1991). It describes a hierarchical structure for pain management clinics. Modality-orientated clinics offer specific treatments such as nerve blocks, acupuncture, and biofeedback. Pain clinics deal with specific pain problems, for instance back pain or headache. Multidisciplinary pain clinics (MPCs) manage a wide range of pain problems utilizing staff of different disciplines. Multidisciplinary pain centers cover the same spectrum of clinical services as MPCs, but they are also actively involved in research, teaching, and training; they are usually associated with a teaching hospital. Staffing of pain treatment facilities should include a range of health care professionals capable of assessing and treating physical, psychosocial, medical, vocational, and social aspects of chronic pain. The clinical team may include physicians of different specialties, physical therapists, occupational therapists, vocational counselors, social workers, and possibly other professionals. Regular communication between members of the team regarding individual patients' assessment and treatment helps to ensure that the care program targets agreed-upon goals and that team members communicate a consistent message to the patient. The IASP guidelines were designed to promote the development of multidisciplinary pain management and to describe desirable characteristics that may be used by credentialing authorities to certify services. The IASP does not offer certification or accreditation of facilities.

Some patients pose special challenges that go beyond the expertise of most pain treatment facilities and may need to be referred elsewhere (Loeser 1991). These patients may include children, persons with major psychiatric illness or drug and alcohol dependency, and elderly persons with complex problems. Most pain facilities have the expertise to manage individuals with age-related pain problems such as postherpetic neuralgia; however, older individuals with major concurrent medical problems such as dementia, those with multiple health problems limiting therapeutic options, and residents of nursing homes are best managed by clinicians with expertise in geriatric care.

Is there a role for MPCs for older people? Helme and colleagues (1996) argued that specific considerations may justify specialized services for older people. First, clinics dealing with older individuals have specialized expertise in age-related pain syndromes and in the assessment and management of concurrent medical problems. Second, such clinics have an appropriate treatment focus, with goals reflecting the population they serve. Third, combining people of similar ages, life experiences, pain problems, and goals is more likely to create a cohesive therapeutic environment. Older people may feel alienated in a clinic where the majority of individuals are younger, particularly those in more intensive programs and those with vocational goals. Finally, as described in Chapter 10, older individuals have decreased tolerance for pharmacological management. Special expertise is required to optimize drug therapy, as there is a delicate balance between drug efficacy and tolerability. Adverse drug reactions may not be immediately recognized by clinicians inexperienced in dealing with older patients, in whom the symptoms are often atypical. On the other hand, fear of causing adverse drug effects may result in undertreatment by less experienced clinicians.

PAIN IN OLDER ADULTS: THE NEED FOR SPECIALIZED CARE

In most instances, the assessment of the older patient does not differ greatly from that in younger patients. However, the strong association between advanced age and chronic diseases and related impairments increases the requirements for specialized skills in the identification and management of age-associated syndromes, including the disease processes and their interactions, as well as impairments, disability, and handicap. Disease presentation often is not organ specific. Aged care medicine is characterized by a predominance of clinical syndromes such as cognitive impairment, mobility disorders, falls and fractures, and incontinence.

It is important to allow adequate time for the assessment of the older patient. Thought processes, verbalization, and movement are often slower. Responses to questions are often cautious, and there is often a reticence to report symptoms such as memory problems, falls, and incontinence. A more flexible interview style is often advantageous. Rather than asking specific questions, it is often helpful to ask patients to describe their daily routine. This approach may assist in eliciting the impact of pain and concurrent medical conditions on the life of the older person. The history may be also unreliable due to cognitive or other impairments such as hearing loss. A corroborative history from a family member or other companion is often helpful. The assessment should be appropriately paced to avoid patient fatigue, and it may need to be spread out over a number of visits.

Medical status is an important factor when assessing and managing older patients with chronic pain. Conditions with high prevalence rates are likely to co-exist. For instance, the prevalence of persistent pain has been estimated to be in the order of 25–50% in community-dwelling older adults (Helme and Gibson 1999; Weiner 2002); the prevalence of dementia is more than 25% in people over 85 years, and more than 50% among nursing home residents regardless of age. Even mild impairment of memory and cognition is likely to have a significant impact on the assessment and management of pain (Farrell et al. 1996).

The altered presentation of disease in the older patient may include the atypical manifestation of pain. In older persons, conditions that typically present with pain in younger adults such as acute myocardial infarction and peritonitis may not have pain as an early or major symptom. The absence of pain in an older person should not be interpreted as indicative of the absence of serious pathology. Symptoms may not occur until a disease is more advanced (Gibson 2003). On the other hand, older individuals are more likely to present with non-organ-specific manifestations of acute disease such as falls, loss of mobility, confusion, and incontinence. Adverse drug reactions are common, particularly in those taking multiple medications. Many of the medications used for pain are associated with an increased risk of adverse events such as falls. These include opioid and non-opioid analgesics, antidepressants, anticonvulsants, and antiarrhythmic drugs (Tinetti 2003; Field et al. 2004). Nonpharmacological approaches, which should be an integral part of the approach to the management of persistent pain at any age, often have particular applicability in the older patient (AGS Panel on Persistent Pain in Older Persons 2002). They may reduce the reliance on medications and hence reduce the risk of adverse drug events.

A multidisciplinary, comprehensive model of care has proliferated over the past 20 years to deal with the complexity of problems that occur in older patients. These programs rely on multifaceted interventions using teams that include geriatricians, primary care physicians, nurses, physical therapists, occupational therapists, social workers, and other professionals. These programs have been subject to extensive evaluation and have been demonstrated to offer improvements in physical functioning and quality of life at no additional cost over usual care (Cohen et al. 2002). The benefit of comprehensive geriatric care is strongest when long-term control is maintained, ensuring that management plans are sustained (Stuck et al. 1993; Elkan et al. 2001).

A PAIN MANAGEMENT CLINIC FOR OLDER ADULTS

There are many similarities in the practices of pain medicine and aged care medicine. Both disciplines rely on a multidisciplinary team approach, which often focuses on reducing the impact of a chronic condition rather than aiming for a cure. In 1986, we established an MPC for older adults in Melbourne, Australia. This clinic, the Pain Management Clinic for the Elderly, brought together the principles of aged care medicine and the multidisciplinary management of pain (Helme et al. 1989). The structure and outcomes of this clinic have been reported elsewhere (Helme et al. 1996).

Ninety-six percent of the patients improved in at least one of three domains: 72% improved in pain scores, 65% in mood, and 53% in level of activity. There are now four multidisciplinary pain management clinics specializing in older adults in the state of Victoria, Australia.

The structure and operation of the clinic has changed over time in response to changes in conditions of funding and staff structure. This chapter outlines our experiences in operating a MPC for older adults and discusses how our program fits in with the IASP guidelines for desirable characteristics for pain management facilities.

The clinic is located within a comprehensive aged care and rehabilitation service, offering inpatient, outpatient, and community-based services. The clinic is one of a range of multidisciplinary aged care clinics including services for the management of continence, memory, falls and balance, and wounds. Another MPC that shares the facilities specializes in adults of working age, usually with vocational goals. Full diagnostic and interventional facilities are available in the major teaching hospital located nearby.

The co-location of two MPCs targeting separate populations has enabled each clinic to become more specialized. Each clinic operates under the conceptual framework of the IASP, yet is quite distinct in approach, reflecting the heterogeneity of other MPCs. The age of the patients is not the major difference between the clinics. Age is used as a surrogate to identify individuals who are likely to have one or more characteristics that require special modifications to a pain management program. These may include non-vocational goals, significant concurrent medical problems, inability to participate in a vigorous physical rehabilitative program, limitations on pharmacological options, and conditions requiring modifications to cognitive-behavioral programs, such as hearing, speech, and cognitive decline. Residents of nursing homes and dementia sufferers are not precluded from entry to the clinic. There are no financial barriers to attendance because the clinic forms part of Australia's universal health system.

Given sufficient staffing levels and patient proximity to the clinic, our preferred procedure is for a member of the team (a nurse or occupational therapist) to perform the initial assessment in the patient's home. This approach allows our staff to obtain the pain history and perform psychometric testing in a relaxed atmosphere, while observing the impact that pain and disability have on the individual in his or her own environment. Whenever possible, a corroborative history is obtained. The need for independent living equipment and supportive services can be evaluated.

A physician undertakes the initial medical assessment in the clinic. Both a standard medical pain evaluation and a comprehensive geriatric medical assessment are performed. The latter includes screening for impaired cognition, mood disturbance, balance, risk of falls, functional status, social supports, response to medications, and adverse drug effects (Table I) (Rubenstein and Rubenstein 2003; Field et al. 2004).

There is a great deal of heterogeneity among older adults referred for pain management (Corran et al. 1997; Weiner et al. 2001). A comprehensive interdisciplinary management program may not be necessary for everyone. Based on this initial evaluation the physician decides whether the patient should proceed to the next stage of assessment.

A feature of the clinic is the time allocated to undertake the comprehensive assessment. It is important to allow enough time for older individuals to relate their history, which often extends over many years with multiple interventions along the way. The physical examination also takes longer, and abnormal physical findings are more common. Even dressing after the assessment takes longer. At least one hour is allowed for the medical assessment. The next stage of the assessment involves patient consultations with a physiotherapist and a clinical psychologist and collection of psychometric data. Many older patients do not have the stamina to complete an evaluation lasting more than 3 hours on a single visit, so appointments are scheduled for a second attendance.

A physiotherapist evaluates the physical factors that may be contributing to the pain, as well as the impact of pain on function. The patient's capacity to participate in and benefit from a program of graded physical activities and/or physical interventions such as transcutaneous electric nerve stimulation is assessed. The assessment by the clinical psychologist utilizes a similar framework to the assessment undertaken in non-age-specific pain clinics. The pain history is often longer, however, since more factors are likely to contribute to the pain experience. The elderly tend to be more reluctant to report psychological issues and more likely to adopt stoic attitudes (Yong et al. 2001). Age-specific issues need to be taken into consideration, including how the individual is coping with aging, as well as concerns about disability and widowhood. Often the simple question: "How would your life be different if you didn't have pain?" reveals insights into the individual's perception about the pain, its prognosis, and the relative impact of concurrent diseases. Hostility, anger, and issues pertaining to litigation and compensation are usually less relevant to this age group than to working-age adults.

Demographic data are collected on all patients, and psychometric testing is performed whenever feasible (Helme et al. 1996). Strategies to encourage compliance and completion of test batteries have included staggering them over several sittings, having a research nurse administer them prior to initial clinician contact, and having each clinician administer one instrument as

Table I

Elements of comprehensive pain assessment for the older adult: a clinical approach

Domain	Construct	Assessment Approach	Comments
Medical	Medical comorbidity	Review of systems	Critical in determination of potential drug-disease interactions
	Medications	Self report/home visit	Assess prescription, over-the-counter, and natural supplements; critical in determination of potential drug-drug interactions
	Geriatric syndromes		
	Dementia	Mini-mental Status Examination (Folstein et al. 1975), clock-drawing test (Wolf-Klein et al. 1989)	Assessment of syndromes is critical as they impact on pain assessment and treatment.
	Mobility and falls	Gait assessment, modified postural stress test, functional reach	For the modified postural stress test, examiner stands behind patient and exerts backward pull at the hips using graded amount of force and judges postural response.
	Incontinence	Clinical question: "Do you sometimes find that it is hard to get to the bathroom in time?"	
	Malnutrition	Weight, appetite, serum albumin, pain-related appetite disruption	
	Insomnia	Clinical question: "Does pain interfere with your sleep?"	For sleep disruption, ask about trouble falling asleep, awakening with pain, abd amount of time in bed versus amount of time sleeping.
	Hearing	Whisper test	
	Vision	Eye chart	

Category	Assessment domain	Instrument/Method	Comment
Social	Living arrangements Marital/children/family issues Home support services Financial assessment Religious affiliations	Visit	
Disability	Impact of concurrent medical conditions and/or pain on function	Personal ADL Katz scale (Katz et al. 1963) Barthel Index Instrumental ADL Lawton scale	The Katz and Barthel scales have low ceilings and are more appropriate for frail and nursing home populations.
		Human Activity Profile (Fix and Daughton 1988)	The Human Activity Profile covers a wide range of physical functions.
Pain	Pain Site Radiation Intensity Quality Duration Unpleasantness	*Unidimensional Instruments:* Body diagram Numerical rating scale Visual analogue scale Present pain intensity Word descriptor	Body diagrams and numerical scales are widely used in clinical practice. Can be completed in a few minutes. The Present Pain Intensity has higher completion rates among cognitively impaired individuals than other instruments listed.
		Multidimensional Instruments: Brief Pain Inventory (Cleeland et al. 1994)	Takes less than 5 minutes to complete. Available in many languages.
Psychological	Depression	Visual analogue scale for mood	
	Anxiety	Clinical question: "Do you often feel anxious?"	
	Attitudes e.g., stoicism, coping	Clinical question: "How are you coping with the pain?"	

part of his or her clinical evaluation. However, difficulties with language and cultural barriers, cognitive impairment, sensory impairments (hearing and vision), and unwillingness to participate in psychometric evaluation cannot always be overcome. Inability to obtain psychometric data does not exclude patients from clinical assessment and management.

The mean age of the patients attending our clinic is 72 years (SD = 10). Only 44.8% are in a current marital relationship, with 38.5% being widowed and 29.5% living alone. Almost half receive social and physical supportive services. Musculoskeletal conditions account for 35% of presentations, neurological conditions 28%, miscellaneous diagnoses 17%, psychiatric disorders 12%, and uncertain 7% (Helme et al. 1996). The majority of patients have multiple concurrent medical conditions that have potential impact on the management and outcome of a pain program. In addition to the pain problem, 57.5% of a sample of 435 patients had two or more other significant medical conditions (Helme and Gibson 1997). It is often difficult to establish which of a number of identified pathologies is principal in leading to presentation to the clinic. Function and independence may be more significantly compromised by concurrent medical conditions than by pain. Under these circumstances, pain may be a proxy for distress and disability caused by a number of factors.

An interdisciplinary case conference is held at the completion of the initial assessments. A consensus formulation is reached regarding the causes of the pain and the relevance of other medical, physical and psychosocial issues. This formulation is the basis for an individualized treatment program targeting the patient's needs. In most cases treatment is provided in the clinic, although this strategy may be modified for patients for whom travel to the clinic is problematic or for nursing home residents. The programs comprise combinations of education, medication, and physical and psychological therapies. Information is provided about the cause of the pain and about what can realistically be expected from the various treatment options. Great emphasis is given to ensuring compliance with therapy, which may require the involvement of family members and other concerned persons.

Clinicians involved in the treatment programs include a geriatrician, pharmacist, physiotherapist, clinical psychologist, occupational therapist, nurse, and dietician. A cognitive-behavioral therapy group, which meets for six to eight one-hour sessions, is run by an occupational therapist supported by a clinical psychologist. The group program has a preferred weekly agenda that may be varied to meet the needs of the participants. Benefit may be enhanced by attendance with a spouse or other individual who is able to reinforce the program outside the clinic. Mild cognitive decline does not preclude the individual from benefiting from a cognitive-behavioral program

(Cook 1998). Some individuals are not suitable for group programs, including those with more severe hearing or cognitive impairment, in which case an individual program can be offered.

Prescription and demonstration of simple exercise programs and other physical therapies is carried out in the clinic. Complex or intensive physical rehabilitation programs and aquatic therapy are available in a community rehabilitation center on the campus. Patients are generally managed on an outpatient basis, but in special circumstances they may be admitted for treatment.

A clinical pharmacist reviews all patients. Older patients are more likely to require ongoing analgesic medications as part of their pain management. The pharmacist plays an important educative role, aiming to enhance the understanding of medications and improve compliance. Patients are instructed in the use of time-contingent analgesia and in the management of drug-related side effects such as opioid-induced constipation. Prepackaged medication dispensing systems are recommended for individuals prescribed multiple medications and for those with cognitive impairment. The clinical pharmacist performs a comprehensive review of all prescribed and over-the-counter medications and supplements, focusing on potential drug-drug and drug-disease interactions.

Treatment programs usually require 8 to 12 visits to the clinic, usually on a weekly basis. Regular progress reports are sent to the patient's primary care physician, who maintains responsibility for other health problems while the patient attends the clinic. On the patient's discharge from the clinic, the primary care physician assumes responsibility for maintaining the pain management program. In special circumstances a patient may be followed in the clinic on a longer-term basis.

The pain management clinic is a collaboration of the hospital and the National Ageing Research Institute (NARI), located on the same campus. The choice of psychometric instruments is determined in collaboration with NARI (Helme et al. 1996; Helme and Gibson 1997; Helme and Katz 2003). Clinicians participate in collecting the data. The instruments cover the domains of demography, pain, mood, and activity. Specific issues related to older individuals include measures of cognition, concurrent medical conditions, and the use of support services. Instruments that have been designed for older adults or validated in this population are preferred, but they are not always available. Patients may be asked to volunteer for research projects. Whether a patient agrees or declines to participate in research does not influence the management in the clinic. Researchers and clinicians meet on a weekly basis for educational purposes and to discuss research.

The staffing structure of the clinic stands in contrast to that suggested for by the IASP for MPCs. The IASP guidelines recommend that at least three different medical specialties should be represented, and if one of these is not a psychiatrist, then a clinical psychologist is a minimum requirement (Loeser 1991). The staffing structure of our clinic, representing one medical specialty, nursing, and four other allied health specialties, including clinical psychology, is more in keeping with established multidisciplinary practice models of health services for older people. All clinicians are trained in geriatric care. The clinic's physicians are geriatricians with training in pain medicine. Access to other medical specialists is readily available upon referral, but they do not constitute part of the core staffing because they do not attend the interdisciplinary team meetings. The absence of an anesthetist as a key staff member is a distinctive feature of the clinic. The small number of patients requiring referral elsewhere for anesthetic interventions may reflect awareness by referring physicians of the services available within the clinic, rather than implying the absence of the need for interventional procedural skills within pain clinics for older persons.

EVIDENCE OF EFFICACY

The comprehensive geriatric assessment emerged as a means to improve the care of frail elderly patients with complex medical, psychosocial, and functional problems who are at risk of cognitive and physical decline, hospitalization, institutionalization, and death. Comprehensive geriatric assessment has been subject to extensive analysis over the past 20 years. Early, single-site evaluations of specialist inpatient units revealed dramatic improvements in survival and functional status when compared with usual care (Rubenstein et al. 1984). A recent study of inpatient and outpatient comprehensive geriatric assessment and management programs reported improvements in physical functioning and the quality of life at no additional cost over usual care, but no significant differences in mortality (Cohen et al. 2002; Kuo et al. 2004). Meta-analysis of 28 controlled trials showed favorable results using a comprehensive multidisciplinary approach in both hospital and outpatient settings (Stuck et al. 1993). The magnitude of benefit of this approach over usual care has become less dramatic over time (Landefeld 2003), which may be related to the adoption of aspects of the practices of geriatric care as an integral part of usual patient care (Cohen et al. 2002; Rubenstein and Rubenstein 2003). The benefit of comprehensive geriatric care is strongest when clinicians maintain long-term control, ensuring that management plans are sustained (Stuck et al. 1993).

The MPC for older adults is an amalgam of the multidisciplinary practices of geriatric care and pain management. Although total eradication of pain is infrequently achieved with multidisciplinary pain programs across all age groups, the evidence suggests that this approach is superior to usual management in reducing the severity of pain. Meta-analysis of multidisciplinary treatment for chronic low back pain revealed a mean pain reduction of 37%, although the majority of patients continued to experience considerable pain (Flor et al. 1992). No single criterion can accurately capture the complexity of persistent pain or adequately measure the outcome of pain management interventions. Evaluation of multidisciplinary pain management requires a broader approach. Several reviews and meta-analyses have evaluated the clinical and cost-effectiveness of multidisciplinary approaches over conventional approaches. Multidisciplinary treatments are reported to be superior to no treatment and to being on a waiting list, as well as to single-discipline treatments such as medical treatment or physical therapy (Flor et al. 1992). The outcome data generally support the validity of employing a range of criteria, including pain intensity, level of function, alleviation of depression, and measures of health care consumption. Decrease in analgesic consumption often accompanies evidence of improvement on these measures (Guzman et al. 2001; Turk 2002). However, many of the published studies do not include subjects older than working age (Guzman et al. 2001).

The limited numbers of publications that include data on older adults attending pain management clinics provide inconsistent results (Gagliese et al. 1999). Some studies report worse outcomes compared with younger patients, whereas others report that the elderly derive substantial benefit. Gibson and colleagues (1996) concluded that 10 out of 13 studies showed some benefit of a multidisciplinary approach for older people with chronic pain. Studies that report a reduced degree of benefit in older compared to younger patients should not be taken as evidence that participation has not been of significant benefit to older individuals. Whether outcomes are worthwhile for older individuals is more relevant than cumulative age-related outcome data relativities. The exclusion of older adults from multidisciplinary pain management programs cannot be supported on the available evidence.

Multidisciplinary pain management programs usually comprise medical, physical, and cognitive-behavioral components. Meta-analysis of 25 controlled trials of cognitive-behavioral therapy (CBT) for chronic pain revealed significant benefits in pain experience, mood/affect, cognitive coping, pain behavior, activity level, and social function when compared with waiting-list controls. The average age in these studies was 48.6 years (Morley et al. 1999). CBT appears equally efficacious whether delivered individually or in a group program (Turner-Stokes et al. 2003). Young and older adults benefit equally from outpatient CBT for chronic pain (Puder 1988; Middaugh and Pawlick 2002). CBT has also been demonstrated to be efficacious for nursing home residents with chronic pain, including those with mild cognitive impairment (Cook 1998). Therefore, age and frailty do not appear to preclude older adults from benefiting from a CBT program.

Age-related physiological changes and concurrent medical conditions limit the ability of older individuals to participate in demanding physical exercise programs. There is some evidence that low-intensity physical programs are of equal effectiveness to intensive physical programs on return-to-work rates among patients with persistent back pain, although this is not a consistent finding (Guzman et al. 2001; Skouen et al. 2002). In older adults, physical exercise programs have been demonstrated to have general health benefits as well as specific benefits for those with chronic pain. Exercise programs not only reduce pain associated with arthritis, but also delay the decline in physical function within an aged population. They reduce the risk of dying from all causes, and specifically from cardiovascular disease; they also improve body composition, lessen the number of falls, and reduce depression (Christmas and Andersen 2000). Exercise programs can be developed with little risk of major injury or of exacerbating joint symptoms (Coleman et al. 1996).

Adverse drug reactions and drug-drug interactions are common in older patients. The employment of nonpharmacological approaches such as physical and psychological therapies may reduce reliance on medications, and hence lower the risk of adverse drug reactions. Nevertheless, older patients with persistent pain tend to be offered fewer treatment options in general, and in particular they are less likely to be offered behavioral and nonpharmacological therapies (Kee et al. 1998). The benefit of programs offering combinations of pharmacological, physical, and cognitive-behavioral therapies is believed to be greater than the sum of the individual components.

DISCUSSION

Persistent pain is common in older people and is associated with numerous consequences including depression, anxiety, decreased socialization, impaired ambulation, and increased health care utilization. It is often unrecognized and undertreated, particularly among residents of nursing homes and in those with dementia and other disorders that impair communication. In most cases, primary care clinicians working in collaboration with other health care professionals can adequately manage pain. Clinical guidelines are available to assist clinicians (AGS Clinical Practice Committee 1997; AGS Panel on Persistent Pain in Older Persons 2002). There remain, however, large numbers of people who continue to suffer with persistent pain for whom referral to a specialist service is indicated.

Recognition that single-modality interventions are often inadequate for dealing with the complexity of persistent pain has led to the proliferation of MPCs. Given the increasing prevalence of pain in older adults, the number of seniors attending MPCs is less than would be expected. Older patients do respond to multidisciplinary pain management approaches. Regardless of the magnitude of benefit when compared with that in younger adults, the gains in pain control, mobility, function, and reduction of unnecessary medications are nevertheless of significant benefit to the older person. Few pain clinics have specifically focused on older adults, and other clinics remain reluctant to admit older patients. Exclusion criteria such as an absence of vocational goals and the presence of concurrent medical problems are powerful barriers against the admission of older patients, particularly the frail elderly.

The amalgamation of the specialties of aged care and pain medicine into one service has created an effective way to deal with the complex interaction of persistent pain, concurrent medical problems, and functional and psychosocial issues, thereby providing a model of care that goes beyond the expertise of the component specialties working in isolation. However, dedicated pain management clinics for older adults have not proliferated in the manner observed following the establishment of the first MPC by Bonica in the 1960s, which raises two rhetorical questions. First, is the MPC the best model for the management of complex pain problems in older adults? Evidence to answer this question definitively is currently not available, so the development of alternate models of care for this population continues to warrant exploration and evaluation. Second, what should be the future direction of pain clinics for older people? The answer to this question may come from the recent history of comprehensive geriatric evaluation services. Initial studies of these services revealed dramatic improvements compared with conventional care. Over time, the techniques of specialized aged care units infiltrated standard care, diminishing the magnitude of differences between specialist aged services and conventional care. Global demographic changes are occurring so rapidly that aged care services are not expanding at the same rate as the growth in numbers of their potential patients. Instead, health services are focusing on the development of new models of care and on education, training, and research. In a similar vein, the expansion of age-specific pain management clinics is not expected to keep pace with the growth of the aged population.

The overwhelming majority of older people with persistent pain will never have access to a specialized pain management clinic. In most cases, primary care clinicians utilizing a multidisciplinary approach will be able to effectively manage these individuals. Specialized pain management clinics for older adults are likely to be beneficial for the management of the sub-population of patients with the most complex problems, including such individuals in nursing homes. Hence, aged care services should consider including multidisciplinary pain management within their portfolio.

In addition, current barriers that hinder older adults from accessing the many well-established MPCs need to be broken down. However, simply accepting older adults into programs designed for a younger, more physically robust population with different goals is bound to fail. These clinics will need to develop expertise and modify their processes to better target the needs of older and frailer patient groups. As well as providing a referral destination for the subpopulation of elderly patients with the most complex problems, specialized pain management clinics for older adults may be capable of offering collaboration and support to assist other MPCs in achieving these ends. In addition, specialized MPCs for older adults offer a crucial capability for education, training, and research.

Future development of pain services for older adults may be as a distinct clinical stream that is a component of a large, non-age-specific MPC, or alternately as a component of an aged care service. Ongoing examination of clinical efficacy and cost-effectiveness should be undertaken using agreed data and outcome measures that are appropriate for use in MPCs for older patients as well as for older patients attending non-age-specific MPCs. The IASP and affiliated national pain societies may need to review the guidelines on the desirable characteristics of pain management facilities to ensure that the needs of older patients can be met. This undertaking would benefit from collaboration with national geriatric medicine societies.

REFERENCES

AGS Clinical Practice Committee. Management of cancer pain in older patients. *J Am Geriatr Soc* 1997; 45:1273–1276.

AGS Panel on Persistent Pain in Older Persons. The management of persistent pain in older persons. *J Am Geriatr Soc* 2002; 50:S205–214.

Bogduk N. Management of chronic low back pain. *Med J Aust* 2004; 180:79–83.

Christmas C, Andersen RA. Exercise and older patients: guidelines for the clinician. *J Am Geriatr Soc* 2000; 48:318–324.

Cleeland CS, Gonin R, Hatfield AK, et al. Pain and its treatment in outpatients with metastatic cancer. *N Engl J Med* 1994; 330:592–596.

Cohen JH, Feussner JR, Weinberger M, et al. A controlled trial of inpatient and outpatient geriatric evaluation and management. *N Engl J Med* 2002; 346:905–912.

Coleman EA, Buchner DM, Cress ME, et al. The relationship of joint symptoms with exercise performance in older adults. *J Am Geriatr Soc* 1996; 44:14–21.

Cook AJ. Cognitive-behavioral pain management for elderly nursing home residents. *J Gerontol C Psychol Soc Sci* 1998; 1:51–59.

Corran TM, Farrell MJ, Helme RD, Gibson SJ. The classification of patients with chronic pain: age as a contributing factor. *Clin J Pain* 1997; 13:207–214.

Elkan R, Kendrick D, Dewey M, et al. Effectiveness of home based support for older people: systemic review and meta-analysis. *BMJ* 2001; 323:1–9.

Farrell MJ, Katz B, Helme RD. The impact of dementia on the pain experience. *Pain* 1996; 67:7–15.

Field TS, Gurwitz JH, Harrold LR, et al. Risk factors for adverse drug events among older adults in the ambulatory setting. *J Am Geriatr Soc* 2004; 52:1349–1354.

Fix A, Daughton D. *Human Activity Profile: Professional Manual.* Odessa, FL: Psychological Assessment Resources, 1988.

Flor H, Fydrich T, Turk DC. Efficacy of multidisciplinary pain treatment centers: a meta-analytic review. *Pain* 1992; 49:221–230.

Folstein MF, Folstein SE, McHugh PR. "Mini-Mental State": a practical method for grading the cognitive state of patients for the clinician. *J Psych Res* 1975; 12:189–198.

Gagliese L, Katz J, Melzack R. Pain in the elderly. In Wall PD, Melzack R (Eds). *Textbook of Pain,* 4th ed. London: Churchill Livingstone, 1999, pp 991–1006.

Gibson SJ. Pain and aging: the pain experience over the adult life span. In: Dostrovsky JO, Carr DB, Koltzenburg M (Eds). *Proceedings of the 10th World Congress on Pain,* Progress in Pain Research and Management, Vol. 24. Seattle: IASP Press, 2003, pp 767–790.

Gibson SJ, Farrell MJ, Katz B, Helme RD. Multidisciplinary management of chronic nonmalignant pain in older adults. In: Ferrell BR, Ferrell BA (Eds). *Pain in the Elderly.* Seattle: IASP Press, 1996, pp 91–99.

Guzman J, Esmail R, Karjalainen K, et al. Multidisciplinary rehabilitation for chronic low back pain: systematic review. *BMJ* 2001; 322:1511–1516.

Harkins SW, Price DD. Assessment of pain in the elderly. In: Turk DC, Melzack R (Eds). *Handbook of Pain Assessment.* New York: Guilford Press, 1992, pp 315–331.

Helme RD, Gibson SJ. Pain in the elderly. In: Jensen TS, Turner JA, Wiesenfeld-Hallin Z (Eds). *Proceedings of the 8th World Congress on Pain,* Progress in Pain Research and Management, Vol. 8. Seattle: IASP Press, 1997, pp 191–944.

Helme RD, Gibson SJ. Pain in older people. In: Crombie IK, Croft PR, Linton SJ, LeResche L, Von Korff M (Eds). *Epidemiology of Chronic Pain.* Seattle: IASP Press, 1999, pp 103–112.

Helme RD, Katz B. Chronic pain in the elderly. In: Jensen TS, Wilson PR, Rice AS (Eds). *Clinical Pain Management, Chronic Pain.* London: Arnold, 2003, pp 649–660.

Helme RD, Katz B, Neufeld M, et al. The establishment of a geriatric pain clinic—a preliminary report of the first 100 patients. *Aust J Ageing* 1989; 8:27–30.

Helme RD, Katz B, Gibson SJ, et al. Multidisciplinary pain clinics for older people. Do they have a role? *Clin Geriatr Med* 1996; 12(3):563–582.

Katz SK, Ford AB, Moskowitz RW, et al. Studies of illness in the aged: the index of ADL: a standardized measure of biological and psychosocial function. *JAMA* 1963; 185:94–99.

Kee WD, Middaugh SJ, Redpath S, Hargadon R. Age as a factor in admission to chronic pain rehabilitation. *Clin J Pain* 1998; 14(2):121–128.

Kuo HK, Scandrett KG, Dave J, Mitchell SL. The influence of outpatient comprehensive geriatric assessment on survival: a meta-analysis. *Arch Gerontol Geriatr* 2004; 39:245–254.

Landefeld CS. Improving health care for older persons. *Ann Intern Med* 2003; 139:421–424.

Lawton MP, Brody E. Assessment of older people: self-maintaining and instrumental activities of daily living. *Gerontologist* 1969; 9:179–186.

Loeser JD. Desirable characteristics for pain treatment facilities: report of the IASP taskforce. In: Bond MR, Charlton JE, Woolf CJ (Eds). *Proceedings of the VIth World Congress on Pain.* Amsterdam: Elsevier, 1991, pp 411–415.

Mahoney FI, Barthel DW. Functional evaluation: the Barthel Index. *Md State Med J* 1965; 14:61–65.

Middaugh SJ, Pawlick K. Biofeedback and behavioural treatment of persistent pain in the older adult: a review and study. *Appl Psychophysiol Biofeedback* 2002; 3:185–202.

Morley S, Eccleston C, Williams A. Systemic review and meta-analysis of randomized controlled trials of cognitive behaviour therapy and behaviour therapy for chronic pain in adults, excluding headaches. *Pain* 1999; 80:1–13.

Puder RS. Age analysis of cognitive-behavioral group therapy for chronic pain outpatients. *Psychol Aging* 1988; 2:204–207.

Rubenstein LZ, Rubenstein LV. Multidimensional geriatric assessment. In: Tallis RC, Fillit HM (Eds). *Brocklehurst's Textbook of Geriatric Medicine and Gerontology,* 6th ed. London: Churchill Livingstone, 2003, pp 291–300.

Rubenstein LZ, Josephson KR, Wieland GD, et al. Effectiveness of a geriatric evaluation unit: a randomized clinical trial. *N Engl J Med* 1984; 311:1664–1670.

Skouen JS, Grasdal AL, Haldorsen EMH, Ursin H. Relative cost-effectiveness of extensive and light multidisciplinary treatment programs versus treatment as usual for patients with chronic low back pain on long-term sick leave. *Spine* 2002; 27:901–910.

Stuck AE, Siu AL, Wieland GD, Adams J, Rubenstein LZ. Comprehensive geriatric assessment: a meta-analysis of controlled trials. *Lancet* 1993; 342:1032–1036.

Tinetti ME. Preventing falls in elderly persons. *N Engl J Med* 2003; 348:42–49.

Turk DC. Clinical effectiveness and cost-effectiveness of treatments for patients with chronic pain. *Clin J Pain* 2002; 18:355–365.

Turner-Stokes L, Erkeller-Yuksel F, Miles A, et al. Outpatient cognitive behavioural pain management programs: a randomized comparison of group-based multidisciplinary versus an individual therapy model. *Arch Phys Med Rehabil* 2003; 84:781–788.

Weiner DK. Improving pain management for older adults: an urgent agenda for the educator, investigator, and practitioner. *Pain* 2002; 97:1–4.

Weiner DK, Rudy TE, Gaur S. Are all older adults with persistent pain created equal? Preliminary evidence for a multiaxial taxonomy. *Pain Res Manage* 2001; 6:133–141.

Wolf-Klein GP, Silverstone FA, Levy AP, Brod MS. Screening for Alzheimer's disease by clock drawing. *J Am Geriatr Soc* 1989; 37:730–736.

Yong HH, Gibson SJ, Horne DJ, Helme RD. Development of a pain attitudes questionnaire to assess stoicism and cautiousness for possible age differences. *J Gerontol B Psychol Sci Soc Sci* 2001; 56:279–284.

Correspondence to: Benny Katz, MBBS, FRACP, FFPMANZCA, 10 Clarke Street, Prahran, Victoria 3181, Australia. Fax: 61-3-9496-2613; email: bkatz@ connexus.net.au.

Part V

Common Painful Disorders in Older Adults: Disorder-Specific Approaches to Evaluation and Treatment

Pain in Older Persons, Progress in Pain
Research and Management, Vol. 35, edited
by Stephen J. Gibson and Debra K. Weiner,
IASP Press, Seattle, © 2005.

16

Low Back Pain and Its Contributors in Older Adults: A Practical Approach to Evaluation and Treatment

Debra K. Weiner and Danelle Cayea

*Division of Geriatric Medicine, Department of Medicine, University
of Pittsburgh; Pain Evaluation and Treatment Institute, University
of Pittsburgh Medical Center, Pittsburgh, Pennsylvania, USA*

Musculoskeletal disorders are responsible for the vast majority of older adults' persistent pain burden worldwide (Helme and Gibson 2001; Leveille 2004). While osteoarthritis (OA) is commonly cited as the main offender, soft tissue disorders such as myofascial pain and fibromyalgia also are extremely common. It is estimated that as many as 1 in 14 women aged 60–79 suffer from fibromyalgia (Wolfe et al. 1995), and myofascial pain occurs in most chronic pain sufferers (Han and Harrison 1997). Despite these facts, primary care providers are poorly trained in musculoskeletal pain evaluation and management (Weiner et al. 2005c), and these disorders often go undiagnosed and untreated, with only a small fraction of older patients being referred to interdisciplinary pain clinics (Harkins et al. 1984; Kee et al. 1998; Helme 2001).

Low back pain (LBP), clearly one of the most therapeutically challenging musculoskeletal disorders from which older adults suffer, is the focus of this chapter. While the Agency for Healthcare Research and Quality has established guidelines for the evaluation and management of acute LBP (Bigos et al. 1994), recommendations about persistent LBP are conspicuously absent. When evaluating the older adult with persistent LBP, the practitioner should keep the following assumptions in mind so as to devise the most effective treatment strategies. (1) LBP in older adults is often caused by more than one pathological contributor. (2) While several musculoskeletal conditions may be identified in the older adult with persistent LBP (e.g., OA, scoliosis, osteoporosis, lumbar spinal stenosis, and leg length discrepancy), it is incumbent upon the practitioner to prioritize treatment efforts by identifying those that are incidental, those that are directly responsible for symptoms, and those that are currently asymptomatic but in need of management in order to avoid future complications. (3) Persistence of pain despite previous treatment efforts in older adults with LBP may be indicative of treatment misguidance as much as treatment recalcitrance.

EPIDEMIOLOGY

Low back pain is prevalent in community-dwelling older adults, is among the leading reasons for physician visits (Hart et al. 1995), and is associated with increased risk of physical disability and psychosocial disruption (Carey et al. 1995; Becker et al. 1997; Gill et al. 2001; Reid et al. 2003). An estimated 36% of community-dwelling older adults have experienced an episode of LBP during the prior year, and 21% of these individuals report experiencing moderate to severe pain that occurs very often or more (Weiner et al. 2003). We recently reviewed U.S. outpatient Medicare claims related to LBP over the past decade, and found a 132% increase in the number of claims, with a 387% increase in associated charges (Weiner et al. 2005a). Studies have estimated that 6 million older adults in the United States alone experience recurrent episodes of LBP (Lawrence et al. 1998), but the prevalence of persistent LBP (i.e., that which persists for at least 3 months) among older adults is unknown.

ETIOLOGY AND EVALUATION

Persistent LBP is complex and is often attributed to idiopathic causes (Jarvik and Deyo 2002). One or more physical contributors, however, can typically be diagnosed. A multitude of pathologies (e.g., osteoporosis, degenerative disk disease, lumbar spinal stenosis, and scoliosis) can often be identified in the older adult with persistent LBP. In order to design cost-effective and clinically effective treatment, the first step in evaluation is separating the wheat from the chaff, that is, differentiating pain-causing pathology from incidental pathology.

An overview of one approach to evaluating and treating the older adult with LBP in provided in Fig. 1. A carefully performed history and physical examination is clearly the first step, and often the only necessary diagnostic step, in evaluating the older adult with persistent LBP. The vast majority of important diagnostic clues can be obtained from a targeted history. The

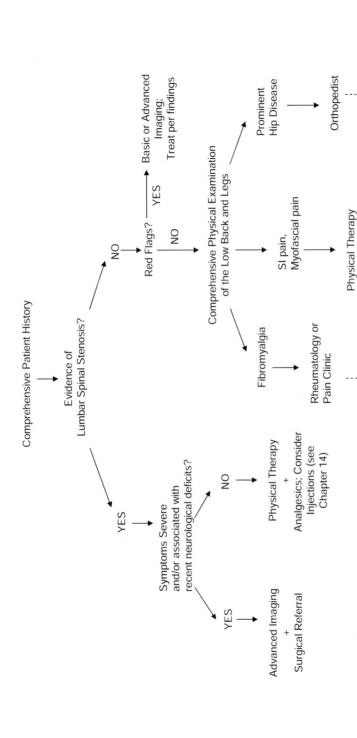

Fig. 1. Evaluation and treatment of the older adult with persistent low back pain.

questions in Table I should be asked routinely of older adults with low back pain with or without accompanying leg pain. The conditions that in our experience can be culled by this series of questions are lumbar spinal stenosis, myofascial pathology of the piriformis and/or tensor fascia lata (with or without pain of the iliotibial [IT] band), sciatica, fibromyalgia, sacroiliac (SI) joint syndrome, and hip arthritis. The approach to treatment of these disorders will be discussed below.

The poor correlation between imaging abnormalities, both basic (i.e., X-ray) and advanced (e.g., magnetic resonance imaging [MRI]), and clinical

Table I
Essential clinic history questions for older adults with persistent
mechanical low back and leg pain

Question	Potential Diagnostic Clue(s) Obtained
1. Can you show me where your back hurts?	If patient places hand to right or left of midline, over sacrum rather than lumbar spine, this suggests sacroiliac joint syndrome (look for associated scoliosis, hip and/or knee disease, leg length discrepancy), inflammatory disorder, or sacral insufficiency fracture.
2. Does the pain get better or worse when you curl up in bed?	Improvement in fetal position suggests spinal stenosis. Worsening in fetal position suggests sacroiliac disease because of joint compression in this position.
3. Does the pain go into your buttocks? If "yes,": Is the pain sharp or dull?	Buttocks involvement can be associated with hip disease, piriformis myofascial pain (often sharp or burning), or spinal stenosis and requires contextual evaluation.
4. Do you have pain in your groin?	Groin pain can be associated with intrinsic hip disease, local myofascial pathology, sacroiliac joint syndrome, or an insufficiency fracture.
5. Does the pain shoot down your leg(s)? If "yes,": In what part of your leg do you feel the pain? Is the pain sharp or dull?	Posterior radiation is consistent with sciatica (sharp) or spinal stenosis (dull). Lateral thigh radiation suggests tensor fascia lata/iliotibial band pain (not past the knee) or gluteus minimus (past the knee "pseudo-sciatica") myofascial pain. Lateral leg pain with paresthesias or numbness suggests L5 radiculopathy. Anterior thigh pain suggests hip disease, meralgia paresthetica, quadriceps strain with knee OA, or L2/3/4 radiculopathy.
6. Is the pain made better or worse with walking?	Worsening with walking suggests spinal stenosis or vasogenic claudication. Improvement with walking suggests myofascial pathology or neuropathic pain. Prolonged walking may worsen myofascial pain. Degenerative disease may be associated with initial pain/stiffness, then improvement and worsening with excessive use.
7. Do you sometimes feel that you have pain all over?	Patients with fibromyalgia syndrome often have prominent axial pain, and may present with a chief complaint of severe low back pain, but in fact LBP is just one of many sites of pain.

symptoms has been well documented. Degenerative lumbosacral pathology is nearly ubiquitous in older adults, whether or not pain is present (Weiner et al. 1994). The finding of central canal stenosis on MRI is also not limited to those with pain, with one small study demonstrating a 21% prevalence of spinal stenosis in pain-free individuals over the age of 60 (Boden et al. 1990). Another study that included those up to age 70 found that age was an independent predictor of degenerative changes, spondylolisthesis, and moderate to severe central stenosis (Jarvik at al., 2001). Thus, premature ordering of imaging studies, with reliance on their often nonspecific findings to guide treatment, may lead to inappropriate utilization of health care resources (e.g., surgical intervention for incidental spinal stenosis) and prolonged patient suffering. Whether this practice has contributed to the substantial incidence of failed back surgery syndrome is unknown. Unless there are red flags regarding the possible presence of ominous pathology such as infection, fracture, or malignancy, or unless surgery is being contemplated (e.g., in the older adult with intractable pain related to lumbar spinal stenosis), imaging should probably be avoided. Practitioners should also be aware that occasionally patients might present with typical symptoms of lumbar spinal stenosis without supportive findings on advanced imaging. In such cases, the use of axial loading techniques may enhance imaging sensitivity (Danielson et al. 1998).

Determining whether red flags exist in the older adult with LBP, that is, serious disorders that require definitive and immediate specialized treatment (e.g., disk space infection, spinal cord compression, or malignancy) is not as straightforward as in younger patients. Weight loss, for example, may be associated with a variety of comorbidities in the older patient such as extraspinal infection (e.g., urinary tract infection), malignancy, depression, failure to thrive, dysgeusia or anorexia associated with new medications, temporal arteritis, and apathetic hyperthyroidism. The same holds true for fever, another potential LBP red flag. It is important, therefore, to determine the temporal relationship between LBP and these other symptoms before embarking on a costly evaluation. Plain films should be obtained if pathology is suspected that does not require advanced imaging (e.g., pathological or nonpathological fracture), or if pathology is suspected that is most appropriately detected with plain radiographs (e.g., multiple myeloma). If the practitioner does not suspect serious nondegenerative, nonbiomechanical pathology or refractory lumbar spinal stenosis that requires surgery, evaluation should focus on a careful and comprehensive physical examination of the back and lower extremities.

Comprehensive physical examination of the older adult with LBP should include examination of the SI joints (direct palpation and Patrick's test), palpation of the lumbar paravertebral muscles, piriformis, and tensor fascia lata for myofascial findings (see below); palpation of the IT band for tightness and pain; palpation for fibromyalgia tender points; evaluation for leg length discrepancy; and assessment of intrinsic hip motion and associated pain. When evaluating the older adult with persistent LBP, the practitioner must also be mindful of the possibility of pain comorbidities, such as knee or hip arthritis, that exacerbate SI joint syndrome. Knee arthritis also contributes to myofascial pain of the tensor fascia lata and pain of the IT band. Only by performing such a comprehensive examination can the clinician prescribe optimal treatment.

We recently surveyed 111 older adults (mean age 74.8 years; 58.6% female) with persistent LBP of at least moderate intensity and a mean duration of 13.2 years. Using a structured physical examination, we found that 77.5% had scoliosis, 83.6% had pain on palpation or maneuver of the SI joint, and 95.5% had myofascial pathology (Weiner et al. 2005b). These findings suggest that soft tissue and biomechanical abnormalities, only detectable by careful physical examination, often underlie persistent LBP. While our observations require corroboration by formal investigation, we believe that overt recognition of contributory biomechanical and soft tissue pathology in older adults with low back pain, with or without leg pain, may save patients from unnecessary imaging studies that lead to misguided and ineffective treatment efforts.

DISORDERS THAT COMMONLY CONTRIBUTE TO LOW BACK PAIN IN OLDER ADULTS

While Occam's razor, i.e., the law of parsimony, is generally sound, its application to the older adult with persistent LBP can be hazardous. According to our experience at the University of Pittsburgh's Older Adult Pain Management Program, LBP in older adults is often caused by a combination of pathologies. For example, we commonly see older patients with a combination of scoliosis, SI joint syndrome, and myofascial pain involving the piriformis with associated sciatica, or involving the tensor fascia lata/IT band with burning pain of the lateral thigh that may be misinterpreted as radicular pathology. Alternatively, the patient with low back and leg pain in the setting of MRI-documented central canal stenosis may have pain attributable to a combination of mechanical low back factors and hip arthritis. Or, consider the 89-year old patient recently seen in our clinic with leg, then back pain, who had a deep venous thrombosis that altered her gait and caused SI pain in the setting of degenerative scoliosis. Thus, comprehensive assessment followed by appropriate treatment tailoring is likely to result in the best therapeutic response, although randomized controlled trials in older adults have not been performed. The most common LBP disorders that we have seen at our center are discussed below. Table II summarizes the treatments for these disorders, with more detailed discussion provided in other chapters of this text.

Table II
Treatment of common disorders that contribute to low back pain
with or without leg pain in older adults

Disorder	Suggested Treatment
Degenerative disk/ facet disease	Oral analgesics (see Chapter 11)
	Physical therapy (see Chapter 12)
	Selected injections (e.g., facets, nerve blocks; see Chapter 14)
	PENS (See Chapter 15)
Lumbar spinal stenosis	Physical therapy (see Chapter 12)
	Oral analgesics (see Chapter 11)
	Consider epidural corticosteroids (no controlled trials)
	PENS (see Chapter 15)
	Surgery for severe, refractory symptoms
Fibromyalgia syndrome	Aerobic exercise
	Oral analgesics
	Tricyclic antidepressants
	Medications for other accompanying symptoms (e.g., fatigue, depression, anxiety)
	Multidisciplinary pain clinic referral for refractory cases to learn activity pacing, cognitive-behavioral therapy techniques (see Chapter 16)
	Acupuncture (see Chapter 15)
Myofascial pain	Physical therapy for gentle stretching, massage, heat, TENS, interferential current, etc. (see Chapter 12)
	Trigger point injections (see Chapter 14)
	Use systemic analgesics sparingly
	Consider gabapentin for neuropathic myofascial pain
	Acupuncture (see Chapter 15)
Sacroiliac (SI) joint syndrome	Physical therapy for stretching, strengthening, and stabilizing pelvic and surrounding musculature
	Oral analgesics (see Chapter 11)
	Injection of SI joint (see Chapter 14)
	Consider shoe lift for leg length discrepancy
Hip and knee arthritis	If mild-moderate, optimize oral analgesics, consider joint injection, physical therapy, assistive device.
	If severe and refractory to other treatment efforts, orthopedic referral for consideration of joint replacement.

AXIAL AND APPENDICULAR OSTEOARTHRITIS

Background and epidemiology.   Degenerative disk and facet disease is nearly universal in people 65 and older, regardless of pain status. One small study demonstrated that 100% of 35 older adults who were pain free and had no history of LBP had radiographic evidence of degenerative disk and/or facet disease (Weiner et al. 1994). Degenerative lumbar spinal stenosis, according to another small study, occurs not uncommonly in pain-free individuals, with a prevalence rate of 21% in adults 60 and older; 36% of these asymptomatic individuals showed herniated nucleus pulposus (Boden et al. 1990).

Because of the generalized nature of OA, non-lumbosacral degenerative pathology such as knee and hip arthritis must be taken into account when evaluating the older adult with LBP. Gait alterations caused by painful lower-extremity arthritis may lead to a variety of adverse consequences including strain of the SI joint and surrounding structures, pain of the tensor fascia lata/IT band, postural instability associated with a risk of falling, and physical disability (Thomas et al. 2004). Thus, clinicians should routinely examine the hips and knees when evaluating the older adult with LBP and/or lower-extremity pain.

Approach to evaluation.   Clinical history, physical examination, and assessment of pain and functional status lie at the core of evaluating older adults with axial and appendicular OA. For patients with hip or knee OA, the American College of Rheumatology (ACR) also recommends X-rays in the setting of worsening pain and/or functional status if none have been performed during the prior 3 months (Pencharz and MacLean 2004). As mentioned above, the evaluation of lumbosacral degenerative disease should be even more conservative, focusing on a thorough history and physical examination. Basic radiographs should be obtained if non-degenerative pathology is suspected (e.g., an osteoporotic compression fracture). Advanced imaging should be avoided unless red flags are uncovered at the time of the history, or if surgery is being contemplated, as the specificity of MRIs is low, with some estimates as low as 72% (Jarvik and Deyo 2002). Investigators have attempted to develop non-radiographic procedures to assist with the diagnosis of lumbar spinal stenosis. One such procedure, the two-stage treadmill test, has been shown to have excellent test-retest reliability (Deen et al. 2000); it correctly classifies patients with lumbar spinal stenosis 76.9% of the time (Fritz et al. 1997).

Approach to treatment.   Treatment of both axial and appendicular OA should be approached in a step care manner, as illustrated in Fig. 2, a scheme that we use to guide treatment at our pain management center for older adults. Details on the pharmacokinetics, dosing, side effects, and drug-

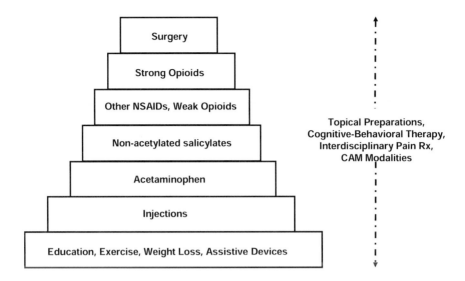

Fig. 2. Stepped care approach to the treatment of axial and appendicular osteoarthritis. CAM = complementary and alternative medicine.

drug and drug-disease interactions of oral analgesics can be found in Chapter 10 and in guidelines published by the American Geriatrics Society Panel on Persistent Pain in Older Persons (2002).

Step 1. At the foundation of OA treatment is patient education as well as prescription of weight loss, exercise, and assistive devices. The American Geriatrics Society Panel on Exercise and Osteoarthritis recently published guidelines on exercise prescription for older adults with OA (2001). For additional information on the benefits of exercise, the reader is also referred to Chapter 11.

Step 2 (injections). (a) For appendicular OA, if the source of pain is well-localized and easily accessible (e.g., in the knee or finger), we feel that corticosteroid injection should be seriously considered as the next step. While studies indicate that corticosteroid efficacy is relatively modest and short-lived (Dieppe et al. 1980; Raynauld et al. 2003), their low side-effect profile and sometimes prolonged efficacy supports their use early on in the course of treatment. The use of local corticosteroids also has scientific underpinnings because of data indicating the underlying inflammatory pathogenesis of OA (Martel-Pelletier et al. 1999; Abramson et al. 2001; Pincus 2001; Hedbom and Hauselmann 2002; Sowers et al. 2002; Haywood et al. 2003). Intra-articular injection of hyaluronic acid has met with mixed results (Brandt et al. 2000; Felson and Anderson 2002). (b) For axial OA, the value of injection procedures for degenerative lumbosacral pathology has not been

rigorously studied, although suggestions regarding how to rationally prescribe these modalities can be found in Chapter 13. Evidence supports the
efficacy of epidural corticosteroid injections for the treatment of acute
radicular pain caused by a herniated disk (Watts and Silagy 1995), although
this scenario represents a very small subset of older adults with LBP.

Step 3 (acetaminophen). In the absence of contraindications, acetaminophen is the first-line oral analgesic for the treatment of OA associated
with pain of mild to moderate severity, and this drug should not be considered a treatment failure until an adequate maximum-dose trial has been
implemented.

Step 4 (non-acetylated salicylates). This class of medications has been
shown to have a superior side-effect profile to nonspecific cyclooxygenase
(COX) agents (Mielants et al. 1984; Bianchi et al. 1989; Lanza et al. 1989;
Roth et al. 1990; Fries et al. 1991; Larkai et al. 1997), although a comparative trial with COX-2 drugs has not been performed. When non-acetylated
salicylates are used in moderate analgesic doses, nephrotoxicity is not an
issue, unless an idiosyncratic hypersensitivity response occurs. Although
they are less potent prostaglandin inhibitors than the COX inhibitors, because of their favorable safety profile, strong consideration should be given
to their use in the event of acetaminophen failure.

Step 5 (other NSAIDs and weak opioids). Medications in this class include propoxyphene, codeine, hydrocodone, and tramadol. The medications
in this class that we use most often are hydrocodone and tramadol. Some
would advocate that other nonsteroidal anti-inflammatory drugs (NSAIDs)
should be tried before opioids and, therefore, included in Step 4. We believe, however, that this decision should be weighed on a case-by-case basis.
Depending upon a particular patient's comorbidities, the potential side-effect profile of weak opioids might well be preferable to that of NSAIDs.

Step 6 (strong opioids). Because of the associated risk of falls (Shorr et
al. 1992; Weiner et al. 1998), a thorough evaluation of mobility should be
performed on all older adults with persistent pain in whom opioid prescription is being considered. A physical therapist should be involved to facilitate
mobility and stability enhancement (e.g., prescription of an assistive device)
for those with impairments. Prescribing details and side effects of opioids
are discussed in Chapter 10.

Step 7 (surgery). A comprehensive discussion of surgical options for
older adults with appendicular and axial OA is beyond the scope of this
chapter. In general, total joint replacement is considered after non-invasive
strategies have failed to control severe pain. Guidelines regarding when to
pursue surgical treatment for refractory LBP are less clear. The number of
spine surgeons in a population strongly predicts spine surgery rates (Deyo

and Tsui-Wu 1987), and the risk of failed back surgery syndrome is substantive, with estimates ranging from 5% to 40% (Hirsch and Nachemson 1963; Law et al. 1963; Davis 1994; Malter et al. 1998; Keskimaki et al. 2000; Yorimitsu et al. 2001; Osterman et al. 2003). Studies to determine the comparative efficacy of physical therapy versus decompressive laminectomy for the treatment of lumbar spinal stenosis are ongoing. Delay of surgery following an initial conservative approach has not been shown to impair ultimate surgical response in elective cases (Johnsson et al. 1991; Amundsen et al. 2000; Simotas et al. 2000). Preliminary data are available that predict poor outcomes following surgery in the case of scoliosis (Frazier et al. 1997); prior surgical intervention, diabetes mellitus, hip arthrosis, preoperative lumbar fracture (Airaksinen et al. 1997); and absence of lower extremity symptoms and symptom duration greater than 4 years (Jonsson et al. 1997). Well-controlled studies are needed to provide better guidance in this area. It has been shown that self-rated health and comorbidity predict response to surgical intervention (Katz et al. 1999) and that age per se does not (Ragab et al. 2003; Vitaz et al. 1999; Hee and Wong 2003). It has also been suggested that severe symptoms generally predict a more favorable response with surgery (Atlas et al. 2000).

Other modalities. A variety of other modalities can be considered for the treatment of pain in the context of axial and appendicular OA, including cognitive-behavioral therapy (see Chapter 12) and complementary and alternative treatments such as glucosamine-chondroitin (see Chapter 14). Topical preparations such as capsaicin and NSAIDs are generally quite safe and can be used alone or along with other nontopical treatments (Rosenstein 1999; Towheed 2002). Well-controlled studies that clearly demonstrate their efficacy, however, are lacking. Interdisciplinary team treatment should always be considered for older adults with refractory pain related to degenerative lumbosacral pathology and to the other pathologies discussed in this chapter (Flor et al. 1992). A full discussion of the role of interdisciplinary pain management programs for older adults can be found in Chapter 15.

MYOFASCIAL PAIN SYNDROMES

Background and epidemiology. Myofascial pain (MP), that is, pain that originates in muscular sites (Gerwin 2001), may be localized or generalized and is characterized by motor and sensory abnormalities, the hallmark being the trigger point. Trigger points are areas of tenderness within taut muscle bands. Pressure applied to an active trigger point should spread and reproduce the patient's pain pattern, unlike fibromyalgia tender points, which are associated with pain only at the site of palpation.

Myofascial pain is a frequently overlooked contributor to chronic LBP, with and without associated leg pain. Estimates of MP prevalence vary, although in our experience, it exists in the majority of chronic pain patients, either as the primary cause of pain or as a pain comorbidity. To date, no large-scale study with rigorous definitions has examined its prevalence in older adults with LBP. In one study, one-third of visits to an internal medicine clinic for pain were found to be related to MP (Skootsky et al. 1989). Among 250 consecutive patients with chronic LBP evaluated at a tertiary referral center, 94 patients were diagnosed with MP (Cassisi et al. 1993).

Myofascial pain syndromes may be primary or secondary. Low back pain related to trigger points in the quadratus lumborum or piriformis muscle is an example of a primary MP syndrome. These muscles become involved because of poor body mechanics or structural asymmetry (e.g., scoliosis), which may cause chronic muscle shortening or strain. Postlaminectomy syndrome, hip or knee OA, and lumbar spondylosis are a few of the many possible causes of secondary MP syndromes.

Several types of MP may contribute to chronic low back and leg pain in older adults. Scoliosis may lead to pelvic rotation and put abnormal forces on the quadratus lumborum, causing LBP. Pelvic asymmetry because of leg length discrepancy associated with knee OA may cause MP in the back musculature and/or the tensor fascia lata. MP of the piriformis may cause piriformis syndrome (Barton 1991; Durrani and Winnie 1991) that mimics radiculopathy. Patients experience buttock pain and posterior leg pain because of irritation of the sciatic nerve as it passes through the piriformis muscle. MP of the tensor fascia lata and associated pain of the IT band may cause a sensation of burning of the lateral thigh. Gluteus medius trigger points can cause referred leg pain in a dermatomal distribution.

The exact pathophysiological mechanism that underlies MP is a subject of debate (Gerwin 2001; Rudin 2003; Wheeler 2004). Proposed etiologies include neuronal sensitization in the spinal dorsal horn after tissue injury, primary muscle spindle dysfunction, and inflammatory changes in the muscle after injury (Rudin 2003). Spontaneous electrical activity, called "end-plate noise," has been demonstrated within the taut bands of trigger points on electromyographic studies (Simons 2001).

Approach to evaluation. A thorough history and physical examination are required for MP diagnosis. Patients may describe MP as dull, achy, or burning. Mild pressure, such as that achieved by lying on the affected side, may relieve pain, and low-level activity also may help to alleviate pain, although excessive activity may worsen pain. Physical examination may reveal both latent and active trigger points. Palpation of latent trigger points may cause tenderness, but it does not necessarily reproduce the radiation of pain that occurs when active trigger points are palpated (Graff-Radford 2004). Local twitch responses, i.e., sharp contractions of the taut band (not the entire muscle) initiated by an intense physical stimulus such as needle insertion or plucking of the band (Gerwin 2001), may also be noted. Sensory abnormalities include hypersensitivity and allodynia of the trigger points. Autonomic phenomena such as temperature change, piloerection, and sweating may be present in the affected area, but they are not required for diagnosis.

Taut bands can be identified by firmly palpating the muscle along the same plane but in the axis that runs perpendicular to the direction of the muscle fibers. The examiner may need to apply pressure in this area for 10–15 seconds before the characteristic pain pattern is reproduced (Gerwin 2001). Reliable identification of trigger points in the low back can be difficult (Nice et al. 1993). Significant reduction in pain with application of vapocoolant spray or local anesthetic injection followed by stretching has been proposed as a diagnostic criterion (Graff-Radford 2004), although this approach has not been validated.

Examination of the piriformis muscle may be aided by directly palpating the muscle under mild stretch. Alternatively, the patient may be asked to lie supine, then flex, adduct, and internally rotate the involved hip; downward pressure is then placed on the knee to reproduce piriformis pain (Fishman et al. 2002). Those affected may have a tender, palpable, sausage-shaped mass over the piriformis (Benzon et al. 2003). Lasègue's sign, defined as 15° reduction in straight-leg raise on the affected side as compared to the unaffected side, may also be seen (Fishman et al. 2002).

Approach to treatment. The cornerstone of MP therapy should be identification and modification of perpetuating factors such as prescription of shoe lifts for leg length discrepancy, together with attention to posture, sleeping position, and body mechanics during activity (Graff-Radford 2004). Several other modalities can be used in the treatment of MP syndromes. Gentle, sustained stretching of involved muscles to reduce focal contractions and inactivate trigger points is a commonly employed technique. Often a vapocoolant spray is applied to the overlying skin before or during the stretch to facilitate completion of the exercise (Rudin 2003). This maneuver is thought to increase pain threshold and range of motion in the short term (Hou et al. 2002). Exercise programs, especially those that include graded stretching and strengthening, are recommended, but have not been systematically evaluated.

Trigger point injections are frequently employed in practice, although definitive data demonstrating their efficacy are lacking (Cummings and White 2001). Needling without injection of anesthetic or steroid, so-called "dry needling," may be just as effective (Garvey et al. 1989; Rudin 2003). At our center, we typically use trigger point injections or deactivation using acupuncture needles along with physical therapy for MP treatment. In the case of piriformis syndrome, as with other types of MP, injections may provide pain relief (Fishman et al. 2002), but stretching and correction of altered biomechanics are the mainstay of therapy (Benzon et al. 2003). Studies investigating the use of botulinum toxin in trigger point injections are ongoing (Lang 2002). For further discussion of trigger point injections, see Chapter 13.

Clonazepam is the only oral medication that has been found, in a double-blind trial, to relieve pain in MP syndromes (Wheeler 2004). There are many risks, however, associated with clonazepam use in older adults. Amitriptyline has been found to have benefit in patients with myofascial or tension-type headache (Rudin 2003). In our experience, oral analgesics are less effective than local modalities and should be used sparingly. We have had some success with low-dose gabapentin (e.g., 300 mg twice a day) for the treatment of neuropathic myofascial pain (Gunn 2001), for example in patients with cervical spondylosis and myofascial pain of the trapezius and paracervical musculature.

Acupuncture may provide short-term relief for patients with lumbar MP (Ceccherelli et al. 2002). Other modalities, such as massage, ultrasound, hot and cold compresses, transcutaneous electrical nerve stimulation, and biofeedback are commonly used to treat MP syndromes. Some of these methods have not been formally studied, and for some there is some evidence that they are no better than placebo (Rudin 2003). Guidelines regarding their practical application are provided in Chapter 11. For some patients with MP syndromes, interdisciplinary team treatment, as described in Chapter 15, may be beneficial.

SACROILIAC JOINT SYNDROME

Background and epidemiology. Sacroiliac joint syndrome (SIJS) is a painful disorder that is thought to be caused by dysfunction of the SI joint (Dreyfuss et al. 1994, 1996), although this point of view is controversial. A minority of patients with symptoms consistent with SIJS may respond to intra-articular injection (Chou et al. 2004), suggesting that periarticular dysfunctions, in large part, may be responsible for pain in the region of the SI joint. No studies of this disorder have been performed exclusively in older adults. In young, healthy individuals, there is a small amount of motion around the SI joint that lessens with aging (Prather 2003). Conclusions drawn about the precipitants of SIJS in younger individuals may or may not be relevant to older adults. In addition, physiological muscular changes that occur with aging, such as decrements in muscle quantity (i.e., sarcopenia) and quality, may affect the SI joint. Data indicate that subclinical changes in responsiveness of pelvic musculature may be causally related to SI joint dysfunction (Hungerford et al. 2003). It should be pointed out that SIJS and sacroiliitis are distinct entities, with sacroiliitis indicating the presence of inflammation in the setting of systemic illness (e.g., inflammatory bowel disease, psoriasis, or ankylosing spondylitis), and SIJS indicating local/regional pathology that may or may not be associated with inflammation.

Approach to evaluation. The function of the SI joint is transmission and dissipation of mechanical forces involving the spine, pelvis, and lower extremities. Evaluation of the older adult with suspected SIJS should include careful evaluation and treatment of all potential contributors, such as scoliosis and kyphosis, leg length discrepancy, and arthritis of the hip and knee, or anatomical derangement that may occur following back surgery, particularly spinal fusion. The currently accepted gold standard diagnostic test is fluoroscopically guided SI intra-articular injection resulting in substantial pain relief, typically 75–80% or greater (Chou et al. 2004). Using this approach, a recent study of 54 patients aged 30–76 years (mean 48.2 years) found that 44% of cases were caused by overt trauma, 21% were caused by cumulative injury (e.g., lifting, running, or lower-extremity disorders) and that 35% were idiopathic (Chou et al. 2004).

The reliability and validity of physical examination maneuvers and historical features have been the focus of a number of studies. The historical features that have literature support for SIJS are the absence of pain in the lumbar region, pain below the level of L5, pain in the region of the posterior superior iliac spine, and groin pain (Freburger and Riddle 2001). The reliability and validity of clinical tests used to assess the symmetry or movement of bony landmarks associated with the SI joint are poor (Freburger and Riddle 2001). Potentially useful pain provocation tests include Patrick's test (Broadhurst and Bond 1998; Slipman et al. 1998), palpation over the sacral sulcus (Slipman et al. 1998), the thigh thrust (Laslett and Williams 1994) or posterior shear test (Broadhurst and Bond 1998), resisted hip abduction (Broadhurst and Bond 1998), and iliac compression and gapping tests (Potter and Rothstein 1985; Laslett and Williams 1994). Evidence indicates that a combination of these tests may be more sensitive than one test alone (Freburger and Riddle 2001). The three tests that we have found the easiest to perform on older adults are (1) direct palpation of the sacral sulcus in the standing position (with the examiner behind the patient, using one hand to brace the patient from the front, using the right hand to palpate the right joint while standing to the left and vice versa for the contralateral side), (2) Patrick's test, and (3) iliac compression in the side-lying position. An important caveat is that Patrick's test may have low specificity in the presence of concomitant intra-articular or periarticular hip restrictions.

Radiographic procedures should not be performed to assist with the diagnosis of SIJS, unless the practitioner suspects a sacral insufficiency fracture. Motion about the SI joint is too small to be detected with radiography (Freburger and Riddle 2001), degenerative changes identified with plain or advanced imaging have poor discriminant validity (Vogler et al. 1984), and bone scans have low sensitivity (Slipman et al. 1996).

Approach to treatment. Because of the complex nature of the SI joint, the approach to treatment should be multidimensional, and thus application of a unidimensional or standardized LBP treatment approach is likely to result in treatment failure. Therapy should be geared toward improving the stability of the surrounding soft tissues and diminishing mechanical stress related to postural abnormalities. Clinicians should consider prescribing orthotics to level the sacral base and using SI joint injection when appropriate (Prather 2003). The existing literature offers no guidelines regarding the timing of SI joint injection relative to other therapies. At our center, we prescribe physical therapy for 4–6 weeks, and then we determine the need for injection. If pain is severe and limits compliance with physical therapy, however, an injection may be beneficial early on. Often myofascial and ligamentous symptoms resolve with physical therapy alone, and injection can be avoided. Other treatment options include oral analgesics and prolotherapy (see Chapter 13).

FIBROMYALGIA

Background and epidemiology. Fibromyalgia syndrome, classically thought of as a disease that primarily afflicts young and middle-aged women, is quite common in older adults. One large epidemiological study found that the group most commonly affected is women aged 60–79 years (Wolfe et al. 1995), although the duration of symptoms in these individuals was not reported. Fibromyalgia is generally poorly recognized by primary practitioners, with one study demonstrating that only 17% of older adults referred to a rheumatologist had previously been accurately diagnosed; 40% of patients had received corticosteroids prior to rheumatology consultation (Yunus et al. 1988). In 1997, the estimated fibromyalgia-related mean yearly medical costs for an individual patient in the United States were U.S.$2,274, similar to the costs of OA (Wolfe et al. 1995). Fibromyalgia, once thought of as an illness with a primarily psychopathological basis, is now recognized as a disorder based on dysregulation of the central nervous system (CNS), including both temporal summation and central sensitization (Gibson et al.

1994; Woolf 1996; Li et al. 1999; Staud et al. 2001). The clinical syndrome is also reported to be a disorder caused by a combination of CNS dysregulation and peripheral pain triggers (Staud 2004). Anecdotally, we have observed that older adults with dementia and localized LBP often have numerous fibromyalgia tender points, which is in keeping with the CNS dysregulation that underlies both dementia and fibromyalgia.

Approach to evaluation. While widespread pain is the sine qua non of fibromyalgia, axial pain is often the chief complaint (Wolfe et al. 1990). Thus, the older adult with fibromyalgia may present with a chief complaint of LBP, and only on further questioning does the generalized nature of the patient's pain become apparent. Criteria for the diagnosis of fibromyalgia, established by the ACR, include widespread pain (that is, pain in three of four body quadrants) in combination with 11 of 18 tender points. Three-quarters of patients also suffer from morning stiffness, fatigue, and nonrestorative sleep. A wide variety of other disorders and symptoms may occur in the older adult with fibromyalgia, including postexertional pain; restless legs or sleep apnea; psychological distress (e.g., anxiety, depression, and general tension); dysesthesias and paresthesias; cognitive difficulties (e.g., impaired memory and concentration); vague auditory, vestibular, and ocular complaints; intolerance or allergies to multiple medications; palpitations and dyspnea; regional pain syndromes (e.g., tension and migraine headaches, atypical chest pain, temporomandibular symptoms, myofascial pain, pelvic pain, and dyspareunia); irritable bowel syndrome; cold intolerance; urinary frequency associated with interstitial cystitis; subjective joint swelling; fluid retention; and unexplained bruising (Russell 2001). The most common fibromyalgia flare precipitants include unaccustomed exertion, soft tissue injuries, lack of sleep, cold exposure, and psychological stressors.

The physical examination sine qua non of fibromyalgia is the finding of at least 11 of 18 tender points. This requirement was developed by the ACR as a means of classifying rather than diagnosing fibromyalgia, that is, differentiating fibromyalgia from other rheumatological syndromes characterized by generalized pain such as systemic lupus erythematosus and rheumatoid arthritis (Wolfe et al. 1995). The requirement for this precise number of tender points, therefore, is not absolute, and patients with a clinical presentation consistent with fibromyalgia who do not have the "correct" number of tender points should still be appropriately treated. In addition to the finding of tender points, patients with fibromyalgia may have tender skin, allodynia, and hyperalgesia (Granges and Littlejohn 1993).

Approach to treatment. The treatment of fibromyalgia requires a multipronged approach. The symptoms that most interfere with patients' quality of life include pain, fatigue, limited exercise tolerance, and sleep disturbance.

Often depression and anxiety coexist in patients with fibromyalgia and also require treatment (pharmacological approaches to depression and anxiety are beyond the scope of this chapter). Tricyclic antidepressants (TCAs) are the best-studied agents for the treatment of fibromyalgia (Arnold et al. 2000; Rao and Bennett 2003). Limited data suggest that selective serotonin reuptake inhibitors (Miller and Kubes 2002), in particular fluoxetine (Goldenberg et al. 1996; Arnold et al. 2002), may be helpful for the treatment of fibromyalgia, but the prolonged half-life of this drug in older adults with age-related decline in renal function makes its use in these patients a low-priority consideration. Cyclobenzaprine has demonstrated efficacy (Tofferi et al. 2004), but because of its CNS sedating effects, its use in older adults is not recommended. Prescription of TCAs should be limited to those with relatively low anticholinergic side-effect potential, i.e., desipramine and nortriptyline (American Geriatrics Society Panel on Persistent Pain in Older Persons 2002). These agents should be used in modest doses for the treatment of fibromyalgia (e.g., 10 mg slowly titrated to 30–50 mg at bedtime) in the absence of depression.

Interdisciplinary team treatment (e.g., physical therapy, occupational therapy, and psychological approaches) for fibromyalgia includes teaching patients a variety of cognitive-behavioral therapy techniques, carefully paced aerobic exercises, flare management techniques, and ways to improve self-efficacy. Nonpharmacological promotion of sleep hygiene is critical for the majority of patients and includes elimination of all chemical stimulants late in the day, elimination of daytime naps, creation of a bedroom characterized by refuge and quiet, and relaxation training.

OSTEOPOROSIS

Background and epidemiology. Approximately 25% of postmenopausal women in the United States will suffer a vertebral compression fracture, and these rates rise substantially with age. In one study, 50% of women aged 80–84 years had radiographically identified vertebral deformities (Melton et al. 1989). Men are also affected, with a vertebral fracture prevalence that is estimated to be equal or greater to that of women (Burgess and Nanes 2002).

Only about one-third of vertebral fractures cause pain (Cooper and Melton 1992). Given the multifactorial nature of chronic LBP, it is difficult to ascertain how much a radiographically identified vertebral compression fracture contributes to an individual's pain. However, several studies have documented higher rates of pain in postmenopausal women with vertebral compression fractures than in those without fractures (Huang et al. 1996; Ross 1997). Pain from acute fractures may resolve in 6–8 weeks. Of those patients suffering from a painful acute vertebral fracture, up to 75% may suffer from persistent back pain (Rapado 1996). Others may develop pain more insidiously with the accumulation of multiple fractures.

While the thoracolumbar junction and midthoracic areas are the most common sites of fractures (Papaioannou et al. 2002), vertebral compression fractures can contribute to chronic lumbar pain through several mechanisms. Lumbar vertebrae themselves may be directly involved. Alternatively, altered spine mechanics may develop because of spinal deformity and pseudoarthroses at involved vertebrae (Phillips 2003). Also, progressive loss of height through multiple fractures can cause paraspinal muscle shortening that in turn leads to prolonged active muscular contraction to maintain posture, resulting in muscular fatigue and pain. Pain can also result from progressive height loss, thoracic kyphosis, and lumbar lordosis, which cause the rib cage to exert pressure on the pelvis (Old and Calvert 2004).

Approach to evaluation. Vertebral compression fractures should be suspected in older adults with kyphosis or back pain of sudden onset. The onset need not have been preceded by significant trauma, as many fractures are precipitated by routine activities such as lifting. Often patients will describe pain over the involved vertebra(e) that can be reproduced with palpation, especially in acute fractures. Patients report variable symptom patterns that occasionally mimic disk herniation, with radiation of pain into the flanks or anterior abdominal wall. These symptoms can usually be differentiated through a careful history, focusing on the pain radiation pattern, and through physical examination (Ross 1997). Plain radiographs should be used to confirm the diagnosis.

Approach to treatment. Older adults with chronic LBP from vertebral compression fractures may require a multidisciplinary treatment approach that focuses on restoration of physical function through strengthening of paraspinal muscles and overall conditioning, pain relief, and prevention of future fractures. Both opioid and non-opioid analgesics may be required. While calcitonin (derived from salmon) has analgesic properties and should be considered in the older adult who has sustained an acute vertebral compression fracture (Maksymowych 1998), studies demonstrate variable efficacy for its use in the treatment of chronic pain from vertebral fractures (Pontiroli et al. 1994; Peichl et al. 1999; Silverman and Azria 2002).

Physical therapy and a regular exercise program should be recommended. In small randomized trials, they have been shown to decrease analgesic use and pain scores, reduce future vertebral fractures, and increase function and bone density (Malmros et al. 1998; Papaioannou et al. 2002; Sinaki et al. 2002). Lumbar supports or back braces have not been specifically studied in patients with chronic pain from vertebral fractures, although there is limited evidence for their efficacy in chronic nonspecific LBP (Jellema et al. 2001). Vertebroplasty or kyphoplasty, minimally invasive techniques in which bone cement is injected into the collapsed vertebral body, result in significant pain reduction in select populations of patients whose pain from acute vertebral fractures does not respond to conservative measures. Published data regarding long-term efficacy are not available (Phillips 2003). For further discussion of these procedures, the reader is referred to Chapter 13.

THE ROLE OF PREVENTION

In addition to treating painful pathology to improve function and quality of life, it is important for practitioners to address prevention. Toward this end, all older adults should have bone density screening, and treatment should be implemented to avoid future painful compression fractures. Balance and mobility also should be carefully assessed, and treatments such as assistive devices or lower-extremity strengthening exercises should be prescribed to avoid falls and fractures. These steps should precede prescription of medications that may impair balance, such as opioids, tricyclic antidepressants, and gabapentin. The patient's existing medication regimen should also be optimized by addressing polypharmacy and substituting medications with fewer side effects when possible. Strategies to enhance exercise compliance should be implemented to optimize functional status and diminish pain flares. In patients with dementia, education of caregivers regarding pain behaviors, the utility of nonpharmacological management techniques to deal with pain flares, and ways to handle the emotional agitation that may accompany such flares is vitally important. Pharmacological strategies to slow cognitive decline should also be implemented.

CONCLUDING REMARKS

Health care expenditure for patients with persistent LBP appears to be excessive due to multiple provider visits and imaging studies, inappropriate specialist referrals and procedures, and ongoing care needs resulting from ineffectively implemented treatments. A change in the paradigmatic approach to evaluating and managing this challenging problem is needed. Our experience suggests that most LBP in older adults arises from multiple pathologies (osteoarthritis, sacroiliac joint syndrome, fibromyalgia, myofascial pain, and osteoporosis) and that a careful history and physical examination are required to identify the causative pathology and prescribe effective treatment.

ACKNOWLEDGMENTS

This work was supported by grants from the National Institutes of Health, R01 AG18299 and R01 AT000985.

REFERENCES

Abramson SB, Attur M, Amin AR, Clancy R. Nitric oxide and inflammatory mediators in the perpetuation of osteoarthritis. *Curr Rheumatol Rep* 2001; 3(6):535–541.

Airaksinen O, Herno A, Turunen V, Saari T, Suomlainen O. Surgical outcome of 438 patient treated surgically for lumbar spinal stenosis. *Spine* 1997; 22(19):2278–2282.

American Geriatrics Society Panel on Persistent Pain in Older Persons. The management of persistent pain in older persons. *J Am Geriatr Soc* 2002; 50(6):S205–S224.

American Geriatrics Society Panel on Exercise and Osteoarthritis. Exercise prescription for older adults with osteoarthritis pain: Consensus practice recommendations. *J Am Geriatr Soc* 2001; 49:808–823.

Amundsen T, Weber H, Nordal HJ, et al. Lumbar spinal stenosis: conservative or surgical management? A prospective 10-year study. *Spine* 2000; 25(11):1424–1436.

Arnold LM, Keck PE Jr, Welge JA. Antidepressant treatment of fibromyalgia: a meta-analysis and review. *Psychosomatics* 2000; 41(2):104–113.

Arnold LM, Hess EV, Hudson JI, et al. A randomized, placebo-controlled, double-blind, flexible-dose study of fluoxetine in the treatment of women with fibromyalgia. *Am J Med* 2002; 112(3):191–197.

Atlas SJ, Keller RB, Robson D, Deyo RA, Singer D E. Surgical and nonsurgical management of lumbar spinal stenosis: four-year outcomes from the Maine lumbar spine study. *Spine* 2000; 25(5):556–562.

Barton PM. Piriformis syndrome: a rational approach to management. *Pain* 1991; 47:345–352.

Becker N, Thomsen AB, Olsen AK, et al. Pain epidemiology and health related quality of life in chronic non-malignant pain patients referred to a Danish multidisciplinary pain center. *Pain* 1997; 73:393–400.

Benzon HT, Katz J, Benzon HA, Iqbal M. Piriformis syndrome, anatomic considerations, a new injection technique, and a review of the literature. *Anesthesiology* 2003; 98:1442–1448.

Bianchi Porro G, Petrillo M, Ardizzone S. Salsalate in the treatment of rheumatoid arthritis: a double-blind clinical and gastroscopic trial versus piroxicam. II. Endoscopic evaluation. *J Int Med Res* 989; 17(4):320–323.

Bigos S, Bowyer O, Braen G, et al. *Acute Low Back Problems in Adults*. Clinical Practice Guideline No. 14, AHCPR Publication No. 95-0642. Rockville, MD: U.S. Department of Health and Human Services, Public Health Service, Agency for Healthcare Policy and Research, 1994.

Boden SD, Davis DO, Dina TS, Patronas NJ, Wiesel SW. Abnormal magnetic-resonance scans of the lumbar spine in asymptomatic subjects—a prospective investigation. *J Bone Joint Surg Am* 1990; 72(3):403–408.

Brandt KD, Smith GN Jr, Simon LS. Intraarticular injection of hyaluronan as treatment for knee osteoarthritis: what is the evidence? *Arthritis Rheum* 2000; 43:1192–1203.

Broadhurst NA, Bond MJ. Pain provocation tests for the assessment of sacroiliac joint dysfunction. *J Spinal Disord* 1998; 11:341–345.

Burgess E, Nanes M. Osteoporosis in men: pathophysiology, evaluation, and therapy. *Curr Opin Rheumatol* 2002; 14:421–428.

Carey TS, Evans A, Hadler N, et al. Care-seeking among individuals with chronic low back pain. *Spine* 1995; 20(3):312–317.

Cassisi JE, Sypert G, Lagana L, Friedman E, Robinson M. Pain, disability, and psychological functioning in chronic low back pain subgroups: myofascial versus herniated disc subgroups. *Neurosurgery* 1993; 33(3):379–386.

Ceccherelli F, Rigoni MT, Gagliardi G, Ruzzante L. Comparison of superficial and deep acupuncture in the treatment of lumbar myofascial pain: a double blind, randomized, controlled study. *Clin J Pain* 2002; 18:149–153.

Chou LH, Slipman CW, Bhagia SM, et al. Inciting events initiating injection-proven sacroiliac joint syndrome. *Pain Med* 2004; 5(1):26–32.

Cooper C, Melton LJI. Vertebral fractures, how large is the silent epidemic? *Br Med J* 1992; 304:793–794.

Cummings TM, White AR. Needling therapies in the management of myofascial trigger point pain: a systematic review. *Arch Phys Med Rehabil* 2001; 82:986–992.

Danielson BI, Willen J, Gaulitz A, Niklason T, Hansson TH. Axial loading of the spine during CT and MR in patients with suspected lumbar spinal stenosis. *Acta Radiol* 1998; 39(6):604–611.

Davis RA. A long-term outcome analysis of 984 surgically treated herniated lumbar discs. *J Neurosurg* 1994; 80:415–421.

Deen HG, Zimmerman RS, Lyons MK, et al. Test-retest reproducibility of the exercise treadmill examination in lumbar spinal stenosis. *Mayo Clin Proc* 2000; 75(10):1002–1007.

Deyo RA, Tsui-Wu YJ. Descriptive epidemiology of low-back pain and its related medical care in the United States. *Spine* 1987; 12(3):264–268.

Dieppe PA, Sathapatayavongs B, Jones HE, et. al. Intra-articular steroids in osteoarthritis. *Rheumatol Rehabil* 1980; 19(4):212–217.

Dreyfuss P, Dreyer S, Griffin J, et al. Positive sacroiliac screening tests in asymptomatic adults. *Spine* 1994; 19:1138–1143.

Dreyfuss P, Michaelsen M, Pauza K, McLarty J, Bogduk N. The value of medical history and physical examination in diagnosing sacroiliac joint pain. *Spine* 1996; (21):2594–2602.

Durrani Z, Winnie AP. Piriformis syndrome: an undiagnosed cause of sciatica. *J Pain Symptom Manage* 1991; 6:374–379.

Felson DT, Anderson JJ. Hyaluronate sodium injections for osteoarthritis: hope, hype, and hard truths. *Arch Intern Med* 2002; 162(3):245–247.

Fishman LM, Dombi G, Michaelsen C, et al. Piriformis syndrome: diagnosis, treatment, and outcome—a 10-year study. *Arch Phys Med Rehabil* 2002; 83:295–301.

Flor H, Fydrich T, Turk DC. Efficacy of multidisciplinary pain treatment centers: a meta-analytic review. *Pain* 1992; 49:221–230.

Frazier DD, Lipson SJ, Fossel AH, Katz JN. Associations between spinal deformity and outcomes after decompression for spinal stenosis. *Spine* 1997; 22(17):2025–2029.

Freburger JK, Riddle DL. Using published evidence to guide the examination of the sacroiliac joint. *Phys Ther* 2001; 81(5):1135–1143.

Fries JF, Williams CA, Bloch DA. The relative toxicity of nonsteroidal antiinflammatory drugs. *Arthritis Rheum* 1991; 34(11):1353–1360.

Fritz JM, Erhard RE, Delitto A, Welch WC, Nowakowski PE. Preliminary results of the use of a two-stage treadmill test as a clinical diagnostic tool in the differential diagnosis of lumbar spinal stenosis. *J Spinal Disord* 1997; 10(5):410–416.

Garvey TA, Marks MR, Wiesel SW. A prospective, randomized, double blind evaluation of trigger-point injection therapy for low-back pain. *Spine* 14:962–964.

Gerwin RD. Classification, epidemiology, and natural history of myofascial pain syndrome. *Curr Pain Headache Rep* 2001; 5:412–420.

Gibson SJ, Littlejohn GO, Gorman MM, Helme RD, Granges G. Altered heat pain thresholds and cerebral event-related potentials following painful CO_2 laser stimulation in subjects with fibromyalgia syndrome. *Pain* 1994; 58(2):185–193.

Gill TM, Desai MM, Gahbauer EA, Holford TR, Williams C. Restricted activity among community-living older persons: incidence, precipitants, and health care utilization. *Ann Intern Med* 2001; 135:313–321.

Goldenberg D, Mayskiy M, Mossey C, et al. A randomized, double-blind crossover trial of fluoxetine and amitriptyline in the treatment of fibromyalgia. *Arthritis Rheum* 1996; 39(11):1852–1859.

Graff-Radford SB. Myofascial pain: diagnosis and management. *Curr Pain Headache Rep* 2004; 8:463–467.

Granges G, Littlejohn GO. A comparative study of clinical signs in fibromyalgia/fibrositis syndrome, healthy and exercising subjects. *J Rheumatol* 1993; 20(2):344–351.

Gunn CC. Neuropathic myofascial pain syndromes. In: Loeser JD, Butler SH, Chapman CR, Turk DC (Eds). *Bonica's Management of Pain,* 3rd ed. Philadelphia: Lippincott Williams Wilkins, 2001.

Han SC, Harrison P. Myofascial pain syndrome and trigger-point management. *Reg Anesth* 1997; 22(1):89–101.

Harkins SW, Kwentus J, Price DD. Pain and the elderly. In: Benedetti C, Chapman CR, Moricca G (Eds). *Recent Advances in the Management of Pain,* Advances in Pain Research and Therapy, Vol. 7. New York: Raven Press, 1984, pp 103–121.

Hart LG, Deyo RA, Cherkin DC. Physician office visits for low back pain. Frequency, clinical evaluation, and treatment patterns from a U.S. national survey. *Spine* 1995; 20(1):11–19.

Haywood L, McWilliams DF, Pearson CI, et al. Inflammation and angiogenesis in osteoarthritis. *Arthritis Rheum* 2003; 48(8):2173–2177.

Hedbom E, Hauselmann HJ. Molecular aspects of pathogenesis in osteoarthritis: the role of inflammation. *Cell Mol Life Sci* 2002; 59(1):45–53.

Hee HT, Wong HK. The long-term results of surgical treatment for spinal stenosis in the elderly. *Singapore Med J* 2003; 44(4):175–180.

Helme RD. Chronic pain management in older people. *Eur J Pain* 2001; 5(Suppl A):31–36.

Helme RD, Gibson SJ. The epidemiology of pain in elderly people. *Clin Geriatr Med* 2001; 17(3):417–431.

Hirsch C, Nachemson A. The reliability of lumbar disc surgery. *Clin Orthop* 1963; 29:189–195.

Hou CR, Tsai LC, Chung KC, Hong CZ. Immediate effects of various physical therapy modalities on cervical myofascial pain and trigger point sensitivity. *Arch Phys Med Rehabil* 2002; 83:1406–1414.

Huang C, Ross P, Wasnich R. Vertebral fractures and other predictors of physical impairment and health care utilization. *Arch Intern Med* 1996; 156(21):2469–2475.

Hungerford B, Gilleard W, Hodges P. Evidence of altered lumbopelvic muscle recruitment in the presence of sacroiliac joint pain. *Spine* 2003; 28(14):1593–1600.

Jarvik JG, Deyo RA. Diagnostic evaluation of low back pain with emphasis on imaging. *Ann Intern Med* 2002; 137:586–597.

Jarvik JJ, Hollingworth W, Heagerty P, Haynor DR, Deyo RA. The longitudinal assessment of imaging and disability of the back (LAIDBack) study: baseline data. *Spine* 2001; 26:1158–1166.

Jellema P, van Tulder M, van Poppel M, Nachemson A, Bouter L. Lumbar supports for prevention and treatment of low back pain. *Spine* 2001; 26(4):377–386.

Johnsson K-E, Uden A, Rosen I. The effect of decompression on the natural course of spinal stenosis—a comparison of surgically treated and untreated patients. *Spine* 1991; 16(6):615–619.

Jonsson B, Annertz M, Sjoberg C, Stromqvist B. A prospective and consecutive study of surgically treated lumbar spinal stenosis: Part II: Five-year follow-up by an independent observer. *Spine* 1997; 22(24):2938–2944.

Katz JN, Stucki G, Lipson SJ, et al. Predictors of surgical outcome in degenerative lumbar spinal stenosis. *Spine* 1999; 24(21):2229.

Kee WG, Middaugh SJ, Redpath S, Hargadon R. Age as a factor in admission to chronic pain rehabilitation. *Clin J Pain* 1998; 14:121–128.

Keskimaki I, Seitsalo S, Osterman H, Rissanen P. Reoperations after lumbar disc surgery. *Spine* 2000; 25:1500–1508.

Lang AM. Botulinum toxin therapy for myofascial pain disorders. *Curr Pain Headache Rep* 2002; 6:355–360.

Lanza F, Rack MF, Doucette M, et al. An endoscopic comparison of the gastroduodenal injury seen with salsalate and naproxen. *J Rheumatol* 1989; 16(12):1570–1574.

Larkai EN, Smith JL, Lidsky MD, Graham DY. Gastroduodenal mucosa and dyspeptic symptoms in arthritic patients during chronic nonsteroidal anti-inflammatory drug use. *Am J Gastroenterol* 1997; 92(2):363–364.

Laslett M, Williams M. The reliability of selected pain provocation tests for sacroiliac joint pathology. *Spine* 1994; 19:1243–1249.

Law JD, Lehman RAW, Kirsch WM. Reoperation after lumbar intervertebral disc surgery. *J Neurosurg* 1963; 29:189–195.

Lawrence RC, Helmick CG, Arnett FC, et al. Estimates of the prevalence of arthritis and selected musculoskeletal disorders in the United States. *Arthritis Rheum* 1998; 41(5):778–799.

Leveille SG. Musculoskeletal aging. *Curr Opin Rheumatol* 2004; 16(2):114–118.

Li J, Simone DA, Larson AA. Windup leads to characteristics of central sensitization. *Pain* 1999; 79:75–82.

Maksymowych WP. Managing acute osteoporotic vertebral fractures with calcitonin. *Can Fam Physician* 1998; 44:2160–2166.

Malmros B, Mortenson L, Jensen MB, Charles P. Positive effects of physiotherapy on chronic pain and performance in osteoporosis. *Osteoporos Int* 1998; 8:215–221.

Malter AD, McNeney B, Loeser JD, et al. 5-year reoperation rates after different types of lumbar spine surgery. *Spine* 1998; 23:814–820.

Martel-Pelletier J, Alaaeddine N, Pelletier JP. Cytokines and their role in the pathophysiology of osteoarthritis. *Front Biosci* 1999; 4:D694–D703.

Melton LJ III, Kan SH, Frye MA, et al. Epidemiology of vertebral fractures in women. *Am J Epidemiol* 1989; 129(5):1000–1111.

Mielants H, Veys EM, Verbruggen G, Schelstraete K. Salicylate-induced occult gastrointestinal blood loss: comparison between different oral and parenteral forms of acetylsalicylates and salicylates. *Clin Rheumatol* 1984; 3(1):47–54.

Miller LJ, Kubes KL. Serotonergic agents in the treatment of fibromyalgia syndrome. *Ann Pharmacother* 2002; 36(4):707–712.

Nice DA, Riddle D, Lamb R, Mayhew T. Rucker K. Intertester reliability of judgements of the presence of trigger points in patients with low back pain. *Arch Phys Med Rehabil* 1993; 73(10):893–898.

Old J, Calvert M. Vertebral compression fractures in the elderly. *Am Fam Physician* 2004; 69:111–116.

Osterman H, Sund R, Seitsalo S, Keskimaki I. Risk of multiple reoperations after lumbar discectomy. *Spine* 2003; 28:621–627.

Papaioannou A, Watts N, Kendler D, et al. Diagnosis and management of vertebral fractures in elderly adults. *Am J Med* 2002; 113:220–228.

Peichl P, Rintelen B, Kumpan W, Broll H. Increase of axial and appendicular trabecular and cortical bone density in established osteoporosis with intermittent nasal salmon calcitonin therapy. *Gynecol Endocrinol* 1999; 13:7–14.

Pencharz JN, MacLean CH. Measuring quality in arthritis care: the Arthritis Foundation's quality indicator set for osteoarthritis. *Arthritis Rheum* 2004; 51(4):538–548.

Phillips F. Minimally invasive treatments of osteoporotic vertebral compression fractures. *Spine* 2003; 28(15S):S45–S53.

Pincus T. Clinical evidence for osteoarthritis as an inflammatory disease. *Curr Rheumatol Rep* 2001; 3(6):524–534.

Pontiroli AE, Pajetta E, Scaglia L, et al. Analgesic effect of intranasal and intramuscular salmon calcitonin in post-menopausal osteoporosis: a double-blind, double-placebo study. *Aging (Milano)* 1994; 6(6):459–463.

Potter NA, Rothstein JM. Intertest reliability for selected clinical tests of the sacroiliac joint. *Phys Ther* 1985; 65:1671–1675.

Prather H. Sacroiliac joint pain: practical management. *Clin J Sport Med* 2003; 13(4):252–255.

Ragab AA, Fye MA, Bohlman HH. Surgery of the lumbar spine for spinal stenosis in 118 patients 70 years of age or older. *Spine* 2003; 28(4):348–353.

Rao SG, Bennett RM. Pharmacological therapies in fibromyalgia. *Best Pract Res Clin Rheumatol* 2003; 17(4):611–627.

Rapado A. General management of vertebral fractures. *Bone* 1996; 18(3):191S–196S.

Raynauld J-P, Buckland-Wright C, Ward R, et al. Safety and efficacy of long-term intraarticular steroid injections in osteoarthritis of the knee. *Arthritis Rheum* 2003; 48(2):370–377.

Reid MC, Williams CS, Concato J, Tinetti M, Gill TM. Depressive symptoms as a risk factor for disabling back pain in community-dwelling older persons. *J Am Geriatr Soc* 2003; 51(12):1710–1717.

Rosenstein ED. Topical agents in the treatment of rheumatic disorders. *Rheum Dis Clin N Am* 1999; 25(4):899–918.

Ross P. Clinical consequences of vertebral fractures. *Am J Med* 1997; 103(2A):30S–43S.

Roth S, Bennett R, Caldron P, et al. Reduced risk of NSAID gastropathy (GI mucosal toxicity) with nonacetylated salicylate (salsalate): an endoscopic study. *Semin Arthritis Rheum* 1990; 19(4 Suppl 2):11–19.

Rudin NJ. Evaluation of treatments for myofascial pain syndrome and fibromyalgia. *Curr Pain Headache Rep* 2003; 7:433–442.

Russell IJ. Fibromyalgia Syndrome. In: *Bonica's Management of Pain,* 3rd ed. Philadelphia: Lippincott Williams Wilkins, 2001, pp 543–555.

Shorr RI, Griffin MR, Daugherty JR, Ray WA. Opioid analgesics and the risk of hip fracture in the elderly: codeine and propoxyphene. *J Gerontol* 1992; 47:M111–M115.

Silverman SL, Azria M. The analgesic role of calcitonin following osteoporotic fracture. *Osteoporos Int* 2002; 13:858–867.

Simons DG. Do endplate noise and spikes arise from normal motor endplates? *Am J Phys Med Rehabil* 2001; 80:134–140.

Simotas AC, Dorey FJ, Hansraj KK, Cammisa F. Nonoperative treatment for lumbar spinal stenosis: clinical and outcome results and a 3-year survivorship analysis. *Spine* 2000; 25(2):197.

Sinaki M, et al. Stronger back muscles reduce the incidence of vertebral fractures: a prospective 10 year follow up of postmenopausal women. *Bone* 2002; 13:858–867.

Skootsky SA, Jaeger B, Oye RK. Prevalence of myofascial pain in general internal medicine practice. *West J Med* 1989; 151(2):157–60.

Slipman CW, Sterenfeld EB, Chou LH, Herzog R, Vresilovic E. The value of radionuclide imaging in the diagnosis of sacroiliac joint syndrome. *Spine* 1996; 21(19):2251–2254.

Slipman CW, Sterenfeld EB, Chou LH, Herzog R, Vresilovic E. The predictive value of provocative sacroiliac joint stress maneuvers in the diagnosis of sacroiliac joint syndrome. *Arch Phys Med Rehabil* 1998; 79:288–292.

Sowers M, Jannausch M, Stein E, et al. C-reactive protein as a biomarker of emergent osteoarthritis. *Osteoarthritis Cartilage* 2002; 10(8):595–601.

Staud R. Fibromyalgia pain: do we know the source? *Curr Opin Rheumatol* 2004; 16(2):157–163.

Staud R, Vierck CJ, Cannon RL, et al. Abnormal sensitization and temporal summation of second pain (wind-up) in patients with fibromyalgia syndrome. *Pain* 2001; 91:165–175.

Thomas E, Peat G, Harris L, Wilkie R, Croft PR. The prevalence of pain and pain interference in a general population of older adults: cross-sectional findings from the North Staffordshire Osteoarthritis Project. *Pain* 2004; 110(1–2):361–368.

Tofferi JK, Jackson JL, O'Malley PG. Treatment of fibromyalgia with cyclobenzaprine: a meta-analysis. *Arthritis Rheum* 2004; 51(1):9–13.

Towheed TE. Published meta-analyses of pharmacological therapies for osteoarthritis. *Osteoarthritis Cartilage* 2002; 10(11):836–837.

Vitaz TW, Raque GH, Shields CB, Glassman SD. Surgical treatment of lumbar spinal stenosis in patients older than 75 years of age. *J Neurosurg* 1999; 91(2 Suppl):181–185.

Vogler JB III, Brown WH, Helms CA, Genant HK. The normal sacroiliac joint: a CT study of asymptomatic patients. *Radiology* 1984; 151:433–437.

Watts R, Silagy C. A meta-analysis of the efficacy of epidural corticosteroids in the treatment of sciatica. *Anaesth Intensive Care* 1995; 23:564–569.

Weiner DK, Distell B, Studenski S, et al. Does radiographic osteoarthritis correlate with flexibility of the lumbar spine? *J Am Geriatr Soc* 1994; 42:257–263.

Weiner D, Hanlon JT, Studenski S. Effects of central nervous system polypharmacy on falls liability in community-dwelling elderly. *Gerontology* 1998; 44:217–221.

Weiner DK, Haggerty CL, Kritchevsky SB, et al. For the Health, Aging, and Body Composition Research Group. How does low back pain impact physical function in independent, well-functioning older adults? Evidence from the Health ABC cohort and implications for the future. *Pain Med* 2003; 4(4):311–320.

Weiner DK, Kim Y-S, Bonino P, Wang T. Low back pain in older adults: are we utilizing health care resources wisely? *Pain Med* 2005a; in press.

Weiner DK, Sakamoto S, Perera S, Breuer P. Chronic low back pain in older adults: prevalence, reliability, and validity of physical examination findings. *J Am Geriatr Soc* 2005b; in press.

Weiner DK, Turner GH, Hennon JG, Perera S, Hartmann S. Chronic pain education in geriatric fellowship training programs: results of a national survey. *J Am Geriat Soc* 2005c; in press.

Wheeler AH. Myofascial pain disorders, theory to therapy. *Drugs* 2004; 64(1):45–62.

Wolfe F, Smythe HA, Yunus MB, et al. The American College of Rheumatology 1990 criteria for the classification of fibromyalgia: report of the multicenter criteria committee. *Arthritis Rheum* 1990; 33:160–172.

Wolfe F, Ross K, Anderson J, Russell IJ, Hebert L. The prevalence and characteristics of fibromyalgia in the general population. *Arthritis Rheum* 1995; 38:19–28.

Woolf CJ. Windup and central sensitization are not equivalent. *Pain* 1996; 66:105–108.

Yorimitsu E, Chiba K, Toyama Y, Hirabayashi K. Long-term outcomes of standard discectomy for lumbar disc herniation. *Spine* 2001; 26:652–657.

Yunus MB, Holt GS, Masi AT, Aldag JC. Fibromyalgia syndrome among the elderly-comparison with younger patients. *J Am Geriatr Soc* 1988; 36:987–995.

Correspondence to: Associate Prof. Debra K. Weiner, MD, Pain Evaluation and Treatment Institute, UPMC Pain Medicine at Centre Commons, 5750 Centre Avenue, Suite 400, Pittsburgh, PA 15206, USA. Tel: 412-665-8051; Fax: 412-665-8067; email: dweiner@pitt.edu.

Pain in Older Persons, Progress in Pain
Research and Management, Vol. 35, edited
by Stephen J. Gibson and Debra K. Weiner,
IASP Press, Seattle, © 2005.

17

Clinical Features and Treatment of Postherpetic Neuralgia and Peripheral Neuropathy in Older Adults

Kenneth E. Schmader[a,b] and Robert H. Dworkin[c]

[a]Division of Geriatrics, Department of Medicine and the Center for the Study of Aging and Human Development, Duke University Medical Center, Durham, North Carolina; [b]Geriatric Research, Education and Clinical Center, Durham VA Medical Center, Durham, North Carolina; [c]Department of Anesthesiology, University of Rochester School of Medicine and Dentistry, Rochester, New York, USA

The International Association for the Study of Pain (IASP) defines neuropathic pain as pain "initiated or caused by a primary lesion or dysfunction in the nervous system" (Merskey and Bogduk 1994). The most common peripheral neuropathic pain states in older adults are postherpetic neuralgia (PHN) and painful diabetic neuropathy (PDN), also called diabetic peripheral neuropathic pain. However, other peripheral neuropathic pain states that may afflict older adults include alcoholic polyneuropathy, chemotherapy-induced polyneuropathy, entrapment neuropathies, post-mastectomy pain, post-thoracotomy pain, nerve compression or infiltration by tumor, phantom limb pain, post-radiation plexopathy, and trigeminal neuralgia. Although it is still a matter of discussion, most experts believe that certain types of chronic back pain have a neuropathic component, for example, cervical, thoracic, or lumbosacral radiculopathy.

Given that PHN is among the most common causes of neuropathic pain in older adults and may serve as a useful model for understanding the pathogenesis and treatment of neuropathic pain in older adults, this chapter will present the epidemiology and clinical features of PHN, including its impact on functional status and health-related quality of life in older adults. We will summarize the evidence for drug and nondrug approaches for the prevention and treatment of PHN as well as for the treatment of peripheral neuropathic pain in general.

EPIDEMIOLOGY OF POSTHERPETIC NEURALGIA

DEFINITION

PHN is a complication of herpes zoster, a neurocutaneous disease that is caused by the reactivation of varicella-zoster virus, a double-stranded DNA herpesvirus, from a latent infection of dorsal sensory or cranial nerve ganglia (Schmader 2001). During herpes zoster, the patient usually experiences a prodrome of pain or discomfort in the affected dermatome followed by the development of a unilateral, dermatomal, maculopapular, vesicular rash and acute pain. The rash heals in 2 to 4 weeks, but the pain may continue beyond rash healing in a large proportion of older persons. PHN has been variably defined as any pain after rash healing or any pain 1 month, 3 months, 4 months, or 6 months after rash onset. Recent analyses of pain trajectories after herpes zoster address this variability and suggest three phases: an acute herpetic neuralgia that lasts for approximately 30 days after rash onset, a subacute herpetic neuralgia that lasts from 30 to 120 days after rash onset, and PHN, defined as pain that persists for at least 120 days after rash onset (Arani et al. 2001; Desmond et al. 2002; Jung et al. 2004). The latter definition of PHN eliminates pain from acute inflammation and ensures a group of patients with true chronic neuropathic pain.

INCIDENCE AND PREVALENCE

The incidence of herpes zoster in persons over 65 years old is estimated to be 7–11 per 1000 per year in European and North American studies. Extrapolating from these studies, the lifetime incidence of herpes zoster has been calculated to be 10–20% in the general population and 50% in a cohort surviving to the age of 85 years (Gnann and Whitley 2002). From these figures, it is easy to see that millions of older adults worldwide are victims of herpes zoster and are at risk for subsequent PHN. However, the incidence and prevalence of PHN are not clear because of variable definitions and because data on PHN are not routinely collected and reported in large population groups. Using the variable definitions of PHN above, investigators have reported that 9–34% of herpes zoster patients developed PHN in community and clinic studies (Dworkin and Schmader 2001). Any study of PHN epidemiology must now take the effects of antiviral therapy for herpes zoster into account. In antiviral trials of adults over 50 years old, 46% of placebo recipients had pain 120 days after rash healing compared to 29% of patients who received antiviral drugs (Dworkin and Schmader 2001). Investigators have estimated that the prevalence of PHN ranges from 500,000 to one million in the United States and 200,000 in the United Kingdom (Bennett 1997; Bowsher 1999).

RISK FACTORS

Increasing age is the strongest predictor of PHN risk. For example, in Rochester, Minnesota, the average age of zoster patients with pain persisting after rash healing was 67 years compared to an average age of 46 years in the remainder of the cohort (Ragozzino et al. 1982). In Boston, patients aged 50 years or older had a 14.7-fold higher prevalence (95% CI = 6.8–32.0) of pain 30 days after rash onset compared to patients younger than 50 years old (Choo et al. 1997). The reason why older age is a very potent and well-replicated risk factor for PHN is not well understood.

The other major risk factors for PHN are greater acute pain severity, presence of a prodrome, and greater rash severity (Dworkin and Schmader 2001). As an example of the importance of greater acute pain severity, an analysis of a large antiviral trial in patients over 50 years old found a hazard ratio for PHN comparing severe acute pain versus mild acute pain to be 3.00 (95% CI = 2.26–3.99) (Whitley et al. 1998). A recent study reported that the major risk factors each make independent contributions to prediction of PHN (Jung et al. 2004). The positive predictive value of each factor alone was low, but together the positive predictive value was almost 50%. Conversely, absence of all these risk factors identified 90 to 95% of patients who did not develop PHN.

NATURAL HISTORY

The natural history of herpes zoster pain for many patients is one of improvement over time even without any treatment. In a combined analysis of major antiviral trials in patients over the age of 50 years who received placebo, 68% of patients had pain 30 days after rash onset, 46% had pain at 120 days, and 35–40% had pain at 180 days (Dworkin and Schmader 2001). Furthermore, some patients with long-lasting PHN will improve over time. In a study of 88 patients with moderate to severe PHN of 1 year or more, 31 (35%) had mild pain and no disability after an average of 2 years of follow-up (Watson et al. 1991). However, a substantial subset of older PHN patients have a poor prognosis and are refractory to treatment. Some patients may develop increased pain intensity over time. In addition, some patients may have pain-free intervals of weeks or months, only to note the return of their pain (Watson et al. 1991).

CLINICAL FEATURES OF POSTHERPETIC NEURALGIA

PHN patients may experience "positive" and "negative" sensory phenomena. The positive sensory phenomena include spontaneous constant or intermittent pain and stimulus-evoked pain such as allodynia or hyperalgesia. Allodynia is a particularly disabling component of the disease. Patients with allodynia suffer from severe pain after the lightest touch of the affected skin by something as trivial as a cold wind or a piece of clothing. Patients with hyperalgesia may suffer from severe pain after a stimulus that would normally be mildly painful or uncomfortable such as a bump against a car door or table. Other positive and underappreciated sensory phenomena in PHN include distracting tingling and severe itching, which has been labeled "postherpetic itch" (Oaklander et al. 2002).

Negative sensory phenomena include sensory loss in the affected dermatome. Although sensory loss may seem like a better problem to have than pain, it can cause substantial functional problems in older adults. When sensory loss accompanies sacral herpes zoster, the patient may not feel the bladder filling, may have difficulty voiding, and may develop urinary retention. Similarly, the patient may lose anorectal sensation and could develop difficulty with defecation or fecal incontinence. Sensory loss in the foot can lead to difficulty with ambulation, whereas sensory loss involving the eye can lead to corneal ulceration.

Several studies have reported on the quality of pain in PHN and compared it to acute herpes zoster pain (Bhala et al 1988; Bowsher 1992). Burning pain appears to be more common in PHN patients than in herpes zoster patients, but sharp, stabbing pain is more common in the latter. The word "tenderness" is used by both groups of patients to describe allodynia. These descriptors illustrate the three different types of pain in PHN—a steady throbbing or burning pain, an intermittent sharp or shooting pain, and allodynia.

Older patients and their clinicians frequently observe a negative impact of PHN on health-related quality of life (HRQL) and functional status contingent on pain intensity. PHN patients can suffer from a variety of constitutional symptoms including chronic fatigue, anorexia, weight loss, physical inactivity, insomnia, depression, and difficulty with concentration. The social activities of PHN patients and their spouses are often curtailed by the illness, and the patient's social role may change from being a vital member of the community to becoming an inactive individual in a household. Furthermore, PHN can interfere with dressing, bathing, grooming, eating, and mobility. For example, the patient with allodynic skin may be forced to avoid bathing or placing clothing around the affected area. Instrumental activities of daily living that are commonly affected include traveling, shopping, cooking, and housework.

However, there are few data to quantify the above clinical observations in a representative sample of PHN patients. In a pain clinic in Liverpool, United Kingdom, 59% of PHN patients were prevented from pursuing their usual activities for up to 16 years, with the average being 1.4 years (Davies et al. 1994). In another study, patients who had PHN for longer than 6 months were found to have greater disability and psychological distress than patients who had PHN for less than 6 months (Graff-Radford et al. 1986). In a large case series of herpes zoster patients from a dermatology clinic, insomnia (25%) and feeling helpless and depressed (20%) were common problems related to herpes zoster pain (Goh and Khoo 1997).

Investigators have reported data on the correlations of zoster pain and its impact on HRQL in clinical trials and instrument validation studies. Using the Nottingham Health Profile in a clinical trial of acyclovir and valacyclovir in 1,141 zoster patients, investigators reported that zoster pain at 8 weeks after rash onset significantly interfered with the energy, sleep, and global quality of life dimensions of the instrument (Mauskopf et al. 1994). The magnitude of interference increased significantly as pain severity increased. For example, there were modest effects on the above dimensions when the pain unpleasantness was rated as annoying but very strong effects when the pain was rated as very distressing or intolerable. In a study comparing the psychometric properties of the Medical Outcomes Study 36-Item Short-Form Health Survey (SF-36) and the Nottingham Health Profile in patients with neuropathic pain that included older adults with PHN, the patients had significantly worse scores on all HRQL dimensions of the two instruments when compared with the general population (Meyer-Rosberg et al. 2001). In a prospective observational study of 121 outpatients 60 or more years of age with herpes zoster, investigators correlated the Zoster Brief Pain Inventory, a zoster-specific measure of pain and interference with activities, with the SF-12 and EuroQoL HRQL measures and an activities of daily living (ADL) questionnaire (Coplan et al. 2004). Using the 0–10 worst pain score, pain at 35 days and 70 days after rash onset significantly interfered with multiple ADLs, reduced HRQL, as measured by the EuroQoL, and impaired mental and physical health, as measured by the SF-12. As with the antiviral study, interference with ADLs and reduced HRQL increased significantly as pain severity increased.

PREVENTION OF POSTHERPETIC NEURALGIA

PHN is difficult to treat, so investigators have pursued antiviral, anti-inflammatory, analgesic, anesthetic, and vaccine strategies during herpes zoster to prevent or reduce this chronic pain syndrome.

ANTIVIRAL THERAPY

Acyclovir, famciclovir, and valacyclovir are guanosine analogues that are phosphorylated by viral thymidine kinase and cellular kinases to a triphosphate form that inhibits varicella-zoster virus DNA polymerase. In general, these drugs are safe and well tolerated in older persons. Randomized controlled trials indicate that oral acyclovir (800 mg five times a day for 7 days), famciclovir (500 mg every 8 hours for 7 days), and valacyclovir (1 g three times a day for 7 days) reduce acute pain and the duration of chronic pain in older herpes zoster patients who are treated within 72 hours of rash onset (Kost and Straus 1996). Unfortunately, 20–30% of treated patients in antiviral trials had pain 6 months from herpes zoster onset, indicating that treated patients can develop PHN. Currently available data suggest that all three drugs are acceptable agents with factors other than efficacy determining the choice, such as cost and dosing schedule.

ANTI-INFLAMMATORY DRUGS

Well-designed randomized controlled clinical trials have shown that corticosteroids do not prevent PHN, whether compared to placebo or when combined with acyclovir (Schmader 2001). Gastrointestinal symptoms (dyspepsia, nausea, and vomiting) and edema were the most common adverse effects in these trials. Current evidence argues against the routine use of corticosteroids in older herpes zoster patients for the purpose of preventing PHN.

ANALGESICS

How effective are opiates, regional anesthetic nerve blocks, anticonvulsants, and tricyclic antidepressants employed during herpes zoster in reducing PHN? The answer to this interesting and important question will require rigorous clinical trials. One small study of amitriptyline or placebo during acute herpes zoster in older patients found no difference between groups at 1 or 3 months after rash onset, but significantly more amitriptyline recipients were pain free 6 months after rash onset (Bowsher 1992). The study was limited by the unequal use of acyclovir between the groups and because the drug is potentially hazardous in older persons. The results suggest that pain treatments during herpes zoster deserve more rigorous study with less toxic alternatives.

HERPES ZOSTER VACCINE

A recent large (n = 38,546), randomized, double-blind, placebo-controlled trial investigated the effect of a high-dose live attenuated varicella-zoster vaccine on herpes zoster and PHN among community-dwelling persons aged 60 years or older (Oxman et al. 2005). Using 90 days from zoster rash onset as the time to define PHN, the investigators reported 107 cases of PHN (27 among vaccine recipients and 80 among placebo recipients). There were 957 confirmed cases of herpes zoster (315 among vaccine recipients and 642 among placebo recipients). The zoster vaccine reduced the incidence of postherpetic neuralgia by 66.5% ($P < 0.001$) and the incidence of herpes zoster by 51.3% ($P < 0.001$). The vaccine also significantly reduced the incidence of neuralgic pain at all time points from zoster rash onset (i.e., 30, 60, 120, and 180 days). Reactions at the injection site were more frequent among vaccine recipients, but they were generally mild. This landmark study showed that the zoster vaccine can markedly reduce morbidity from PHN and herpes zoster among older adults.

TREATMENT OF POSTHERPETIC NEURALGIA AND NEUROPATHIC PAIN

ORAL AND TOPICAL PHARMACOTHERAPY

Most randomized controlled drug trials for neuropathic pain address PHN and PDN. The U.S. Food and Drug Administration (FDA) has approved medications for the treatment of only trigeminal neuralgia (carbamazepine), PHN (gabapentin, topical lidocaine patch 5%), and PDN (duloxetine). Whether the results of clinical trials in one neuropathic pain state can be extrapolated to others is not clear. Furthermore, clinical trials in neuropathic pain often include relatively small numbers of patients, so the magnitude of benefit and risk may not be nearly as precise as in clinical trials that include large numbers of patients. In addition, none of these trials include complex geriatric patients who have multiple comorbidities and take multiple medications and are therefore at risk for adverse drug events. As a result, clinicians need to carefully consider the risks of drugs for neuropathic pain in older adults, particularly in frail elders, before prescribing for potential benefits, especially when efficacy has not been established. Pharmacotherapy should be part of a more comprehensive approach to treatment that

includes education, support, and reassurance. Multidisciplinary team treatment often has a role in the treatment of neuropathic pain (please see Chapter 15 for a comprehensive discussion of multidisciplinary pain clinics).

Tricyclic antidepressants, gabapentin, lidocaine patches, and opioids are
considered first-line therapies because one or more high-quality, randomized
controlled trials have demonstrated efficacy with these agents (Table I).
These agents are discussed below along with selected second-line drugs.
One important caveat is that carbamazepine is the drug of choice for trigeminal
neuralgia. Pregabalin will likely be a first-line agent, but it is awaiting FDA
approval. Duloxetine and venlafaxine may be effective in PDN.

Pharmacotherapy for PHN and neuropathic pain is discussed in more
detail in recently published guidelines (Dworkin et al. 2003a; Dubinsky et
al. 2004). When reading any treatment recommendations for neuropathic
pain agents, it is imperative to remember that starting doses and maximum
doses of drugs are generally lower in older adults than in younger adults.
The upward titration of drug doses often needs to be slower in older adults
as well. These principles of geriatric pharmacotherapy apply most to the use
of drugs in complex older patients.

Tricyclic antidepressants (TCAs). Multiple randomized controlled trials of TCAs have demonstrated significant pain relief in patients with PHN
and PDN (Max 1995). In PHN trials, 44–67% of patients treated with TCAs
reported moderate to good pain relief compared to 5–19% of placebo or
control drug recipients. Although amitriptyline was tested in many of these
trials and is widely used for neuropathic pain syndromes, it is often poorly
tolerated in older adults because of its high anticholinergic activity. Nortriptyline demonstrated equivalent efficacy to amitriptyline in a PHN trial, but
was better tolerated (Watson et al. 1998). Nortriptyline should be considered
a preferred TCA for the treatment of PHN and neuropathic pain in older
adults; desipramine is a reasonable alternative.

TCAs have several potentially significant adverse effects in older adults.
They may cause cardiac toxicity in patients with a history of cardiovascular
disease (Roose et al. 1998). A screening EKG to check for cardiac conduction abnormalities is recommended before beginning TCA treatment in older
persons. TCAs are contraindicated in patients with QT prolongation or familial histories of long-QT syndromes, with atrioventricular block or bundle-
branch block, and with a recent acute myocardial infarction. Other important
adverse effects include dry mouth, constipation, dizziness, orthostatic hypotension, disturbed vision, drowsiness, cognitive impairment, and balance
problems. All TCAs must be used cautiously in patients with a history of
cardiovascular disease, glaucoma, urinary retention, and autonomic neuropathy. TCAs are metabolized by the cytochrome P450 D26 enzyme system.

Table I
First-line medications for neuropathic pain in older adults

Medication Class	Medication	Pharmacokinetics	Key Drug-Drug Interactions	Key Drug-Disease Interactions	Important Adverse Effects
Tricyclic antidepressants	Nortriptyline, desipramine, (amitriptyline)	Hepatic metabolism; higher levels of active metabolites in the elderly	Antipsychotics, anticholinergics, SSRIs, sedative-hypnotics, antiarrhythmics, MAO inhibitors, clonidine, antiretrovirals	Myocardial infarction, QT prolongation, AV block, bundle branch block, ileus, prostatic hypertrophy, glaucoma, seizure disorder, dementia	Arrhythmia, cardiac conduction block, orthostatic hypotension, urinary retention, constipation, cognitive impairment; adverse withdrawal events after abrupt discontinuation; death if torsades de pointes arrhythmia
Anticonvulsants	Gabapentin	Renal elimination; prolonged half-life with renal impairment	Opioids	Dementia, ataxia	Somnolence, dizziness, peripheral edema, increased appetite and weight gain, adverse withdrawal events after abrupt discontinuation
Opioids and opioid-like drugs	Oxycodone, morphine, tramadol	Hepatic metabolism and renal elimination; plasma levels may be higher in the elderly	Anticholinergics, sedative-hypnotics, anxiolytics, CYP2D6 inhibitors, SSRIs, TCAs, muscle relaxants	Ileus, chronic obstructive pulmonary disease, dementia, prostatic hypertrophy	Constipation, sedation, nausea/vomiting, respiratory depression, nervous system symptoms, pruritis, adverse withdrawal events after abrupt discontinuation
Topical anesthetics	Topical lidocaine patch 5%	Very little systemic absorption	Class I antiarrhythmics		Skin rash

Abbreviations: AV = atrioventricular; MAO = monoamine oxidase; SSRIs = selective serotonin reuptake inhibitors; TCAs = tricyclic antidepressants.

Because all selective serotonin reuptake inhibitors (SSRIs) inhibit P450 D26, caution is necessary in the concomitant administration of TCAs and SSRIs so as to prevent toxic TCA plasma concentrations. The patient should understand that TCAs have an analgesic effect independent of their antidepressant effect. Dosages are listed in Table II.

Anticonvulsants. Anticonvulsant medications have been employed for the treatment of neuropathic pain for years. Gabapentin was associated with a statistically significant reduction in daily pain ratings as well as improvements in sleep, mood, and quality of life at daily dosages of 1800–3600 mg in clinical trials in PHN and PDN (Backonja et al. 1998; Rowbotham et al. 1998; Rice et al. 2001). In the PHN trials, 41–43% of patients on gabapentin reported moderate or much pain improvement compared to 12–23% of those on placebo. Using a 0–10-point numerical rating scale, average pain ratings decreased approximately 2 points in one study (Rowbotham et al. 1998) compared to a 0.5–1 point change in the placebo group over an 8-week period (i.e., 6.3–4.2 points in the treated group compared to 6.5–6.0 points in the placebo group, $P < 0.001$, in one study).

The adverse effects of gabapentin included somnolence, dizziness, and peripheral edema, which in one trial occurred in 27%, 23%, and 10% of participants, respectively (Rowbotham et al. 1998). These adverse effects require monitoring and possibly dosage adjustment, but usually not treatment discontinuation. In frail older adults, gabapentin may cause or exacerbate gait and balance problems and cognitive impairment that can require discontinuation of therapy. Dosage adjustment is necessary in patients with renal insufficiency (Table II).

Pregabalin is an α_2-δ calcium channel ligand that has demonstrated efficacy in randomized controlled trials of PHN and PDN (Dworkin et al. 2003b; Rosenstock et al. 2004; Sabatowski et al. 2004). In a multicenter trial of 173 PHN patients, pregabalin-treated patients had greater decreases in pain than patients treated with placebo (endpoint mean scores of 3.60 versus 5.29 on a 0–10-point VAS of pain intensity; $P = 0.0001$) (Dworkin et al. 2003b). The proportions of patients with greater than 50% decreases in mean pain scores were greater in the pregabalin group than in the placebo group (50% versus 20%, $P = 0.001$). Dizziness, somnolence, peripheral edema, amblyopia, dry mouth, and gait disturbances were the most common adverse effects of the medication. The drug can be given once a day, has few drug interactions, and has a relatively rapid onset of action. Pregabalin was recently approved by the FDA for PHN and PDN.

Regarding other anticonvulsants, carbamazepine is effective in trigeminal neuralgia, and lamotrigine has demonstrated efficacy in relatively small trials in patients with HIV sensory neuropathy, PDN, and central post-stroke

Table II

Dosage of first-line medications for neuropathic pain

Medication	Beginning Dosage	Titration	Maximum Dosage	Duration of Adequate Trial
Gabapentin	100–300 mg at bedtime	Increase by 100–300 mg a day every 1–7 days as tolerated in divided doses up to t.i.d.	3600 mg daily (1200 mg tid); reduce if creatinine clearance is less than 60 mL/min	3–8 weeks for titration plus 1–2 weeks at maximum tolerated dosage
Lidocaine patch 5%	Maximum of 3 patches daily for a maximum of 12 hours	None needed	Maximum of 3 patches daily for a maximum of 12 hours	2 weeks
Opioid analgesics (dosages given are for morphine)	2.5–15 mg every 4 hours as needed	After 1–2 weeks, convert total daily dosage to a long-acting opioid analgesic and continue short-acting medication as needed	No maximum with careful titration; consider evaluation by pain specialist at dosages exceeding 120–180 mg daily	4–6 weeks
Tramadol	25 mg once daily	Increase by 25–50 mg daily in divided doses every 3–7 days as tolerated	400 mg daily (100 mg q.i.d.); in patients over 75 years of age, 300 mg daily in divided doses	4 weeks
Tricyclic antidepressants, especially nortriptyline or desipramine	10–25 mg at bedtime	Increase by 10–25 mg daily every 3–7 days as tolerated	75–150 mg daily; if blood level of active drug and its metabolite is below 100 ng/mL, continue titration with caution	6–8 weeks with at least 1–2 weeks at maximum tolerated dosage

Source: Adapted with permission from Dworkin et al. (2003a).

pain (Dworkin et al. 2003a). Lamotrigine should be used very cautiously in older adults because it requires careful dosing and poses the risk of a severe rash and Stevens-Johnson syndrome. The risk-benefit profile of phenytoin is not clear in neuropathic pain in older adults because available data do not meet current methodological standards. Other second-generation anticonvulsants (e.g., levetiracetam, oxcarbazepine, tiagabine, topiramate, zonisamide, and valproate) cannot be considered first-line agents for the treatment of neuropathic pain in older adults at this time because of limited data and/or significant adverse effects, although these agents are under active investigation. Available anticonvulsants have different and often multiple mechanisms, so non-response to one anticonvulsant may not predict non-response to the category as a whole. For further discussion of anticonvulsants for the treatment of neuropathic pain, see Chapter 10.

Topical agents. Three randomized, vehicle-controlled trials of the 5% topical lidocaine patch in PHN patients demonstrated statistically significantly greater pain relief with the lidocaine patch compared with control patches containing no lidocaine (Rowbotham et al. 1996; Galer et al. 1999; Meier et al. 2003). One study involved patients with PHN and many other focal peripheral neuropathic pain syndromes in a cross-over trial of 7-day application periods (Meier et al. 2003). The percentage of patients who obtained 50% reduction in ongoing pain was 31% with the lidocaine patch compared to 8% with placebo patch. Although the exact percentage was not reported, fewer patients with allodynia obtained 50% reduction of pain with the lidocaine patch than did similarly treated patients with ongoing pain, illustrating the importance of recognizing allodynia and the difficulty in treating it. An open-label study of the topical lidocaine patch in PDN indicated that up to four patches were well tolerated and significantly improved pain and HRQL, but the results need to be confirmed in a randomized controlled trial (Barbano et al. 2004). For PHN, up to three patches should be applied over the painful area. The adverse effects of the 5% lidocaine patch involve skin reactions (e.g., erythema, rash). Systemic absorption is minimal but must be considered in patients receiving oral class I antiarrhythmic drugs. Table II details the use of the patch.

Many other topical agents have been used by patients with PHN and other neuropathic pain states, but few have been studied in controlled clinical trials save capsaicin and topical anti-inflammatory drugs. However, the trials with these agents have significant methodological limitations. Most clinical trials of capsaicin in PHN and PDN showed greater pain relief with capsaicin compared to vehicle control (Bernstein et al. 1989; Watson et al. 1993; Zhang and Li Wan Po 1994; Mason et al. 2004). In one trial, topical capsaicin showed the same pain relief as oral amitriptyline in PDN

(Biesbroeck et al. 1995). However, topical capsaicin often causes burning in the area of the application. The burning sensation limits interpretation of the clinical trials because they were not truly blinded. Furthermore, the burning interferes with adherence to therapy. Of the topical anti-inflammatory drugs, aspirin in cream showed mild pain reduction in PHN compared to no pain reduction with indomethacin or diclofenac in cream (De Benedittis and Lorenzetti 1996). Topical capsaicin and aspirin in cream may be considered as a therapeutic option in PHN and PDN because it may occasionally be effective in individual circumstances. All topical therapies may be impractical when the involved area of skin is too large or difficult to reach.

Opioid and opioid-like analgesics. Multiple randomized controlled trials of oral opioids in PHN, PDN, and phantom limb pain in older adults demonstrated significant pain relief compared to placebo (Watson and Babul 1998; Huse et al. 2001; Raja et al. 2002; Gimbel et al. 2003; Watson et al. 2003). Depending on the trial, improvements in mood, sleep, and functional status were also demonstrated with opioids compared to placebo. In a notable PHN crossover trial, mean pain intensity on a 100-mm visual analogue scale (VAS) was lower on controlled-release oxycodone than with placebo (35 mm versus 54 mm, $P = 0.0001$) after 4 weeks of treatment. At the completion of the two treatments, 67% of patients preferred oxycodone, 11% preferred placebo, and 22% had no preference (Watson and Babul 1998). In a crossover study of PHN comparing opioid analgesics, TCAs, and placebo, controlled-release morphine and TCAs provided statistically significant benefits on pain (Raja et al. 2002). In this trial, patients preferred treatment with opioid analgesics compared to TCAs and placebo despite a greater incidence of side effects and more dropouts during opioid treatment.

The well-known adverse effects of opioids may preclude their use in some older adults. Constipation, sedation, and nausea are very common adverse effects of opioid analgesics in older persons. Constipation is so common that patients should be educated about stimulant laxatives at the same time that an opioid is prescribed, and these agents should be started at the first sign of constipation. Cognitive impairment and falls and fractures can occur in older patients. Opioid analgesics must be used very cautiously in patients with a history of substance abuse or suicide. Patients treated with opioid analgesics may develop analgesic tolerance. All patients will develop physical dependence (i.e., withdrawal symptoms develop with abrupt discontinuation or rapid dose reduction) and must be advised that they should not abruptly discontinue their medication. The risk that abuse will develop in patients who do not have a history of substance abuse is not known but is thought to be low in the older patient with neuropathic pain. Numerous short- and long-acting opioid analgesics are available, and one dosing approach is shown in Table II.

Tramadol has a major metabolite that is a μ-opioid agonist, and it is also a norepinephrine and serotonin reuptake inhibitor. Three randomized controlled trials of tramadol in PHN, PDN, and painful polyneuropathy of different etiologies showed significant relief of pain and allodynia compared to placebo (Harati et al. 1998; Sindrup et al. 1999; Boureau et al. 2003). In the PHN trial, 77% of subjects on tramadol versus 56% on placebo reported greater than 50% reduction in pain after 6 weeks of treatment. The average difference in pain intensity on the 100-mm VAS was 9 mm in favor of tramadol. The adverse effects of tramadol include dizziness, nausea, constipation, somnolence, and orthostatic hypotension. Other important adverse effects unique to tramadol compared to opioids are the increased risk of seizures in patients who have a history of seizures or who use drugs that can reduce the seizure threshold, as well as an increased risk of serotonin syndrome in patients who use serotonergic medications, especially SSRIs and monoamine oxidase inhibitors. Tramadol may cause or exacerbate cognitive impairment in older patients. Dosage adjustment is necessary in patients with renal or hepatic disease (Table II).

Other agents. Duloxetine is a serotonin and norepinephrine reuptake inhibitor that is effective in treating depression and painful symptoms associated with depression (Fava et al. 2004). The drug showed significant pain reduction in two placebo-controlled trials of PDN patients according to an FDA report (Anonymous 2004), although the publications are pending. Based on these trials, the FDA recently approved duloxetine specifically for PDN. The most common adverse effects are nausea, dizziness, fatigue, and somnolence. The recommended dose is 60 mg a day, although in older adults it may be prudent to start at 30 mg a day.

Venlafaxine is a serotonin and norepinephrine reuptake inhibitor that may be effective in neuropathic pain (Tasmuth et al. 2002; Sindrup et al. 2003; Rowbotham 2004). In a randomized, placebo-controlled 6-week study in patients with PDN, the percentage reduction from baseline on a 100-mm VAS of pain intensity was 27% for placebo and 50% for treatment with a daily dose of 150–225 mg of venlafaxine ($P < 0.001$). The percentage of patients with 50% or more pain reduction from baseline was 34% placebo versus 56% for treatment ($P < 0.01$). The most common adverse effects include drowsiness, weakness, dizziness, dry mouth, anxiety, and tremor. The starting dose is 75 mg a day, aiming toward 150–225 mg a day.

Sequential and combination pharmacological treatment. Clinical observations and data from the few clinical trials comparing medications in neuropathic pain indicate that patients may respond to one drug but not to another, even within the same class of drug. There is no way to reliably predict which patient will respond to a given drug. Unfortunately, some patients with PHN and other neuropathic pain states may not respond to *any* drug. Therefore, the choice of initial and sequential therapy will require weighing the potential benefits, adverse effects, costs, and patient preferences for an individual patient. Furthermore, non-response to single drug therapy often leads to combination therapy, but there are no data regarding the additive or synergistic benefits of combination treatment. Also, it is not known which patients are most likely to benefit from which combinations. Disadvantages of combination therapy in older adults include an increased risk of adverse effects and difficulty in determining which medication is responsible for which adverse effects.

OTHER TREATMENTS

A considerable percentage of older patients with neuropathic pain will not respond to medications. For these patients, there are numerous non-drug treatments that deserve consideration. A clinically useful way to approach non-drug treatments is to divide them into non-invasive and invasive treatments. Invasive treatments may be considered when patients have failed to obtain adequate relief from non-invasive treatment approaches. Patients who require complex drug combinations, risky second-line treatments, or invasive treatments should be referred to a pain management center. A detailed review of each intervention is beyond the scope of this chapter, but we will briefly summarize the available evidence.

Non-invasive treatments. Non-invasive treatments include physical modalities such as cold application or transcutaneous electrical nerve stimulation (TENS), psychological treatments, and acupuncture. Anecdotally, some patients with PHN report a decrease in pain with application of a cold pack over the painful area, while others note an increase in pain with this treatment. TENS has been reported in PHN case series to be beneficial in some patients (Nathan and Wall 1974). Likewise, authors have reported that biofeedback and other psychological treatments are successful in case series of neuropathic pain patients such as those discussed in Chapter 12 of this text (Haythornthwaite and Benrud-Larson 2000). These interventions have little risk and may be useful in some patients, but whether they are truly effective in a population of patients with PHN and other neuropathic pain states is unknown, and they must be tested in controlled clinical trials.

Acupuncture has been reported to be effective in reducing pain in PHN, PDN, and other neuropathic pain states in case reports and case series. The only randomized controlled trial of acupuncture in PHN compared acupuncture with placebo (mock transcutaneous nerve stimulation) in 62 patients (Lewith et al. 1983). The amount of pain relief was no different in the two groups during or after treatment. At the end of treatment, 22% of patients in the acupuncture group and 22% of patients in the placebo group had significant improvement in their pain. A modality related to TENS and acupuncture is percutaneous electrical nerve stimulation (PENS). PENS was compared to sham (needles only) in a 3-week randomized controlled crossover trial of 50 patients with PDN (Hamza et al. 2000). Compared with the 10-cm VAS scores before PENS (6.2 ± 1.0) and sham (6.4 ± 0.9) treatments, pain scores after treatment were reduced to 2.5 ± 0.8 and 6.3 ± 1.1, respectively. Physical activity and HRQL also significantly improved with the PENS treatment compared to the sham treatment.

Invasive treatments. The categories of invasive treatments include peripheral and central neural blockade, central nervous system (CNS) drug delivery, spinal cord stimulation, and neurosurgical techniques. These interventions represent rational approaches to pain relief, but they have not been proven effective in controlled trials, partly because the design and conduct of such trials are difficult, and they carry procedural risks in older persons. In general, these interventions have a limited role in neuropathic pain treatment and should be contemplated only in patients who have failed other treatments and continue to have disabling pain. Neurosurgical techniques will not be discussed further because they are particularly risky in older persons. Some procedures, such as dorsal root entry zone lesions, have been abandoned because of pain recurrence and significant complications (Friedman and Bullitt 1988).

Neural blockade techniques include sensory nerve, plexus, and sympathetic nerve blocks as well as epidural and intrathecal blockade with lidocaine-like drugs and/or corticosteroids. The level of evidence for the effectiveness of these techniques in neuropathic pain is limited to case reports and case series. In most studies, many patients note initial relief of pain, but few experience long-lasting relief (Abram 2000). In PHN, the greater the duration of pain, the less likely it is that neural blockade will provide pain relief. In a widely publicized case series of patients with intractable PHN for more than a year, investigators reported good or excellent pain relief for up to 2 years in 90% of patients treated with intrathecal methylprednisolone plus lidocaine compared to 6% of patients treated with intrathecal lidocaine alone and 4% in a no-injection control group (Kotani et al. 2000). This treatment has significant risks, including neurological complications and adhesive arachnoiditis, so before this treatment modality can be recommended its safety and feasibility will need to be confirmed in other studies and in clinical practice.

Central nervous system drug delivery attempts to place drug as close as possible to central pain receptors in the spinal cord corresponding to the affected dermatome(s). The intrathecal administration of opioids, especially morphine, has been reported to provide significant pain relief in case series that included neuropathic pain states (Bennett et al. 2000). Other agents reported in CNS delivery systems include bupivacaine, clonidine, and baclofen. These interventions have not been studied in older patients nor in controlled trials, and they have the same risks mentioned above for intrathecal procedures. Neural blockade and CNS drug delivery systems are discussed in more detail in Chapter 13.

Spinal cord stimulation requires implantation of an electrode in the thoracic or lumbar epidural space and the placement of a percutaneous electrical stimulator. This technique has been reported to provide pain relief in uncontrolled studies of neuropathic pain (Cameron 2004). For example, in one study of 28 patients with intractable PHN (median age 70 years), 23 patients demonstrated long-term pain relief of pain and improvements in daily functioning (Harke et al. 2002). The authors reported that pain recurred after the stimulator was turned off, arguing against spontaneous improvement. This procedure has not been well studied in older persons.

CONCLUSION

Neuropathic pain afflicts millions of older persons worldwide, lowering quality of life and interfering with functional status. The most common types of neuropathic pain in older persons are PHN and PDN. The clinical features of neuropathic pain include spontaneous constant or intermittent pain, stimulus evoked-pain such as allodynia or hyperalgesia, itching or tingling, and sensory loss. The treatment of PHN, PDN, and other neuropathic pain states is challenging. These conditions require a comprehensive approach to management that includes education and counseling, together with a balanced consideration of pharmacotherapeutic and alternative options depending on the pain's intensity, its impact on functional status, comorbidity, and the patient's drug regimen and preferences. Available evidence indicates that anticonvulsants, topical lidocaine, tricyclic antidepressants, and opioids effectively reduce pain in a significant proportion of neuropathic pain patients. Tricyclic antidepressants and opioids generally require more caution in older adults because of their adverse effect profile. Gabapentin, pregabalin, and topical lidocaine are considered agents of first choice. Nortriptyline or desipramine are, however, a reasonable first choice in a healthy senior without heart disease. Non-invasive treatments that do not involve drugs (e.g., TENS) may be useful in some patients and carry little risk. Invasive treatments (e.g., spinal cord stimulators) have a more limited role due to limited evidence for efficacy and potential adverse effects. These interventions should only be contemplated in patients who have failed other treatments and continue to have disabling pain. Undoubtedly, these recommendations will need to be refined as investigations with newer treatments and with combination and sequential drug strategies become available. Nonetheless, patient and clinicians have several options to better manage neuropathic pain in older patients than ever before.

ACKNOWLEDGMENTS

Dr. Schmader was supported by a Mid-Career Investigator Award in Patient-Oriented Research (K24-AI-51324-01) from the National Institute of Allergy and Infectious Diseases. Dr. Dworkin has received support, consulting fees, or lecture honoraria in the past year from Abbott Laboratories, Cephalon, Eli Lilly & Co., Endo Pharmaceuticals, EpiCept Corporation, Neurogesix, Novartis Pharmaceuticals, Organon, Ortho-McNeil Pharmaceutical, Pfizer, Ranbaxy Corporation, UCB Pharma, Wyeth, and Yamanouchi Europe.

REFERENCES

Abram SE. Neural blockade for neuropathic pain. *Clin J Pain* 2000; 16:S56–61.

Anonymous. New drug for neuropathic pain. *FDA Consumer* 2004; 38:2.

Arani RB, Soong SJ, Weiss HL, et al. Phase specific analysis of herpes zoster associated pain data: a new statistical approach. *Stat Med* 2001; 20:2429–2439.

Backonja M, Beydoun A, Edwards KR, et al. Gabapentin Diabetic Neuropathy Study Group. Gabapentin for the symptomatic treatment of painful neuropathy in patients with diabetes mellitus. *JAMA* 1998; 280:1831–1836.

Barbano RL, Herrmann DN, Hart-Gouleau S, et al. Effectiveness, tolerability, and impact on quality of life of the 5% lidocaine patch in diabetic polyneuropathy. *Arch Neurol* 2004; 61:914–918.

Bennett GJ. Neuropathic pain: an overview. In: Borsook D (Ed). *Molecular Neurobiology of Pain,* Progress in Pain Research and Management, Vol. 9. Seattle: IASP Press, 1997, pp 109–113.

Bennett G, Serafini M, Burchiel K, et al. Evidence-based review of the literature on the intrathecal delivery of pain medication. *J Pain Symptom Manage* 2000; 20:S12–36.

Bernstein JE, Korman NJ, Bickers DR, Dahl MY, Millikan LE. Topical capsaicin treatment of chronic postherpetic neuralgia. *J Am Acad Dermatol* 1989; 21:265–270.

Biesbroeck R, Bril V, Hollander P, et al. A double blind comparison of topical capsaicin and oral amitriptyline in painful diabetic neuropathy. *Adv Ther* 1995; 12:111–120.

Bhala BB, Ramamoorthy C, Bowsher D, et al. Shingles and postherpetic neuralgia. *Clin J Pain* 1988; 4:169–174.

Boureau F, Legallicier P, Kabir-Ahmadi M. Tramadol in post-herpetic neuralgia: a randomized, double-blind, placebo-controlled trial. *Pain* 2003; 104:323–331.

Bowsher D. Acute herpes zoster and postherpetic neuralgia: effects of acyclovir and outcome of treatment with amitriptyline. *Br J Gen Pract* 1992; 42:244–246.

Bowsher D. The lifetime occurrence of herpes zoster and prevalence of postherpetic neuralgia: a retrospective survey in an elderly population. *Eur J Pain* 1999; 3:335–342.

Cameron T. Safety and efficacy of spinal cord stimulation for the treatment of chronic pain: a 20 year literature review. *J Neurosurg Spine* 2004; 100:254–267.

Choo PW, Galil K, Donahue JG, et al. Risk factors for postherpetic neuralgia. *Arch Intern Med* 1997; 157:1217–1224.

Coplan PM, Schmader K, Nikas A, et al. Development of a measure of the burden of pain due to herpes zoster and postherpetic neuralgia for prevention trials: adaptation of the brief pain inventory. *J Pain* 2004; 5:344–356.

Davies L, Cossins L, Bowsher D, Drummond M. The cost of treatment for post-herpetic neuralgia in the UK. *PharmacoEconomics* 1994; 6:142–148.

De Benedittis G, Lorenzetti A. Topical aspirin/diethyl ether mixture versus indomethacin and diclofenac/diethyl ether mixtures for acute herpetic neuralgia and postherpetic neuralgia: a double-blind crossover placebo-controlled study. *Pain* 1996; 65:45–51.

Desmond RA, Weiss HL, Arani RB, et al. Clinical applications for change-point analysis of herpes zoster pain. *J Pain Symptom Manage* 2002; 23:510–516.

Dubinsky RH, Kabbani H, El-Chami Z, Boutwell C, Ali H. Practice parameter: treatment of postherpetic neuralgia. *Neurology* 2004; 63:959–965.

Dworkin RH, Schmader KE. Epidemiology and natural history of herpes zoster and postherpetic neuralgia. In: Watson CPN, Gershon AA (Eds). *Herpes Zoster and Postherpetic Neuralgia*, 2nd ed, New York: Elsevier Press, 2001, pp 39–64.

Dworkin RH, Allen RR, Argoff CR, et al. Guidelines for the pharmacologic management of chronic neuropathic pain. *Arch Neurol* 2003a; 60:1524–1534.

Dworkin RH, Corbin AE, Young JP Jr, et al. Pregabalin for the treatment of postherpetic neuralgia: a randomized, placebo-controlled trial. *Neurology* 2003b; 60:1274–1283.

Fava M, Mallinckrody CH, Detke MJ, Watkin JG, Wohlreich MM. The effect of duloxetine on the painful physical symptoms in depressed patients: do improvements in these symptoms result in higher remission rates? *J Clin Psychiatry* 2004; 65(4):521–530.

Friedman AH, Bullitt E. Dorsal root entry zone lesions in the treatment of pain following brachial plexus avulsion, spinal cord injury and herpes zoster. *Appl Neurophysiol* 1988; 51:164–169.

Galer BS, Rowbotham MC, Perander J, et al. Topical lidocaine patch relieves postherpetic neuralgia more effectively than a vehicle topical patch: results of an enriched enrollment study. *Pain* 1999; 80:533–538.

Gimbel JS, Richards P, Portenoy RK. Controlled-release oxycodone for pain in diabetic neuropathy: a randomized controlled trial. *Neurology* 2003; 60:927–934.

Gnann JW Jr, Whitley RJ. Herpes zoster. *N Engl J Med* 2002; 347:340–346.

Goh CL, Khoo L. A retrospective study of the clinical presentation and outcome of herpes zoster in a tertiary dermatology outpatient referral clinic. *Int J Dermatol* 1997; 36:667–672.

Hamza MA, White PF, Craig WF, et al. Percutaneous electrical nerve stimulation: a novel analgesic therapy for diabetic neuropathic pain. *Diabetes Care* 2000; 23:365–370.

Harati Y, Gooch C, Swenson M, Edelman S, et al. Double-blind randomized trial of tramadol for the treatment of the pain of diabetic neuropathy. *Neurology* 1998; 50:1842–1846.

Harke H, Gretenkort P, Ladleif HU, et al. Spinal cord stimulation in postherpetic neuralgia and in acute herpes zoster pain. *Anesth Analg* 2002; 94:694–700.

Haythornthwaite JA, Benrud-Larson LM. Psychological aspects of neuropathic pain. *Clin J Pain* 2000; 16:S101–105.

Huse E, Larbig W, Flor H, Birbaumer N. The effect of opioids on phantom limb pain and cortical reorganization. *Pain* 2001; 90:47–55.

Jung BF, Johnson RW, Griffin DR, Dworkin RH. Risk factors for postherpetic neuralgia in patients with herpes zoster. *Neurology* 2004; 62:1545–1551.

Kost RG, Straus SS. Postherpetic neuralgia - pathogenesis, treatment, and prevention. *N Engl J Med* 1996; 335:32–42.

Kotani N, Kushikata T, Hashimoto H, et al. Intrathecal methylprednisolone for intractable postherpetic neuralgia. *N Engl J Med* 2000; 343:1514–1519.

Lewith GT, Field J, Machin D. Acupuncture compared with placebo in post-herpetic pain. *Pain* 1983; 17:361–368.

Mason L, Moore RA, Derry S, Edwards JE, McQuay HJ. Systematic review of topical capsaicin for the treatment of chronic pain. *BMJ* 2004; 328(7446):991.

Mauskopf J, Austin R, Dix L, Berzon R. The Nottingham Health Profile as a measure of quality of life in zoster patients: convergent and discriminant validity. *Qual Life Res* 1994; 3:431–435.

Max MB. Thirteen consecutive well-designed randomized trials show that antidepressants reduce pain in diabetic neuropathy and postherpetic neuralgia. *Pain Forum* 1995; 4:248–253.

Meier T, Wasner G, Faust M, Kuntzer, et al. Efficacy of lidocaine patch 5% in the treatment of focal peripheral neuropathic pain syndromes: a randomized, double-blind, placebo-controlled study. *Pain* 2003; 106:151–158.

Merskey H, Bogduk N (Eds). *Classification of Chronic Pain: Descriptions of Chronic Pain Syndromes and Definitions of Pain Terms,* 2nd ed. Seattle: IASP Press, 1994, p 212.

Meyer-Rosberg K, Burckhardt CS, Huizar K, et al. A comparison of the SF-36 and Nottingham Health Profile in patients with chronic neuropathic pain. *Eur J Pain* 2001; 5:391–403.

Nathan PW, Wall PD. Treatment of post-herpetic neuralgia by prolonged electrical stimulation. *Br Med J* 1974; 3:645–647.

Oaklander AL, Cohen SP, Raju SV. Intractable postherpetic itch and cutaneous deafferentation after facial shingles. *Pain* 2002; 96:9–12.

Oxman MN, Levin MJ, Johnson GR, et al. Shingles Prevention Study Group. A vaccine to prevent herpes zoster and postherpetic neuralgia in older adults. *N Engl J Med* 2005; 352:2271–2284.

Ragozzino MW, Melton LF III, Kurland LT. Population-based study of herpes zoster and its sequelae. *Medicine (Baltimore)* 1982; 61:310–316.

Raja SN, Haythornthwaite JA, Pappagallo M, et al. Opioids versus antidepressants in postherpetic neuralgia: a randomized, placebo-controlled trial. *Neurology* 2002; 59:1015–1021.

Rice ASC, Maton S, Postherpetic Neuralgia Study Group. Gabapentin in postherpetic neuralgia: a randomised, double blind, placebo controlled study. *Pain* 2001; 94:215–224.

Roose SP, Laghrissi-Thode F, Kennedy JS, et al. Comparison of paroxetine and nortriptyline in depressed patients with ischemic heart disease. *JAMA* 1998; 279:287–291.

Rosenstock J, Tuchman M, LaMoreaux, Sharma U. Pregabalin for the treatment of painful diabetic peripheral neuropathy: a double-blind, placebo-controlled trial. *Pain* 2004; 110:628–638.

Rowbotham MC, Davies PS, Verkempinck C, et al. Lidocaine patch: double-blind controlled study of a new treatment method for post-herpetic neuralgia. *Pain* 1996; 65:39–44.

Rowbotham MC, Harden N, Stacey B, et al. Gabapentin for the treatment postherpetic neuralgia: a randomized controlled trial. *JAMA* 1998; 280:1837–1842.

Rowbotham MC, Goli V, Kunz NR, Lei D. Venlafaxine extended release in the treatment of painful diabetic neuropathy: a double-blind, placebo controlled study. *Pain* 2004; 110(3):697–706.

Sabatowski R, Galvez R, Cherry DA, et al. Pregabalin reduces pain and improves sleep and mood disturbances in patients with post-herpetic neuralgia: results of a randomised, placebo-controlled clinical trial. *Pain* 2004; 109:26–35.

Schmader KE. Herpes zoster in older adults. *Clin Infect Dis* 2001; 32(10):1481–1486.

Sindrup SH, Andersen G, Madsen C, et al. Tramadol relieves pain and allodynia in polyneuropathy: a randomised, double-blind, controlled trial. *Pain* 1999; 83:85–90.

Sindrup SH, Bach FW, Madsen C, Gram LF, Jensen TS. Venlafaxine versus imipramine in painful polyneuropathy: a randomized, controlled trial. *Neurology* 2003; 60:1284–1289.

Tasmuth T, Hartel B, Kalso E. Venlafaxine in neuropathic pain following treatment of breast cancer. *Eur J Pain* 2002; 6:17–24.

Watson CPN, Babul N. Efficacy of oxycodone in neuropathic pain: a randomized trial in postherpetic neuralgia. *Neurology* 1998; 50:1837–1841.

Watson CPN, Watt VR, Chipman M, et al. The prognosis with post-herpetic neuralgia. *Pain* 1991; 46:195–199.

Watson CPN, Tyler KL, Bickers DR, et al. A randomized, vehicle-controlled trial of topical capsaicin in the treatment of postherpetic neuralgia. *Clin Ther* 1993; 15:510–526.

Watson CPN, Vernich L, Chipman M, Reed K. Nortriptyline versus amitriptyline in postherpetic neuralgia: a randomized trial. *Neurology* 1998; 51:1166–1171.

Watson CPN, Moulin D, Watt-Watson J, Gordon A, Eisenhoffer J. Controlled-release oxycodone relieves neuropathic pain: a randomized controlled trial in painful diabetic neuropathy. Pain 2003; 105:71–78.

Whitley RJ, Shukla S, Crooks RJ. The identification of risk factors associated with persistent pain following herpes zoster. *J Infect Dis* 1998; 178:S71–S75.

Zhang WY, Li Wan Po A. The effectiveness of topically applied capsaicin. A meta-analysis. *Eur J Clin Pharmacol* 1994; 46:517–522.

Correspondence to: Kenneth E. Schmader, MD, 182 GRECC, 508 Fulton Street, Durham VA Medical Center, Durham, NC 27705, USA. Tel: 919-286-6932; Fax: 919-286-6823; email: schma001@mc.duke.edu.

Pain in Older Persons, Progress in Pain Research and Management, Vol. 35, edited by Stephen J. Gibson and Debra K. Weiner, IASP Press, Seattle, © 2005.

18

Postoperative Pain Management in the Older Adult

Chris Pasero,[a] Barbara Rakel,[b] and Margo McCaffery[c]

[a]Clinical Consultant, El Dorado Hills, California, USA; [b]John A. Hartford Foundation Building Academic Geriatric Nursing Capacity Scholar, Iowa City, Iowa, USA; [c]Clinical Consultant, Los Angeles, California, USA

PREVALENCE OF POSTOPERATIVE PAIN IN THE OLDER ADULT

In 2000, the National Center for Health Statistics documented more than 27.7 million inpatient surgeries, of which one-third (8.9 million) were performed on persons 65 years of age or older (Hall and Owings 2002). This proportion is increasing with advancements in surgical technology and techniques aimed at improving function and quality of life for elders. Types of surgery commonly performed in older adults include a host of eye, orthopedic, thoracic, cardiac, vascular, gastrointestinal, urologic, and cancer procedures. Some are life-saving, while others are performed to improve quality of life or reduce chronic pain (Pasero et al. 1999c).

BARRIERS TO EFFECTIVE POSTOPERATIVE PAIN MANAGEMENT IN OLDER ADULTS

Despite improvements in surgical techniques and methods for controlling pain, a proliferation of guidelines, and over 10 years of extensive educational efforts, postoperative pain in older patients is often undertreated (Feldt and Oh 2000; Morrison and Siu 2000; Feldt and Finch 2002; Titler et al. 2003; Yorke et al. 2004). Older adults receive less analgesia and are refused pain medication more often than younger patients (Yorke et al. 2004), and those with cognitive impairment receive significantly less pain medication than do cognitively intact older individuals with similar painful conditions (Morrison and Siu 2000; Titler et al. 2003).

Administration of opioids via the intramuscular (i.m.) route and use of the p.r.n. ("as needed") approach persist in the postoperative setting, despite studies showing a direct relationship with ineffective pain control (Feldt and Oh 2000; Morrison and Siu 2000; Ardery et al. 2003a; Titler et al. 2003) and recommendations against these practices (Pasero et al. 1999b,c; American Geriatric Society 2002; American Pain Society 2003). The i.m. route is particularly dangerous in elders, who have more muscle wasting and less fatty tissue than younger adults. Because i.m. opioid absorption is unreliable, patients may be unattended at the peak effect, making them vulnerable to undetected adverse events such as respiratory depression (Sinatra 1998; Pasero et al. 1999b).

The p.r.n. approach consistently results in poor pain control because it requires patients to request pain medication, something many elders are reluctant to do (Pasero et al. 1999c). The lag time between the report or detection of pain and analgesic administration is significant, and doses are often inadequate. Duggleby and Lander (1992) reported over 10 years ago that nurses administered roughly a mere 25% of available p.r.n. prescribed analgesic doses. Four recent studies of older patients following surgery for repair of hip fracture showed that there has been no improvement in this statistic (Feldt and Oh 2000; Morrison and Siu 2000; Morrison et al. 2003; Titler et al. 2003). Around-the-clock analgesic dosing or intravenous (i.v.) patient-controlled analgesia (PCA) is indicated for hip fracture pain, yet in all of these studies most of the patients received prescriptions for p.r.n. analgesics. Although 60% of elders in one study were cognitively intact, only two received i.v. PCA (Morrison and Siu 2000). When analgesics are prescribed p.r.n., nurses must offer them regularly and should consider establishing around-the-clock dosing once a safe dose and interval have been established.

Fears of side effects and addiction continue to cause undertreatment of pain. Clinicians must assume that patients fear addiction and should routinely explain that its occurrence is rare when opioids are taken for pain relief (Pasero et al. 1999c; American Pain Society 2003). Adequate time must also be taken preoperatively and throughout the postoperative course to discuss fears of side effects and explain the use of self-administration devices.

Ultimately, the failure to recognize pain treatment as a universal right underlies many of the barriers to effective pain management. It is, therefore, extremely important that clinicians emphasize this right during the preoperative interview (American Pain Society Quality of Care Committee 1995).

This interview should include explaining the pain treatment plan and the patient's and family's roles in implementing it, setting pain relief goals, and emphasizing the relationship between adequate pain relief and recovery (Pasero et al. 1999b,c). See Table I for a summary of the barriers to effective postoperative pain management in older patients.

IMPACT OF UNRELIEVED POSTOPERATIVE PAIN

The adverse effects of unrelieved postoperative pain are numerous, and older patients are among the most vulnerable (Pasero et al. 1999a; Cook and Rooke 2003). Poorly managed pain in the immediate postoperative period can prolong a patient's stay in the post-anesthesia care unit (Buss and Melderis 2002). Reluctance to deep breathe, cough, and ambulate postoperatively because of poorly controlled pain can result in atelectasis and pneumonia (Shea et al. 2002), muscle wasting, and fatigue (Kehlet 1997, 1998). Immobility and poor tissue oxygenation during the postoperative period may be a

Table I
Barriers to effective postoperative pain management in older patients

Barriers Related to the Patient
Fear of bothering, distracting, or angering caregivers
Belief that caregivers know pain is present and are doing all they can to relieve it
Hesitation or confusion using unfamiliar equipment, such as patient-controlled analgesia
    pumps
Tendency not to report pain until it is moderate to severe
Feeling unworthy; depression

Barriers Related to the Health Care Team
Belief that pain perception decreases with age
Belief that failure to report pain means absence of pain
Belief that elders cannot tolerate opioids
Persistent use of ineffective methods of controlling postoperative pain, such as
    inappropriate analgesics, intramuscular injections, and the p.r.n. approach
Failure to use effective methods of minimizing and controlling postoperative pain, such
    as preemptive analgesia, patient-controlled analgesia, perineural infusion, and
    intraspinal techniques
Persistent use of general, rather than regional/local, anesthetic techniques

Barriers Related to the Patient, Family, and Health Care Team
Belief that postoperative pain is an inevitable consequence of aging, surgery, and
    hospitalization
Belief in the value of stoicism
Fear of addiction and tolerance
Fear of side effects
Failure to recognize pain treatment as a patient right

Source: Copyright 1995 by M. McCaffery and C. Pasero; used with permission.

precursor to other complications such as wound infection and delayed healing (Kehlet 1997, 1998). Undertreated pain has also been cited as a factor in the development of postoperative confusion and delirium (Duggleby and Lander 1994; Parikh and Chung 1995; Miller et al. 1996; Lynch et al. 1998) and may "tip the balance toward delirium in borderline patients" (Parikh and Chung 1995). All of these complications have the potential to increase hospital stay (Shea et al. 2002; Manku and Leung 2003; Morrison et al. 2003).

Immobility is one of the most detrimental effects of unrelieved postoperative pain in elders. Morrison and colleagues (2003) studied 411 patients (median age 82 years) admitted to four metropolitan hospitals for repair of hip fractures over a one-year period. A score of 2.5 or higher on a scale of 1 (no pain) to 5 (very severe pain) was reported by 50% of the patients during rest, by 83% during transfer, and by 91% during physical therapy. Patients with high pain scores had more difficulty ambulating, missed their physical therapy sessions or had shorter sessions, and had longer hospital stays than patients with lower pain scores.

Unrelieved postoperative pain can cause pulmonary complications, a source of significant morbidity and mortality in older patients. One study showed that elders with postoperative atelectasis had significantly more pain at rest and with deep breathing, walked less, and had longer hospital stays than those who had no atelectasis (Shea et al. 2002). A correlation between increased pain and walking was noted, suggesting that unrelieved pain contributed to decreased mobility and subsequent pulmonary dysfunction in these patients.

Studies have also shown an association between poorly managed postoperative pain and long-term adverse effects, including prolonged convalescence (Kehlet 1997, 1998), functional disability (Feldt and Oh 2000; Manku and Leung 2003; Morrison et al. 2003), development of chronic pain syndromes (Bach et al. 1988; Gotoda et al. 2001; Senturk et al. 2002; Bruce et al. 2003; Goldstein et al. 2004), increased reliance on the health care system (Manku and Leung 2003; Morrison et al. 2003), and increased mortality (Manuku et al. 2003).

PRINCIPLES OF PERIOPERATIVE PAIN ASSESSMENT

Other chapters in this volume extensively discuss pain assessment and tools for use in older adults. This section summarizes general principles that apply specifically to perioperative pain assessment in older adults.

HIERARCHY OF IMPORTANCE OF PAIN INTENSITY MEASURES

The most reliable indicator of the existence and intensity of pain is the patient's self-report (McCaffery and Pasero 1999a; American Pain Society 2003; Ardery et al. 2003b). When obtaining a self-report of pain after surgery, clinicians should understand that older adults may use other terms to express their pain. In a study of 417 postoperative orthopedic patients, 16% scored their pain as zero on verbal rating and visual analogue scales; however, when asked to *describe* what they felt, these patients used words such as "ache," "sore," or "stabbing" rather than "pain" (Closs and Briggs 2002).

It is also important to assess the patient's pain in the present. Cognitively impaired patients can report reliably in the present, but they have difficulty remembering past pain experiences (Miller et al. 1996; Feldt et al. 1998). Older adults who had undergone cardiac surgery later recalled pain as less severe than they had reported at the time (Valdix and Puntillo 1995).

When older adults are not able to provide a self-report of pain, the next best measure of pain is the presence of factors that cause pain. Postoperatively, when self-report is absent, clinicians can assume the presence of pain due to the obvious tissue injury associated with surgery and can record it using the acronym "APP" (Pasero and McCaffery 2001). This pain should be treated with appropriate analgesics even in the absence of pain behaviors. Behavioral indicators may be used to assess pain in patients who cannot self-report and to evaluate the effect of interventions to relieve pain. A valuable source of information about behaviors that may indicate pain in patients who are unable to self-report is a family member or someone else who knows the patient well.

Physiological measures such as blood pressure or heart rate are the least sensitive indicators of pain and may be normal or below normal in the presence of moderate to severe pain. Absence of a specific pain behavior or physiological indicator does not mean absence of pain (McCaffery and Pasero 1999a).

PAIN ASSESSMENT SCALES

Most hospitalized elders, including those with mild-to-moderate cognitive impairment, can use some type of pain intensity rating scale (Chibnall and Tait 2001). The most commonly used tool in the postoperative environment, the 0–10 numeric rating scale, is a valid measure of pain intensity in older patients and should be attempted (McCaffery and Pasero 1999a; Herr et al. 2004a). For patients with moderate-to-severe cognitive deficits or those who have difficulty with abstract thinking, the pain thermometer (Herr and

Mobily 1993) or simple verbal descriptor scale is preferred, such as one with the words "none," "mild," "moderate," and "severe" (Closs et al. 2004).

Two of the most important aspects of pain assessment are to find a tool that the patient can easily understand and then consistently use it with each assessment. Having a choice of scales is ideal so that selection can be based on individual preferences and abilities. Many institutions use a combination of the horizontal numeric 0–10 scale along with the Wong-Baker FACES scale, composed of six faces numbered with even numbers 0 through 10 (McCaffery and Pasero 1999a).

A recent review of existing tools for assessment of pain in nonverbal elders (Herr et al. 2004c) found that only one, the Checklist of Nonverbal Pain Indicators, had been evaluated in cognitively impaired elders with acute pain (Feldt 2000). The paucity of behavioral tools for assessing pain in cognitively impaired older adults being treated in acute care settings and the desire to have a tool that can be scored has tempted clinicians to use behavioral checklists or tools that have been developed for infants or children, such as the Faces, Legs, Activity, Cry and Consolability (FLACC) behavioral pain assessment scale (Merkel and Voepel-Lewis 1997). However, some components of the FLACC, such as crying and consolability, are not applicable to older adults (Odhner et al. 2003).

PREOPERATIVE ASSESSMENT AND TEACHING

Since older adults commonly present with chronic conditions and other etiologies for pain, a first step in pain assessment is obtaining a thorough preoperative baseline assessment. It helps to have family members or caregivers present to provide information about the patient's ongoing pain and cognitive and physical functioning if the patient displays impaired cognition or communication (Hanks-Bell et al. 2004).

Use of the pain intensity scale should be taught preoperatively if at all possible. Teaching older patients preoperatively how to communicate their pain after surgery may increase their reporting of pain and achieve better pain relief (McDonald and Molony 2004). Time constraints do not always allow clinicians to do comprehensive preoperative teaching, and provision of written materials helps to reinforce important points. For example, the patient teaching brochure "Understanding Your Pain: Using a Pain Rating Scale" by McCaffery et al. (2001) teaches the 0–10-point numeric and faces pain rating scales and explains how to establish a comfort-function goal.

COMFORT-FUNCTION GOALS

A comfort-function goal that can be used postoperatively to achieve and maintain adequate pain control should be established preoperatively by asking the patient to identify a level of pain that makes it easy to perform needed recovery activities (Pasero and McCaffery 2003, 2004c). Clinicians should describe the most important and possibly most painful postoperative recovery activities the patient may have to perform, such as coughing and deep breathing. The patient is then asked to select the pain rating on a scale of 0 to 10 that will make it easy to cough and breathe deeply. Explaining that ratings above 3 interfere significantly with function and that those above 5 adversely affect quality of life helps patients set realistic goals (McCaffery and Pasero 1999a).

PAIN WITH MOVEMENT

Pain should be assessed in relation to the comfort-function goal. In the above example, patients would be asked what their pain rating is when they cough and breathe deeply. If pain exceeds the goal, a pain relief intervention is implemented. Studies that measure both pain at rest and pain with movement frequently report differences in the effect of various treatments on these two aspects of pain (Bouchier-Hayes et al. 1990; Plummer et al. 1996; Rakel and Frantz 2003). Pain with movement is often not as well controlled as pain at rest and may require supplemental pain treatments.

SYSTEMATIC ASSESSMENT

The most important components of pain assessment in older adults are regular assessment; assessment after a relief intervention, such as an analgesic; consistent use of a standardized tool; and documentation (Hanks-Bell et al. 2004). In one study showing undertreated hip fracture pain in 709 older adults from 12 acute care settings (Titler et al. 2003), pain assessment practices were well below optimal standards (Herr et al. 2004b), suggesting that the lack of regular assessments contributed to the undertreatment of pain in these patients. Most patients do not take the initiative in reporting unrelieved pain to clinicians after surgery (Yorke et al. 2004), and elders in particular underreport pain for a variety of reasons. Health care providers are often unaware when elderly patients have pain because their perceptions of postoperative pain differ significantly from those of the patients (Carr 1990; Bowman 1994).

PERIOPERATIVE OPTIMIZATION

Optimal postoperative pain relief begins before surgery with what has been called perioperative optimization (Cooke and Rook 2003). This process involves evaluating patients for morbidity and mortality risk factors and implementing measures to reduce the surgical stress response and minimize or prevent postoperative complications (Jin and Chung 2001; Zakriya et al. 2002). Kehlet (1997) recommends identifying concomitant disease and organ dysfunction and correcting deficiencies preoperatively. This process includes maximizing pulmonary function, insuring adequate hydration and nutritional status, and identifying use of alcohol and medications that may produce adverse intraoperative and postoperative events. Clinicians should also ensure that underlying chronic pain is well controlled.

MULTIMODAL ANALGESIA

Multimodal analgesia is the recommended approach for managing postoperative pain in the older patient (Pasero et al. 1999b,c; Pasero 2003). This approach combines analgesic regimens to allow lower doses of each analgesic, thereby producing fewer side effects and achieving comparable or better pain relief than is possible with any single analgesic. The regimen may include several of the drugs commonly used to manage postoperative pain, including acetaminophen (paracetamol), nonsteroidal anti-inflammatory drugs (NSAIDs), opioids, and local anesthetics. A major benefit of multimodal analgesia is that each drug works on a different part of the pain pathway; acetaminophen may inhibit a third isoform of cyclooxygenase (COX-3) found in the central nervous system (American Pain Society 2003), NSAIDs reduce sensitization of nociceptors by inhibiting prostaglandin production, local anesthetics block sensory input, and opioids work centrally to inhibit the transmission of pain (Woolf and Chong 1993). Many of the drugs work synergistically, and non-opioids and local anesthetics produce significant opioid-sparing effects (Pasero et al. 1999b; Kehlet and Holte 2001).

HISTORY OF PREEMPTIVE ANALGESIA

Early research by Bach and colleagues (1988) showed that preoperative epidural blockade 72 hours prior to surgery in patients undergoing elective lower-limb amputation resulted in a lower incidence of phantom limb pain. This finding led to a flurry of research on preemptive analgesic techniques involving preoperative administration of NSAIDs, opioids, and local anesthetics. Many studies reported reductions in pain, postoperative complications, and length of hospital stay. However, a wide range of variables has made it difficult to compare trials, and the design of many of the studies has been criticized (Siddall and Cousins 1998). Nevertheless, experts emphasize the need for further research, pointing out that preemptive analgesia may have the potential to prevent the development of chronic pain syndromes (Siddall and Cousins 1998). Despite the lack of conclusive research, implementation of interventions aimed at preempting central sensitization are worthy of consideration (Woolf and Chong 1993; Pasero et al. 1999a).

NON-OPIOID ANALGESICS

The non-opioid analgesic group includes acetaminophen (paracetamol) and the NSAIDs. This group of analgesics is widely underused in the management of postoperative pain despite accepted guidelines recommending their administration to all patients, unless there is a contraindication (Agency for Health Care Policy and Research 1992; American Pain Society 2003). The non-opioids are considered appropriate alone for the treatment of mild to some moderate postoperative pain and in combination with opioids or local anesthetics for more severe postoperative pain (McCaffery and Portenoy 1999; Pasero et al. 1999b).

Major benefits for postoperative elders are that non-opioids do not produce sedation or respiratory depression or slow gastric motility (Souter 1994). Perhaps the greatest contribution, however, is their opioid-sparing effect (McCaffery and Portenoy 1999; Basto et al. 2001; Hyllested et al. 2002; Iohom et al. 2002; Ng et al. 2002; Romsing et al. 2002). A disadvantage of the non-opioids is that they all have a ceiling on analgesic dose. There is great variability among patients in response to non-opioids, which warrants asking patients what has worked well previously and using that non-opioid whenever possible postoperatively. See Table II for perioperative use of non-opioid analgesics.

OPIOID ANALGESICS

The μ-opioid analgesics are the cornerstone of moderate-to-severe postoperative pain in all populations (Pasero et al. 1999b). Long-standing principles of safely administering opioids in older patients are to decrease the starting dose by 25–50% and titrate upward slowly, based on patient response (Pasero and McCaffery 1997; Pasero et al. 1999b,c).

Studies have shown that elders may require lower opioid doses during the course of treatment after titration (Woodhouse and Mather 1997; Jin and Chung 2001; Aubrun et al. 2004); however, there is as much as a 10-fold

Table II

Considerations in the perioperative use of analgesics in the older adult

Drug/Group	Indications	Dosing Comments	General Comments
Acetaminophen (paracetamol, propacetamol)	Alone for mild pain; add NSAID for moderate pain; add opioid to above for more severe pain; opioid-sparing effect	*Oral:* Less effective analgesia than NSAIDs with regular dosing; high single doses (e.g., 1000 mg) may be more effective (Hyllested et al. 2002). *Rectal:* 40–60 mg/kg (single doses) = improved analgesia; 14–20 mg/kg (repeat doses) = reduction in analgesic intake (Romsing et al. 2002).	Viable alternative to NSAIDs (Hyllested et al. 2002); low adverse GI effect profile (McCaffery and Portenoy 1999); no antiplatelet effects (McCaffery and Portenoy 1999); can be coadministered with any analgesic; parenteral form (propacetamol) = up to 50% opioid-sparing effect (Romsing et al. 2002).
Nonselective NSAIDs, e.g., ibuprofen, ketoprofen, diclofenac, ketorolac	Alone or with acetaminophen for mild to moderate pain; add opioid to above for more severe pain; opioid-sparing effect	Administer lowest effective dose for shortest time necessary; maximum ketorolac dose should not exceed 60 mg/day (McCaffery and Portenoy 1999).	GI adverse effects limit usefulness in elders (McCaffery and Portenoy 1999); avoid in patients with history of GI complications, renal dysfunction, concomitant anticoagulant use, or hypovolemia (McCrory and Lindahl 2002); GI adverse effects are dose related (McCaffery and Portenoy 1999); do not use ketorolac after spinal fusion (McCaffery and Portenoy 1999); coadministration of two NSAIDs does not improve analgesia and increases GI adverse effects (McCaffery and Portenoy 1999).
COX-2-selective NSAIDs, e.g., celecoxib, valdecoxib, parecoxib	Alone or with acetaminophen for mild to moderate pain; add opioid to above for more severe pain; opioid-sparing effect	Administer lowest effective dose for shortest time necessary.	Avoid in patients with cardiovascular risk factors and for postoperative analgesia after coronary artery bypass graft and other vascular surgeries (Peck 2004; Topol 2005); less pronounced GI adverse effects than nonselective NSAIDs; lack of antiplatelet effect is major perioperative benefit (Leese et al. 2002; Reuben et al. 2002); may be administered preoperatively (Reuben et al. 2002); single-dose analgesia similar to nonselective NSAIDs (Chen et al. 2004); parecoxib analgesia comparable to ketorolac and morphine (Kranke et al. 2004).

Dipyrone	Mild to moderate pain; add opioid to above for more severe pain; opioid-sparing effect	5 g infusion intraoperatively (Braun et al. 1999) or over 24-hour periods postoperatively (Lempa and Kohler 1999).	Alternative when NSAIDs are contraindicated (Braun et al. 1999; Lempa and Kohler 1999); elevated risk of agranulocytosis with use (Braun et al. 1999); lacks GI, renal, and hepatic adverse effects (Braun et al. 1999); more effective than acetaminophen (Braun et al. 1999; Lempa and Kohler 1999).
Tramadol	Mild to moderate pain	Titrate slowly; do not exceed 300 mg/day in patients older than 75 years (American Geriatric Society 2002); lower doses may be necessary in patients with renal and hepatic disease (Dworkin et al. 2003).	Use with caution in patients with a history of seizure disorder or those taking medications that lower seizure threshold (American Geriatric Society 2002); serotonin syndrome can occur when used with serotonergic agents, such as some antidepressants and MAO inhibitors (Dworkin et al. 2003).
Opioid plus non-opioid formulations, e.g., hydrocodone or oxycodone plus acetaminophen or ibuprofen	Mild to moderate pain	Do not exceed maximum recommended daily non-opioid dose (McCaffery and Portenoy 1999).	Check for potential non-opioid overdosing when home medications are resumed (Pasero et al. 1999b).
Mu-agonist opioids, e.g., morphine, hydromorphone, fentanyl, oxycodone	Moderate to severe pain	Consider reducing recommended adult starting dose by 25%, then titrate slowly based on response (Pasero et al. 1999b); no analgesic ceiling (Pasero et al. 1999b); combine with acetaminophen and an NSAID to facilitate administration of lowest effective dose (Pasero et al. 1999b).	*Morphine:* Acceptable in patients with satisfactory renal function (Pasero et al. 1999b). *Hydromorphone:* Good alternative to morphine; short-term use in renal failure and after organ transplantation (Quigley and Wiffen 2003). *Fentanyl:* Fewer adverse hemodynamic effects; no clinically relevant metabolites; best choice for renal failure (Pasero and Montgomery 2002). *Oxycodone:* No clinically relevant metabolites; controlled-release formulation allows uninterrupted sleep (Pasero and McCaffery 2004a).

interindividual difference in analgesic requirements during the postoperative period (Benedetti 1990). Therefore, opioid therapy must be systematically assessed and individualized based on patient response rather than on a pre-conceived notion of what dose a patient will require (Pasero et al. 1999b; Woodhouse and Mather 2000). See Table II for perioperative use of opioid analgesics; see Chapter 10 for analgesics and other drugs that should be avoided or used cautiously in older adults.

OPIOID-INDUCED SIDE EFFECTS

Diligence is required to effectively manage opioid-induced side effects. Appropriate steps include prophylactic treatment when indicated, careful opioid drug and dose selection, and slow and steady dose titration. Since most opioid side effects are dose related, the use of multimodal analgesia is critical because it allows lower doses of each agent and thus results in fewer side effects (Pasero et al. 1999b). After initiation of opioid therapy, the severity of side effects is minimized with systematic assessment, prompt treatment, and adjustment of the pain management plan based on patient response.

An important consideration, particularly in postoperative patients, is that a simple decrease in dose often eliminates a side effect or makes it tolerable without jeopardizing pain control (Pasero et al. 1999b). This approach is preferable to repeatedly treating side effects with drugs that can produce more side effects or by changing opioid medications. Doses can be de-creased by 25% for treatment of mild side effects and by 50–75% for more severe side effects, or the opioid can be discontinued if necessary (Pasero et al. 1999b). Adding or increasing the dose of a non-opioid facilitates de-creases in opioid dose.

GASTROINTESTINAL DISTURBANCES

Opioids delay gastric emptying, slow bowel motility, and decrease peri-stalsis; therefore, unless there are contraindications, all patients receiving opioids postoperatively should be given a laxative and stool softener for the duration of opioid therapy (Pasero et al. 1999b). Administering non-opioids, local anesthetics, and the lowest effective opioid dose is also recommended to prevent or minimize the severity of gastrointestinal (GI) disturbances (Liu et al. 1995; Groudine et al. 1998; Steinbrook 1998; Kehlet 1999, 2000; Pasero et al. 1999b).

The risk of postoperative nausea and vomiting decreases as age increases; high risk factors include female gender, prior history of motion sickness or postoperative nausea and vomiting, nonsmoking status, and use of postoperative opioids (Apfel et al. 1999; Sinclair et al. 1999; Gan et al. 2003). However, prophylaxis may be cost effective in an older patient who has two or more high risk factors or when avoiding postoperative nausea and vomiting is crucial to outcome. Many clinicians routinely administer a serotonin receptor ($5HT_3$) antagonist intraoperatively as part of a multimodal rehabilitation program that includes early enteral feeding after major surgery (Kehlet and Morgensen 1999; Basse et al. 2000, 2002a,b).

Ileus (GI paralysis) is a major cause of postoperative morbidity (Liu et al. 1995), and older patients are at risk for the development of this complication for a variety of reasons, including age-related alterations in GI function and exposure to surgical procedures associated with a high incidence of ileus, such as colorectal surgery. Multimodal analgesia and regimens that enhance normalization of GI function, such early oral feeding and aggressive ambulation, are widely recommended (Liu et al. 1995; Kehlet 1997, 1998, 2000; Mythen 2005).

MENTAL STATUS CHANGES

Mild cognitive impairment can be expected in postoperative patients, whether or not they are given opioids for pain relief. Age is identified as a risk factor in the development of postoperative cognitive impairment (Liu et al. 1995; Scott et al. 1995; Moller et al. 1998; Jin and Chung 2001), but the exact incidence in this population is unknown (Wheeler et al. 2002). Although opioids are often blamed for the development of postoperative confusion in elders, numerous other potential causes should be ruled out, including polypharmacy and drug interaction, alcohol withdrawal, sleep deprivation, endocrine and metabolic compromise (Jin and Chung 2001), fluid disturbances (Rosenberg and Kehlet 1993), and infectious and respiratory complications (Moller et al. 1998).

Studies have shown that pain, not analgesic intake, predicts postoperative mental status decline (Duggleby and Lander 1994; Lynch et al. 1998). This finding suggests that improving pain management may be an important step in reducing postoperative mental confusion. Intravenous PCA has been shown to produce less mental confusion than i.m. opioids in older men (Egbert et al. 1990), and epidural analgesia is associated with less sedation than parenteral opioids and may have the potential for reduced postoperative cognitive dysfunction (Liu et al. 1995).

RESPIRATORY DEPRESSION

Advanced age has been cited as a risk factor for developing clinically significant respiratory depression (Pasero et al. 1999b; Macintyre and Ready 2001). Tolerance to the respiratory depressant effects of opioids develops within a few days of regular opioid dosing; therefore, opioid-naive elders are among those at risk for developing opioid-induced respiratory depression (Pasero et al. 1999b).

An important clinical observation is that patients with opioid-induced respiratory depression are rarely awake and alert (Pasero et al. 1999b; American Pain Society 2003). Excessive sedation precedes and is a hallmark of this complication; therefore, systematic monitoring of sedation is critical so that opioid doses can be decreased when increased sedation is detected (Pasero et al. 1999b; Pasero and McCaffery 2002). Table III presents a popular scale for assessing opioid-induced sedation and lists appropriate interventions at each level of sedation.

Nursing observation is the best and most commonly used method for monitoring sedation and respiratory status (Pasero et al. 1999b). Frequent assessment (every one to two hours) of opioid-naive patients is recommended, especially during the first 24 hours of opioid therapy (Pasero and McCaffery 2002). Close monitoring of sedation and respiratory status during sleep and nighttime hours is especially important for older patients, as they are at higher risk for nocturnal episodes of desaturation (Stone et al. 1999; Browdle 2004). Supplemental oxygen may be beneficial (Stone et al. 1999).

Pulse oximetry and apnea monitors in patients receiving opioids can be unreliable and give a false sense of security (Mulroy 1996; Pasero et al. 1999b; Institute for Safe Medication Practices 2003). Capnography may more accurately detect respiratory decline and apnea (Soto et al. 2004); however, further research is required to recommend widespread use of this method

Table III
Sedation scale for assessment of opioid-induced sedation

S = Sleep, easy to arouse (acceptable; no action necessary; safe to increase opioid dose)

1 = Awake and alert (acceptable; no action necessary; safe to increase opioid dose)

2 = Slightly drowsy, easily aroused (acceptable; no action necessary; safe to increase opioid dose)

3 = Frequently drowsy, arousable, drifts off to sleep during conversation (unacceptable; decrease opioid dose by 25–50%, add an opioid-sparing analgesic, such as an NSAID, and monitor level of sedation and respiratory status closely)

4 = Somnolent, minimal or no response to physical stimulation (unacceptable; stop opioid, consider administering naloxone to reverse sedation and adding acetaminophen or an NSAID to control pain)

Source: Copyright 1994 by C. Pasero; used with permission.

outside of the operating room and post-anesthesia care unit. Mechanical monitoring is warranted if a patient has a pre-existing condition such as chronic obstructive pulmonary disease or sleep apnea (Pasero et al. 1999b).

If it is necessary to use naloxone to reverse clinically significant respiratory depression, the drug should be diluted and titrated very slowly while observing patient response (Pasero et al. 1999b; American Pain Society 2003). Giving too much naloxone too fast can precipitate severe pain and increase sympathetic nervous system activity, leading to hypertension, ventricular dysrhythmias, and even cardiac arrest (Brimacombe et al. 1991).

PATIENT-CONTROLLED ANALGESIA

Patients aged 65 years old or older are reportedly at risk for hypoxemia and respiratory depression during i.v. PCA therapy (Sidebotham et al. 1997). Despite this finding, numerous studies and vast clinical experience have shown i.v. PCA to be safe and effective in older adults (Egbert et al 1990; Bedder et al. 1991; Duggleby and Lander 1992; Pasero et al. 1999c; Mann et al. 2000; Mcintyre 2001). Elders should not be denied access to this modality simply because of their age. Following careful screening, PCA should be considered for use in anyone who is cognitively and physically able to use the PCA equipment and understand the relationships between pain, pressing a button, and pain relief (Pasero et al. 1999b).

Regularly reinforcing patient-only use of PCA to patients and visitors is important (Ashburn et al 1994; Pasero 1996; Joint Commission on Accreditation of Healthcare Organizations 2004). The principle behind PCA is that only the patient knows how much pain is present and how much analgesic is needed to relieve it (Pasero 1996). PCA is considered safe because overly sedated patients are likely to drop the PCA button, thereby preventing delivery of more opioid. However, this built-in safeguard is circumvented when family members decide to activate PCA for the patient (Pasero 1996).

Ashburn and colleagues (1994) reported the occurrence of 14 critical events in 3,785 patients receiving i.v. PCA; three of these events involved unauthorized family members pressing the PCA button. In 2004, the Joint Commission on Accreditation of Healthcare Organizations, a private organization that surveys U.S. health care facilities, issued an alert stating that 15 out of 460 reports, collected over a 5-year period, of PCA-related errors resulting in death or serious injury to patients were the result of unauthorized family or staff pressing the PCA button.

When patients are unable or unwilling to use PCA, safe alternative methods have been found for using PCA technology to deliver analgesia, such as family-controlled analgesia and nurse-activated dosing (Pasero et al. 1999b). Family-controlled analgesia designates *one* family member to be the patient's pain manager and authorizes only that person to press the PCA button for the patient. Keys to safe use of this method are appropriate selection and education (pain and side effect assessment) of the pain manager and frequent follow-up to ensure safe use (Pasero et al. 1999b). The patient's primary nurse is responsible for using the PCA technology to manage pain when nurse-activated dosing is implemented (Pasero and McCaffery 2001).

USE OF A CONTINUOUS INFUSION WITH I.V. PCA

The use of a continuous infusion (basal rate) with i.v. PCA helps patients maintain a steady analgesic level and enjoy undisturbed sleep at night; however, basal rates must be used with caution in opioid-naive patients (Pasero et al. 1999c; Mcintyre 2001; American Pain Society 2003). The decision to add a basal rate to i.v. PCA in these patients should be based on patient response, rather than on a preconceived notion that they cannot tolerate continuous infusions (Pasero et al. 1999c; Pasero and McCaffery 2004b).

A conservative approach is to begin PCA therapy without a basal rate and assess response to treatment. If the patient has inadequate pain control with the bolus-only mode and is otherwise tolerating the therapy well with no adverse effects, a low basal rate, such as 0.5 mg/hour for morphine, may be added (Pasero and McCaffery 2004b). Hourly nurse monitoring of sedation and respiratory status is recommended, and the basal rate should be stopped if increasing sedation is noted; the use of a continuous infusion in opioid-naive patients is discouraged if this level of care is not possible (Pasero and McCaffery 2004b).

INTRASPINAL ANALGESIA

Epidural analgesia has a long history of safety and effectiveness in older patients (de Leon-Casasola et al. 1994; Pasero et al. 1999b,c). The opioids morphine and fentanyl and the local anesthetics bupivacaine and ropivacaine are the analgesics most commonly administered epidurally. They are most often combined to produce a synergistic effect, allowing lower doses of each and thus fewer side effects (Pasero et al. 1999b).

Epidural analgesia offers numerous benefits to elders following major surgery. Research comparing epidural analgesia and traditional pain management after major surgery in older patients showed that epidural analgesia provided better pain relief (Boylan et al. 1998; Wulf et al. 1999; Mann et al.

2000; Park et al. 2001), reduced opioid requirements (Boylan et al. 1998), shortened the intubation time (Boylan et al. 1998; Park et al. 2001), reduced the stay in the intensive care unit (Mann et al. 2000; Park et al. 2001), improved mental status and bowel function (Mann et al. 2000), and improved the overall outcome (Park et al. 2001).

Epidural analgesia is a key component of multimodal rehabilitation programs that include early ambulation and feeding following major surgery in high-risk older patients. One study evaluated 60 high-risk patients (median age 74 years) undergoing colon resection; only 18 had normal preoperative mobility and no complicating disease (Basse et al. 2000). Continuous epidural infusion of opioid and local anesthetic was administered postoperatively. Most (95%) of the patients regained normal bowel function within 48 hours, and the median hospital stay was 2 days. Similarly dramatic findings have been reported in other studies (Kehlet and Morgensen 1999; Kehlet 1999; Basse et al. 2002a,b).

Although epidural analgesia is used more often for postoperative pain, single-dose intrathecal morphine (100 µg) is also safe and effective in older adults (Slappendel et al. 1999; Murphy et al. 2003). It is appropriate for pain that is expected to be severe for 24 hours after surgery, such as hip or knee arthroplasty (Pasero et al. 1999b).

PERINEURAL LOCAL ANESTHETIC INFUSION

Local anesthetics administered via PCA or continuous infusion near nerves that innervate the surgical site is a relatively new technique for managing severe postoperative pain (Pasero 2004). A randomized study of older patients following knee arthroplasty evaluated extended femoral block with bupivacaine and clonidine via continuous infusion, continuous infusion with PCA boluses, or PCA boluses only (Singelyn and Gouverneur 2000). Pain was mild during both rest and movement, and supplemental analgesia and side effects were similar among the groups. The PCA bolus-only modality was recommended because it required the smallest amount of local anesthetic, an important consideration in older patients with altered drug clearance because they are at risk for systemic local anesthetic toxicity (Pasero et al. 1999c).

Advances in technology have made it possible to deliver perineural infusions via portable, disposable pumps, making this a practical method for controlling severe postoperative pain in the home setting. A case report described a 77-year-old woman who managed her pain at home following rotator cuff repair using PCA perineural infusion of ropivacaine (Ilfeld and

Enneking 2002). She experienced mild pain during rest and physical therapy sessions. Although this technique has been shown to significantly reduce opioid requirements, patients should be provided with oral opioid analgesia and advised to take it p.r.n. for breakthrough pain (Pasero 2004).

NONPHARMACOLOGICAL INTERVENTIONS FOR POSTOPERATIVE COMFORT

Nonpharmacological interventions are appropriate for the management of postoperative pain only when used to supplement pharmacological treatments (McCaffery and Pasero 1999b; Titler and Rakel 2001; Rakel and Herr 2004). Evidence of the effect of many of these strategies on postoperative pain is conflicting and inconclusive. They tend to be most effective at decreasing anxiety and distress and improving comfort and sleep (Richards et al. 2000; Titler and Rakel 2001). When studied in older adults, massage significantly decreased the unpleasantness of postoperative pain after major surgery (Piotrowski et al. 2003), significantly improved calmness scores following cardiac surgery (Hattan et al. 2002), and significantly improved sleep in critically ill men (Richards 1998). Music was reported to improve sleep (Zimmerman et al. 1996) and to promote comfort, familiarity in a strange environment, and distraction from fear, pain, and anxiety after surgery (McCaffery and Good 2000; Dunn 2004). Guided imagery significantly reduced anxiety in older adults after cardiac surgery (Deisch et al. 2000; Halpin et al. 2002).

The application of nonpharmacological interventions in the postoperative setting presents numerous challenges because of competing demands for nursing time and the severity of patient illness. Older surgical patients are less likely to use complementary and alternative techniques than their younger counterparts (Wang et al. 2003). Therefore, selection of nonpharmacological interventions should depend on the older patient's preference and be individualized rather than provided generally to all patients, with the possible exception of splinting the incision with a pillow during coughing.

Nonpharmacological interventions that require active participation, such as imagery and rhythmic breathing, may be less desirable than passive techniques, such as music and cold or heat application, in the postoperative setting when patients, especially elders, are exhausted from surgery. Audiocassettes with earphones, cold packs, and heating pads can be made available. When using music, it is essential to allow patients to select their preferred type of music (Good et al. 2000).

PREPARATION FOR DISCHARGE

The transition from parenteral or epidural analgesia to oral analgesia should be made when the patient is able to take oral medications. Prescriptions for oral analgesics other than the traditional non-opioid-opioid formulations may be necessary for patients with moderate postoperative pain. For example, oral morphine 15 to 30 mg, oxycodone 10 to 20 mg, or hydromorphone 4 to 8 mg would provide better pain relief than the combination analgesics. Oral analgesics should be administered before discontinuing parenteral or epidural analgesia so that patients remain comfortable during the transition.

The discharge plan should include documenting that the patient is not experiencing any side effects and can ambulate (if applicable) while taking oral analgesics. Careful attention must be paid to possible drug incompatibilities and overdoses. For example, excessive amounts of acetaminophen could be consumed if a patient was taking this drug before admission, received a prescription for acetaminophen plus hydrocodone upon discharge, and took both at home. The importance of maintaining adequate pain control during convalescence must be stressed, and patients and their families should know whom to contact and when if pain relief is inadequate after discharge (Pasero et al. 1999bc).

SUMMARY

Advances in surgical technology, combined with growth in the older adult population, have resulted in this age group experiencing increasing numbers of surgical procedures to save their lives or improve their quality of life. Yet, despite over a decade of extensive educational efforts aimed at improving postoperative pain relief, this population is grossly undertreated for such pain. The numerous adverse effects of poorly managed postoperative pain make it imperative that clinicians address this issue.

The provision of effective postoperative pain relief begins with a thorough assessment, use of a pain rating scale, and relating pain relief to recovery. Cognitively impaired elders who cannot report pain require careful selection of assessment tools that reflect their developmental status.

Multimodal analgesia is ideal for older patients because it combines analgesics, allowing lower doses of each. A preventive approach is recommended whenever possible for opioid-induced side effects. Nonpharmacological interventions may be considered if the patient desires them. An individualized plan for tapering analgesics prior to discharge and a prescription for an appropriate analgesic for use after discharge help to ensure optimal convalescence.

ACKNOWLEDGMENT

C. Pasero is on the speakers bureau for Endo Pharmaceuticals, Baxter Healthcare Corporation, Purdue Pharma, Pfizer, and Janssen Pharmaceuticals.

REFERENCES

Agency for Health Care Policy and Research Acute Pain Management Guideline Panel. *Acute Pain Management: Operative or Medical Procedures and Trauma, Clinical Practice Guideline,* AHCPR Publication No. 92-0032. Rockville, MD: Department of Health and Human Services, Public Health Service, Agency for Health Care Policy and Research, 1992.

American Geriatric Society Panel on Persistent Pain in Older Persons. The management of persistent pain in older patients. *J Am Geriatr Soc* 2002; 46:635–651.

American Pain Society. *Principles of Analgesic Use for the Treatment of Acute Pain and Cancer Pain,* 5th ed. Glenview, IL: American Pain Society, 2003.

American Pain Society Quality of Care Committee. Quality improvement guidelines for the treatment of acute pain and cancer pain. *JAMA* 1995; 274:1874–1880.

Apfel CC, Laadra E, Koivuranta M, Greim C-A, Roewer N. A simplified risk score for predicting postoperative nausea and vomiting. *Anesthesiology* 1999; 91:693–700.

Ardery G, Herr K, Hannon BJ, Titler MG. Lack of opioid administration in older hip fracture patients. *Geriatr Nurs* 2003a; 24:343–359.

Ardery G, Herr K, Titler M, Sorofman B, Schmitt M. Assessing and managing acute pain in older adults: a research base to guide practice. *Medsurg Nurs* 2003b; 12:7–18.

Ashburn MA, Love G, Pace NL. Respiratory-related critical events with intravenous patient-controlled analgesia. *Clin J Pain* 1994;10:52–56.

Aubrun F, Bunge D, Langeron O, et al. Postoperative morphine consumption in the elderly patient. *Anesthesiology* 2004; 99:160–165.

Bach S, Noreng MF, Tjellden NU. Phantom limb pain in amputees during the first 12 months following limb amputation. *Pain* 1988; 33:297–301.

Basse L, Hjort Jakobsen D, Billesbolle P, Werner M, Kehlet H. A clinical pathway to accelerated recovery after colonic resection. *Ann Surg* 2000; 232:51–57.

Basse L, Billesbolle P, Kehlet H. Early recovery after abdominal rectopexy with multimodal rehabilitation. *Dis Colon Rectum* 2002a; 45:195–199.

Basse L, Raskov HH, Hjort Jakobsen D, et al. Accelerated postoperative recovery programme after colonic resection improves physical performance, pulmonary function and body composition. *Br J Surg* 2002b; 89:446–453.

Basto ER, Waitrop C, Mourey FD, et al. Intravenous ketoprofen in thyroid and parathyroid surgery. *Anesth Analg* 2001; 92:1052–1057.

Bedder MD, Soifer BE, Mulhall JJV. A comparison of patient-controlled analgesia and bolus PRN intravenous morphine in the intensive care environment. *Clin J Pain* 1991; 7:205–208.

Benedetti C. Acute pain: a review of its effects and therapy with systemic opioids. In: Benedetti C, Chapman CR, Giron G (Eds). *Opioid Analgesia: Recent Advances in Systemic Administration,* Advances in Pain Research and Therapy, Vol. 14. New York: Raven Press, 1990, pp 367–424.

Bouchier-Hayes T, Rotman H, Darekar B. Comparison of the efficacy and tolerability of diclofenac gel (Voltarol Emulgel) and felbinac gel (Traxam) in the treatment of soft tissue injuries. *Br J Clin Pract* 1990; 44:319–320.

Bowman J. Perception of surgical pain by nurses and patients. *Clin Nurs Res* 1994; 3:69–76.

Boylan JF, Katz J, Kavanaugh BP, et al. Epidural bupivacaine-morphine analgesia versus patient-controlled analgesia following abdominal aortic surgery. *Anesthesiology* 1998; 89:585–593.

Braun R, Buche I, Maier P, Thiele H. Perioperative analgesia with intraoperatively started infusion of high-dose dipyrone in orthopaedic and trauma surgery. *Acute Pain* 1999; 2:167–171.

Brimacombe J, Archdeacon J, Newell S, et al. Two cases of naloxone-induced pulmonary oedema: the possible use of phentolamine in management. *Anaesth Intensive Care* 1991; 19:578–580.

Browdle TA. Nocturnal arterial oxygen desaturation and episodic airway obstruction after ambulatory surgery. *Anesth Analg* 2004; 99:70–76.

Bruce J, Drury N, Poobalan AS, et al. The prevalence of chronic chest and leg pain following cardiac surgery: a historical cohort study. *Pain* 2003; 104:265–273.

Buss HE, Melderis K. PACU pain management algorithm. *J Perianesth Nurs* 2002; 17:11–20.

Carr E. Postoperative pain: patients' expectations and experiences. *J Adv Nurs* 1990; 15:89–100.

Chen L-C, Elliott RA, Ashcroft DM. Systematic review of the analgesic efficacy and tolerability of COX-2 inhibitors in post-operative pain control. *J Clin Pharm Ther* 2004; 29:215–229.

Chibnall J, Tait R. Pain assessment in cognitively impaired and unimpaired older adults: a comparison of four scales. *Pain* 2001; 92:173–186.

Closs SJ, Briggs M. Patients' verbal descriptions of pain and discomfort following orthopaedic surgery. *Int J Nurs Stud* 2002; 39:563–572.

Closs SJ, Barr B, Briggs M, et al. A comparison of five pain assessment scales for nursing home residents with varying degrees of cognitive impairment. *J Pain Symptom Manage* 2004; 27:196–206.

Cook DJ, Rooke GA. Priorities in perioperative geriatrics. *Anesth Analg* 2003; 96:1823–1836.

Deisch P, Soukup S, Adams P, Wild M. Guided imagery: replication study using coronary artery bypass graft patients. *Nurs Clin North Am* 2000; 35:417–425.

de Leon-Casasola, Parker B, Lema MJ, Harrison P, Massey J. Postoperative epidural bupivacaine-morphine therapy. *Anesthesiology* 1994; 81:368–375.

Duggleby W, Lander J. Patient-controlled analgesia for older adults. *Clin Nurs Res* 1992; 1:107–113.

Duggleby W, Lander J. Cognitive status and postoperative pain: older adults. *J Pain Symptom Manage* 1994; 9:19–27.

Dunn K. Music and the reduction of post-operative pain. *Nurs Stand* 2004; 18:33–9.

Dworkin RH, Backonja M, Rowbotham MC, et al. Advances in neuropathic pain. *Arch Neurol* 2003; 60:1524–1534.

Egbert AM, Parks LH, Short LM, Burnett ML. Randomized trial of postoperative patient-controlled analgesia vs intramuscular narcotics in frail elderly men. *Arch Intern Med* 1990; 150:1897–1903.

Feldt KS. The checklist of nonverbal pain indicators (CNPI). *Pain Manage Nurs* 2000; 1:13–21.

Feldt KS, Finch M. Older adults with hip fractures: treatment of pain following hospitalization. *J Gerontol Nurs* 2002; 28:27–35.

Feldt KS, Oh HL. Pain and hip fracture outcomes for older adults. *Orthop Nurs* 2000; 19:35–44.

Feldt KS, Ryden M, Miles S. Treatment of pain in cognitively impaired compared with cognitively intact older adult patients with hip-fracture. *J Am Geriatr Soc* 1998; 46:1079–1085.

Gan TJ, Meyer T, Apfel CC, et al. Consensus guidelines for managing postoperative nausea and vomiting. *Anesth Analg* 2003; 97:62–71.

Goldstein DH, Ellis J, Brown R, et al. Meeting proceedings: recommendations for improved acute pain services: Canadian collaborative acute pain initiative. *Pain Res Manage* 2004; 9:123–130.

Good M, Picot B, Salem S. Cultural differences in music chosen for pain relief: five pain studies. *J Holist Nurs* 2000; 18:245–260.

Gotoda Y, Kambara N, Sakai T, et al. The morbidity, time course and predictive factors for persistent post-thoracotomy pain. *Eur J Pain* 2001; 5:89–96.

Groudine SB, Fisher HAG, Kaufman RP, et al. Intravenous lidocaine speeds the return of bowel function, decreases postoperative pain, and shortens hospital stay in patients undergoing radical retropubic prostatectomy. *Anesth Analg* 1998; 86:235–239.

Hall M, Owings M. *2000 National Hospital Discharge Survey,* Vol. 329. Hyattsville, MD: National Center for Health Statistics, 2002.

Halpin L, Speir A, CapoBianco P, Barnett S. Guided imagery in cardiac surgery. *Outcomes Manag* 2002; 6:132–137.

Hanks-Bell M, Halvey K, Paice J. Pain assessment and management in aging. *Online J Issues Nurs* 2004.

Hattan J, King L, Griffiths P. The impact of foot massage and guided relaxation following cardiac surgery: a randomized controlled trial. *J Adv Nurs* 2002; 37:199–207.

Herr K, Mobily P. Comparison of selected pain assessment tools for use with the elderly. *Appl Nurs Res* 1993; 6:39–46.

Herr K, Decker S, Bjoro K. *State of the Art Review of Tools for Assessment of Pain in Nonverbal Older Adults.* City of Hope, 2004a. Available at: www.cityofhope.org/prc/elderly.asp.

Herr K, Spratt K, Mobily P, Richardson G. Pain intensity assessment in older adults: use of experimental pain to compare psychometric properties and usability of selected pain scales with younger adults. *Clin J Pain* 2004b; 20:331–340.

Herr K, Titler M, Schilling M, et al. Evidence-based assessment of acute pain in older adults: current nursing practices and perceived barriers. *Clin J Pain* 2004c; 20:331–340.

Hyllested M, Jones S, Pederson JL, Kehlet H. Comparative effect of paracetamol, NSAIDs, or their combination in postoperative pain management; a qualitative review. *Br J Anaesth* 2002; 88:199–214.

Ilfeld BM, Enneking FK. A portable mechanical pump providing over four days of patient-controlled analgesia by perineural infusion at home. *Reg Anesth Pain Med* 2002; 27:100–104.

Institute for Safe Medication Practices. Safety issues with patient-controlled analgesia. *ISMP Medication Safety Alert* 2003; 8:1–3. Available at: www.ismp.org.

Iohom G, Walsh M, Higgins G, Shorten G. Effect of perioperative administration of dexketoprofen on opioid requirements and inflammatory response following elective hip arthroplasty. *Br J Anaesth* 2002; 88:520–526.

Jin F, Chung F. Minimizing perioperative adverse events in the elderly. *Br J Anaesth* 2001; 87:608–624.

Joint Commission on Accreditation of Healthcare Organizations. Patient controlled analgesia by proxy. *Sentinel Event Alert* 2004; 33 (December 20). Available at: www.jcaho.org; accessed January 7, 2005.

Kehlet H. Multimodal approach to control postoperative pathophysiology and rehabilitation. *Br J Anaesth* 1997; 78:606–617.

Kehlet H. Modification of stress responses to surgery by neural blockade. In: Cousins MJ, Bridenbaugh PO (Eds). *Neural Blockade.* Philadelphia: Lippincott-Raven, 1998, pp 129–175.

Kehlet H. Acute pain control and accelerated postoperative surgical recovery. *Surg Clin North Am* 1999; 79:431–443.

Kehlet H. Postoperative ileus. *Gut* 2000; 47(Suppl IV):85–86.

Kehlet H, Holte K. Effect of postoperative analgesia on surgical outcome. *Br J Anaesth* 2001; 87:62–72.

Kehlet H, Morgensen T. Hospital stay of 2 days after open sigmoidectomy with a multimodal rehabilitation programme. *Br J Surg* 1999; 86:227–230.

Kranke P, Morin AM, Roewer N, Eberhart LH. Patients' global evaluation of analgesia and safety of injected parecoxib for postoperative pain: a quantitative systematic review. *Anesth Analg* 2004; 99:797–806.

Leese PT, Talwalker S, Kent JD, Recker DP. Valdecoxib does not impair platelet function. *Am J Emerg Med* 2002; 20:275–281.

Lempa M, Kohler L. Postoperative pain relief in the morbidly obese patient: feasibility study of a combined dipyrone/tramadol infusion. *Acute Pain* 1999; 2:172–175.

Liu SS, Carpenter RL, Neal J. Epidural anesthesia and analgesia. *Anesthesiology* 1995; 82:1474–1506.

Lynch EP, Lazor MA, Gellis JE, et al. The impact of postoperative pain on the development of postoperative delirium. *Anesth Analg* 1998; 86:781–785.

Manku K, Leung JM. Prognostic significance of postoperative in-hospital complications in elderly patients. II. Long-term quality of life. *Anesth Analg* 2003; 96:589–594.

Mann C, Pouzeratte Y, Boccara G, et al. Comparison of intravenous or epidural patient-controlled analgesia in the elderly after major abdominal surgery. *Anesthesiology* 2000; 92:433–441.

McCaffery RG, Good M. The lived experience of listening to music while recovering from surgery. *J Holist Nurs* 2000; 18:378–390.

McCaffery M, Pasero C. Assessment: underlying complexities, misconceptions, and practical tools. In: McCaffery M, Pasero C. *Pain: Clinical Manual*, 2nd ed. St. Louis: Mosby, 1999a, pp 35–102.

McCaffery M, Pasero C. Practical nondrug approaches to pain. In: McCaffery M, Pasero C. *Pain: Clinical Manual*, 2nd ed. St. Louis: Mosby, 1999b, pp 399–427.

McCaffery M, Portenoy RK. Nonopioid analgesics. In: McCaffery M, Pasero C. *Pain: Clinical Manual*, 2nd ed. St. Louis: Mosby, 1999, pp 129–160.

McCaffery M, Pasero CL, Portenoy RK. *Understanding Your Pain: Using a Pain Rating Scale*. 2001. Chadds Ford, PA: Endo Pharmaceuticals. Available at: www.endo.com.

McCrory CR, Lindahl SGE. Cyclooxygenase inhibition for postoperative analgesia. *Anesth Analg* 2002; 95:169–176.

McDonald D, Molony S. Postoperative pain communication skills for older adults. *West J Nurs Res* 2004; 26:836–852.

Merkel SI, Voepel-Lewis T. The FLACC: a behavioral scale for scoring postoperative pain in young children. *Pediatr Nurs* 1997; 23(3):293–297.

Miller J, Meelon V, Dalton J, et al. The assessment of discomfort in elderly confused patients: a preliminary study. *J Neurosci Nurs* 1996; 28:175–182.

Moller JT, Cluitmans P, Rasmussen LS, et al. Long-term postoperative cognitive dysfunction in the elderly. International study of postoperative cognitive dysfunction. *Lancet* 1998; 351:857–861.

Morrison RS, Siu AL. A comparison of pain and its treatment in advanced dementia and cognitively intact patients with hip fracture. *J Pain Symptom Manage* 2000; 19:240–248.

Morrison RS, Magaziner J, McLaughlin MA, et al. The impact of post-operative pain on outcomes following hip fracture. *Pain* 2003; 103:303–311.

Mulroy MF. Monitoring opioids. *Reg Anesth* 1996; 21:89–93.

Murphy PM, Stack D, Kinirons B, Laffery JG. Optimizing the dose of intrathecal morphine in older patients undergoing hip arthroplasty. *Anesth Analg* 2003; 97:1709–1715.

Mythen MG. Postoperative gastrointestinal tract dysfunction. *Anesth Analg* 2005; 100:196–204.

Ng A, Parker J, Toogood L, Cotton BR, Smith G. Does the opioid-sparing effect of rectal diclofenac following total abdominal hysterectomy benefit the patient? *Br J Anaesth* 2002; 88:714–716.

Odhner M, Wegmen D, Freeland N, et al. Assessing pain control in nonverbal critically ill adults. *Dimens Crit Care* 2003; 22:260–267.

Parikh SS, Chung F. Postoperative delirium in the elderly. *Anesth Analg* 1995; 80:1223–1232.

Park WY, Thompson JS, Lee KK. Effect of epidural anesthesia and analgesia on perioperative outcome: a randomized, controlled Veterans Affairs cooperative study. *Ann Surg* 2001; 234:560–569.

Pasero C. PCA: for patients only. *Am J Nurs* 1996; 96(9):22–23.

Pasero C. Multimodal balanced analgesia in the PACU. *J Perianesth Nurs* 2003;18:265–268.

Pasero C. Perineural local anesthetic infusion. *Am J Nurs* 2004; 104(7):89, 91–93.

Pasero C, McCaffery M. Postoperative pain management in the elderly. In: Ferrell BR, Ferrell BA (Eds). *Pain in the Elderly*. Seattle: IASP Press, 1997.

Pasero C, McCaffery M. Multimodal balanced analgesia in the critically ill. *Crit Care Nurs Clin North Am* 2001; 13(2):195–206.

Pasero C, McCaffery M. Monitoring sedation. *Am J Nurs* 2002; 102(2):67–68.

Pasero C, McCaffery M. Accountability for pain relief. *J Perianesth Nurs* 2003; 18:50–52.

Pasero C, McCaffery M. Controlled-release oxycodone. *Am J Nurs* 2004a; 104(1):30–32.

Pasero C, McCaffery M. Safe use of continuous infusion with IV PCA. *J Perianesth Nurs* 2004b; 19(1):42–45.

Pasero C, McCaffery M. Comfort-function goals. *Am J Nurs* 2004c; 104(9):77–78.

Pasero C, Montgomery R. IV fentanyl. *Am J Nurs* 2002; 102(4):73, 75, 76.

Pasero C, Paice JA, McCaffery M. Basic mechanisms underlying the causes and effects of pain. In: McCaffery M, Pasero C. *Pain: Clinical Manual*, 2nd ed. St. Louis: Mosby, 1999a, pp 15–34.

Pasero C, Portenoy RK, McCaffery M. Opioid analgesics. In: McCaffery M, Pasero C. *Pain: Clinical Manual*, 2nd ed. St. Louis: Mosby, 1999b, pp 161–299.

Pasero C, Reed BA, McCaffery M. Pain in the elderly. In: McCaffery M, Pasero C. *Pain: Clinical Manual*, 2nd ed. St. Louis: Mosby, 1999c, pp 674–710.

Peck P. Valdecoxib meta-analysis suggests increased cardiovascular risk. Available at: http://medscape.com. Accessed November 12, 2004.

Piotrowski M, Paterson C, Mitchinson A, et al. Massage as adjuvant therapy in the management of acute postoperative pain: a preliminary study in men. *J Am Coll Surg* 2003; 197:1037–1046.

Plummer J, Owen H, Ilsley A, Tordoff K. Sustained-release ibuprofen as an adjunct to morphine patient-controlled analgesia. *Anesth Analg* 1996; 83:92–96.

Quigley C, Wiffen P. A systematic review of hydromorphone in acute and chronic pain. *J Pain Symptom Manage* 2003; 25:169–178.

Rakel BA, Frantz R. Effectiveness of transcutaneous electrical nerve stimulation (TENS) on postoperative pain with movement. *J Pain* 2003; 4:455–464.

Rakel B, Herr K. Assessment and treatment of postoperative pain in older adults. *J Perianesth Nurs* 2004; 19:194–208.

Reuben SS, Fingerothe R, Krushell R, Maciolek H. Evaluation of the safety and efficacy of the perioperative administration of rofecoxib for total knee arthroplasty. *J Arthroplasty* 2002; 17:26–31.

Richards K. Effect of a back massage and relaxation intervention on sleep in critically ill patients. *Am J Crit Care* 1998; 7:288–299.

Richards K, Gibson R, Overton-McCoy A. Effects of massage in acute and critical care. *AACN Clin Issues* 2000; 11:77–96.

Romsing J, Moiniche S, Dahl JB. Rectal and parenteral paracetamol in combination with NSAIDs, for postoperative analgesia. *Br J Anaesth* 2002; 88:315–226.

Rosenberg J, Kehlet H. Postoperative mental confusion: association with postoperative hypoxemia. *Surgery* 1993; 114:76–81.

Scott DA, Beilby DSN, McClymont C. Postoperative analgesia using epidural infusion of fentanyl with bupivacaine. *Anesthesiology* 1995; 14:727–737.

Senturk M, Ozcan PE, Talu GK, et al. The effects of three different analgesia techniques on long-term post-thoracotomy pain. *Anesth Analg* 2002; 94:11–15.

Shea RA, Brooks JA, Dayhoff NE, Keck J. Pain intensity and postoperative pulmonary complications among the elderly after abdominal surgery. *Heart Lung* 2002; 31:440–449.

Siddall PJ, Cousins MJ. Introduction to pain mechanisms: implications for neural blockade. In: Cousins MJ, Bridenbaugh PO (Eds). *Neural Blockade*. Philadelphia: Lippincott-Raven, 1998, pp 675–713.

Sidebotham D, Dijkhuizen MRJ, Schug SA. The safety and utilization of patient-controlled analgesia. *J Pain Symptom Manage* 1997; 14:202–209.

Sinatra RS. Acute pain management and acute pain services. In: Cousins MJ, Bridenbaugh PO (Eds). *Neural Blockade*. Philadelphia: Lippincott-Raven, 1998, pp 793–835.

Sinclair DR, Chung F, Mezel G. Can postoperative nausea and vomiting be predicted? *Anesthesiology* 1999; 91:109–118.

Singelyn FJ, Gouverneur J-MA. Extended "three-in-one" block after total knee arthroplasty: continuous versus patient-controlled techniques. *Anesth Analg* 2000; 91:176–180.

Slappendel R, Weber EWG, Dirksen R, et al. Optimization of the dose of intrathecal morphine in total hip surgery: a dose-finding study. *Anesth Analg* 1999; 88:822–826.

Soto RG, Fu ES, Vila H, Miguel RV. Capnography accurately detects apnea during monitored anesthesia care. *Anesth Analg* 2004; 99:379–382.

Souter AJ, Fredman B, White PF. Controversies in the perioperative use of nonsteroidal antiinflammatory drugs. *Anesth Analg* 1994; 79:1178–1190.

Steinbrook RA. Epidural anesthesia and gastrointestinal motility. *Anesth Analg* 1998; 86:837–844.

Stone JG, Cozine KA, Wald A. Nocturnal oxygenation during patient-controlled analgesia. *Anesth Analg* 1999; 89:104–110.

Titler M, Rakel BA. Non-pharmacologic treatment of pain. *Crit Care Nurs Clin North Am* 2001; 13:221–232.

Titler MG, Herr K, Schilling ML, et al. Acute pain treatment for older adults hospitalized with hip fracture: current nursing practices and perceived barriers. *Appl Nurs Res* 2003; 16:1–227.

Topol EJ. Arthritis medicines and cardiovascular events—"house of coxibs." *JAMA* 2005; 293:366–369.

Valdix S, Puntillo K. Pain, pain relief and accuracy of their recall after cardiac surgery. *Prog Cardiovasc Nurs* 1995; 10:3–11.

Wang S, Caldwell-Andrews A, Kain Z. The use of complementary and alternative medicines by surgical patients: a follow-up survey study. *Anesth Analg* 2003; 97:1010–1015.

Wheeler M, Oderda GM, Ashburn MA, Lipman AG. Adverse events associated with postoperative opioid analgesia: a systematic review. *J Pain* 2002; 3:159–180.

Woodhouse A, Mather LE. The influence of age upon opioid analgesic use in the patient-controlled analgesia (PCA) environment. *Anaesthesia* 1997; 52:949–955.

Woodhouse A, Mather LE. The minimum effective concentration of opioids: a revisitation with patient controlled analgesia fentanyl. *Reg Anesth Pain Med* 2000; 25:259–267.

Woolf CJ, Chong M-S. Preemptive analgesia—treating postoperative pain by preventing the establishment of central sensitization. *Anesth Analg* 1993; 77:362–379.

Wulf H, Biscoping J, Beland B, et al. Ropivacaine epidural anesthesia and analgesia versus general anesthesia and intravenous patient-controlled analgesia with morphine in the perioperative management of hip replacement. *Anesth Analg* 1999; 89:111–116.

Yorke J, Wallis M, McLean B. Patients' perceptions of pain management after cardiac surgery in an Australian critical care unit. *Heart Lung* 2004; 33:33–41.

Zakriya KJ, Christmas C, Wenz J, et al. Preoperative factors associated with postoperative change in confusion assessment method score in hip fracture patients. *Anesth Analg* 2002; 94:1628–1632.

Zimmerman L, Nieveen J, Barnason S. The effects of music interventions on postoperative pain and sleep in coronary artery bypass graft (CABG) patients. *Sch Inq Nurs Pract* 1996; 10:153–170.

Correspondence to: Chris Pasero, MS, RN, FAAN, 1252 Clearview Drive, El Dorado Hills, CA 95762, USA. Tel: 916-933-2023; Fax: 916-933-2024; email: cpasero@aol.com.

Pain in Older Persons, Progress in Pain Research and Management, Vol. 35, edited by Stephen J. Gibson and Debra K. Weiner, IASP Press, Seattle, © 2005.

19

Cancer Pain and End-of-Life Issues

Linda A. King and Robert Arnold

Section of Palliative Care and Medical Ethics, Division of General Internal Medicine, University of Pittsburgh, Pittsburgh, Pennsylvania, USA

CANCER PAIN

BACKGROUND

Each year over 10 million people develop cancer worldwide, and 6.2 million die as a result of this disease (Stewart and Kleihues 2003). The majority of cancer patients are older adults; in the United States and Europe 60% of all cancers and 69% of cancer deaths occur in patients over age 65 (Balducci 2003). Unfortunately, a cancer diagnosis is often accompanied by significant pain. Studies suggest that between 28% and 80% of cancer patients experience pain, with the prevalence of pain increasing during active anticancer treatments and as the disease advances (Bernabei et al. 1998; Patrick et al. 2004). Cancer pain is often undertreated, especially in older adults. Multiple studies reveal an inverse relationship between age and opioid dose prescribed for cancer pain (Vigano et al. 1998; Hall et al. 2003). Older adults are less likely to be prescribed a strong opioid for cancer pain, and they receive a lower dose compared with younger adults if a strong opioid is prescribed (Bernabei et al. 1998; Hall et al. 2003).

Several comprehensive clinical guidelines detail strategies for the assessment and management of cancer pain in adults (Jacox et al. 1994; Benedetti et al. 2000). Unfortunately, these clinical practice guidelines and most of the available studies do not focus specifically on cancer pain in older adults. Currently, insufficient data exist to guide cancer pain management in older adults (Patrick et al. 2004). Clinicians are left to extrapolate from the available studies and guidelines addressing cancer pain management in general populations.

APPROACH TO CANCER PAIN MANAGEMENT

Fig. 1 depicts a flowchart for managing pain in patients with cancer (Jacox et al. 1994). Pain in patients with cancer may be related to the malignant disease itself, to the treatments aimed at controlling the cancer, or to exacerbations of other coexisting benign conditions. Pain is treated based on its most likely etiology, with frequent reassessment and adjustment of the treatment plan. The assessment methods and pharmacological and nonpharmacological pain management strategies discussed throughout this volume are relevant in the older adult with cancer and will not be reviewed in detail here.

Established clinical practice guidelines for the management of cancer pain describe the World Health Organization (WHO) analgesic ladder for titrating analgesics for cancer pain (Jacox et al. 1994). While the WHO analgesic ladder has been validated by several studies (Ventafridda et al. 1987; Grond et al. 1991), one systematic review found inadequate evidence to confirm its effectiveness for the management of cancer pain (Jadad and Browman 1995). A recent randomized trial compared the efficacy of strong opioids as first-line therapy for cancer pain with a pain regimen based on the WHO analgesic ladder (Marinangeli et al. 2004). This study found that patients started on a strong opioid experienced significantly better pain control, required fewer changes in therapy, and reported greater satisfaction with treatment than did patients treated according to the WHO analgesic ladder. More recent guidelines for cancer pain management (Miaskowski et al. 2005) support a role for opioids as first-line therapy for any patient with cancer pain.

PRESCRIPTION INDICATIONS FOR VARIOUS CANCER PAIN TREATMENTS

Opioid therapy. Benefits of early opioid therapy include effective analgesia, ease of titration, and lack of a ceiling effect. However, use of opioid analgesics requires balancing these benefits with the potential for significant side effects including sedation, constipation, mental cloudiness, and nausea. Often, the clinician must compromise between achieving optimal analgesia and minimizing toxicities in designing an opioid regimen for a given patient. Individual patients and their caregivers vary in how they weigh the importance of achieving pain relief versus avoiding side effects and should be involved in such determinations.

Adjuvant analgesics. The use of adjuvant analgesics, such as nonsteroidal anti-inflammatory drugs (NSAIDs) and corticosteroids for bone and musculoskeletal pain and tricyclic antidepressants, anticonvulsants, and topical

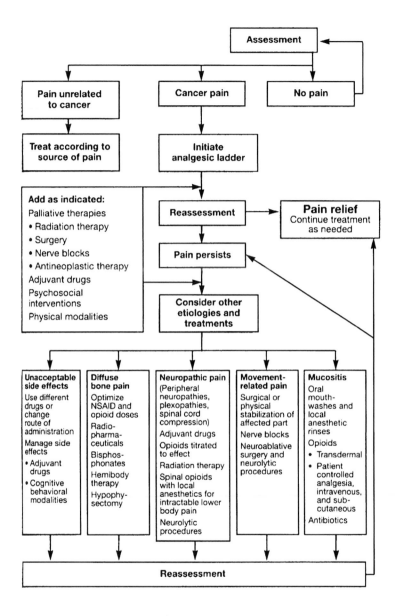

Fig. 1. Flow chart for the management of cancer pain. From Jacox et al. (1994).

agents (e.g., capsaicin, lidocaine) for neuropathic pain can enhance the analgesic efficacy of opioids and also provide independent analgesic efficacy for specific types of pain. Evidence supporting the use of many of these agents either alone or in combination with opioids is limited and is mostly derived from noncancer patient populations. For example, a systematic review of the role of anticonvulsants for pain found only one controlled study in cancer patients and overall found insufficient evidence to strongly support the use of these agents in cancer (Wiffen et al. 2000). A recent randomized controlled trial of gabapentin for neuropathic pain in cancer patients did confirm improved analgesia with gabapentin in patients already receiving opioids (Caraceni et al. 2004). For further discussion of drug prescribing for neuropathic pain, the reader is referred to Chapters 10 and 17 in this volume.

Invasive therapies (neurolytic blockade of peripheral nerves, intraspinal delivery of analgesics) have traditionally been reserved for patients who do not respond to a well-designed analgesic regimen. However, a randomized controlled trial of the use of implantable pumps for the delivery of opioid analgesics in cancer patients (Smith et al. 2002) showed improved pain control, reduced toxicities, and longer survival compared with an oral analgesic regimen, suggesting an earlier role for such interventions.

Nonpharmacological therapies. While much of the literature on cancer pain management focuses on the early role of opioid analgesics and other pharmacological and interventional strategies, attention to psychological, behavioral, and environmental contributors to cancer pain and the role of nonpharmacological therapies (described in more detail in Chapter 12) is essential. The evidence supporting the use of nonpharmacological modalities including heat, cold, massage, transcutaneous electrical nerve stimulation, acupuncture, relaxation, and imagery is quite limited in elderly cancer patients and must be extrapolated from the evidence available from the study of chronic nonmalignant pain populations (see Chapter 11). Two studies in older adults with cancer do suggest that educational interventions for older adults and their caregivers can help prevent and manage cancer pain (Ferrell et al. 1995; Clotfelter 1999).

Often, improvement in cancer pain can best be achieved by reducing cancer burden and controlling tumor growth. Even if life is not prolonged, patients may benefit if tumor control decreases pressure on a visceral or neurological structure. Therefore, consideration of the role of chemotherapy, radiation therapy, and other disease-specific therapies is relevant in the evaluation of the cancer patient with pain. Clinicians are often concerned about the ability of older adults to tolerate cancer treatments; they may not offer treatment or may offer less aggressive treatments to older adults with cancer. However, decisions regarding ability to tolerate cancer treatments should be based on factors other than age. A comprehensive geriatric assessment, adapted for use with oncology patients, can identify patients who are too frail to benefit from certain cancer therapies, can lead to treatment of unsuspected coexisting conditions, and can help eliminate social barriers to cancer treatment (Repetto et al. 2003).

Pain from cancer or its treatment, associated with specific characteristics and physical signs, defines cancer pain syndromes. Cancer can result in both acute and chronic pain syndromes. Two of the most common and important cancer-related chronic pain syndromes—bone pain and back pain—will be discussed in further detail below.

METASTATIC BONE PAIN

Bone metastases are the most common cause of chronic pain in patients with cancer (Foley 1985; Mercadante 1997). Any tumor type can metastasize to bone, with multiple myeloma, breast, prostate, lung, thyroid, and kidney cancers being the most frequent. The most typical sites for bone metastases include the pelvis, vertebrae, femur, ribs, and skull, although metastasis to any bone is possible. Recent studies examining the mechanism of pain caused by bone metastases suggest inflammatory, neuropathic, and tumor-related components (Mantyh 2004; Roodman 2004; Urch 2004).

CLINICAL PRESENTATION

Bone pain from metastatic cancer usually presents as a localized, constant, dull ache that may be worse with weight-bearing and activity. Patients typically experience days to weeks of pain that gradually increases in intensity. Pain that worsens acutely may indicate a pathological fracture or neural impingement. Up to 25% of patients with bone metastases are pain-free, and patients with multiple sites of bone metastases may experience pain at only one or a few sites (Wagner 1984). The factors that determine whether a particular lesion will result in pain are not well understood.

ASSESSMENT

Plain X-rays represent the first diagnostic test for a cancer patient presenting with localized bone pain. For long bones, assessment of cortical integrity is useful in determining the risk of pathological fracture. The risk of pathological fracture is high if more than 50% of the cortex is destroyed by the tumor (Leggon et al. 1988; Hipp et al. 1995). Technetium bisphosphonate bone scan is very sensitive for identifying bone lesions, but its specificity is low, making it difficult to distinguish between benign and malignant processes, especially when evaluating solitary lesions. Bone scans are most valuable in evaluating patients with multifocal pain and to determine the overall extent of bony spread. However, in some tumors such as multiple myeloma and melanoma (which evoke less reactive bone turnover), false negative scans can occur, and plain X-rays may be more reliable. Computed tomography (CT) scans better define the morphology of bone lesions and are helpful for assessing cortical integrity and the presence of pathological fractures. Magnetic resonance imaging (MRI) is usually reserved to better define lesions that are suspicious on plain radiography or bone scan, to evaluate for spinal cord compression, and to detect marrow lesions.

TREATMENT

Treatment of pain from bone metastases involves multiple complementary approaches based on the needs of the individual patient. NSAIDs and opioids have traditionally been the mainstay of drug therapy for cancer pain.

Anti-inflammatory drugs. A systematic review confirms the efficacy of NSAIDs for cancer pain in general (though not specifically for bone pain), but few of the individual studies suggested a clinically greater effect of NSAIDs combined with opioids (McNicol et al. 2005). The relatively low therapeutic ceiling of NSAIDs as well as their gastrointestinal and renal toxicity may limit their use in older adults with cancer, especially those with abnormal renal function, a history of peptic ulcer disease, or a tendency to bleed (Eisenberg et al. 1994; Gloth 1996; American Geriatrics Society 2002). Corticosteroids may also be effective in relieving bone pain, but the ideal dose, frequency, and duration of therapy are not well-established. The analgesic effect of corticosteroids may be short-lived and their use complicated by serious side effects (including thrush, glucose intolerance, edema, and dyspepsia); therefore, their use should be limited to as short a course as possible. Some would limit their use to patients with neurological emergencies or those with a very short life expectancy (Berger and Koprowski 2002).

Opioid analgesics are effective for bone pain and are indicated for most patients and certainly for any patient with moderate to severe pain. Patients with bone metastases typically experience both continuous pain and incident pain with movement or activity. A regimen of a long-acting opioid on a scheduled basis supplemented with a short-acting opioid used for episodes of breakthrough pain is most effective. When bone metastases invade adjacent neural structures, treatment for neuropathic pain is indicated.

Radiation therapy is perhaps the most effective treatment for local metastatic bone pain. A systematic review confirms that radiation therapy produced at least 50% pain relief in more than two-thirds of treated patients, with one-quarter obtaining complete pain relief (McQuay et al. 2000). Most patients achieved maximal pain relief within 4 weeks, and the median duration of complete relief was 12 weeks. The specific treatment regimen (number and size of fractions) is individualized based on the patient's prognosis and tumor type and location, but simple, short schedules may be most appropriate for palliative treatments in patients with advanced disease. A systematic review of single-fraction radiotherapy for bone metastases suggests similar pain relief compared with multifraction radiotherapy, but patients treated with a single fraction had a slightly greater rate of retreatment and pathological fracture (Wai et al. 2004). Patients with diffuse bone metastases and multiple sites of bone pain may benefit from treatment with radiopharmaceuticals. A systematic review of four trials of radioisotopes for metastatic bone pain suggested improved pain control at both 1 and 6 months (Roque et al. 2003). These bone-seeking radioactive isotopes (samarium-153 are strontium-89) are administered intravenously, with pain relief occurring within 1–2 weeks. The main toxicity is bone marrow suppression, which occurs after 3–4 weeks and is usually mild and self-limited.

Bisphosphonates are potent inhibitors of bone resorption that have been studied for the treatment of bone metastases in various cancers. In breast cancer and multiple myeloma, regular administration of intravenous pamidronate or zoledronate has resulted in decreased pain, decreased skeletal complications, and delayed progression of bone disease (Berenson et al. 1996; Hortobagyi et al. 1996). Similar studies looking at bone metastases from prostate cancer, and especially from other solid tumors, have been less compelling, and the role for bisphosphonate administration for bone pain is less clear in these malignancies. A systematic review of 30 randomized, controlled studies of bisphosphonates for pain from bone metastases suggested some degree of pain relief but found insufficient evidence to recommend their use as first-line therapy. The authors suggested the addition of bisphosphonates when analgesics and/or radiation therapy have been inadequate (Wong and Wiffen 2002). Side effects from bisphosphonate infusions include renal failure, hypocalcemia, and a transient increase in pain.

In summary, management of pain from bone metastases requires a multimodal strategy aimed at optimizing analgesia, avoiding complications, and maximizing functional outcomes.

BACK PAIN IN CANCER PATIENTS

Back pain in a cancer patient can occur from a variety of etiologies, but the most worrisome are bone or epidural metastases resulting in spinal cord compression. Up to one-third of cancer patients develop metastases to the spine (Posner 1987). Untreated metastases may encroach upon the spinal

cord or cauda equina with devastating and irreversible neurological consequences. Epidural compression of the spinal cord or cauda equina occurs in
up to 10% of patients and can be the initial presenting symptom of malignancy in a patient not known to have cancer (Stark et al. 1982; Grant et al.
1991). The prevalence of spinal cord compression varies with tumor type.
Multiple myeloma in adults and osteogenic sarcoma are the most common
primary spinal tumors. Breast, lung, and prostate cancer frequently spread to
the spinal column. Spinal metastases are less common in renal cell carcinoma, head and neck carcinoma, soft tissue sarcomas, and neoplasms of the
liver, pancreas, and bladder.

The goal of the initial evaluation of a cancer patient with back pain is to
identify those patients at highest risk for epidural spinal cord compression.
Since the most important determinant of the patient's ultimate neurological
outcome is the extent of neurological impairment at the time therapy is
initiated, prompt evaluation and diagnosis are essential. If a patient is treated
while still ambulatory, the probability of remaining ambulatory is 89–94%
(Abrahm 1999). Back pain usually precedes neurological signs by a significant period, so prompt evaluation can result in an earlier diagnosis and a
more favorable neurological outcome.

The initial evaluation begins with a thorough history and physical examination with particular attention to the temporal progression of the pain
and to any evidence of neurological symptoms and findings. Rapid progression of back pain in a crescendo pattern is especially concerning. Radicular
pain, especially if exacerbated by lying down, coughing, sneezing, or strain-
ing, suggests epidural compression (Ruff and Lanska 1989). Pain may be
unilateral in the cervical or lumbosacral region. Thoracic involvement is
often bilateral and experienced as a tight, belt-like band across the chest or
abdomen (Helweg-Larsen and Sorensen 1994). Neurological symptoms, such
as weakness, sensory loss, and autonomic abnormalities usually occur after
a period of progressive pain.

Fig. 2 depicts an algorithm for evaluating a cancer patient with back
pain (Cherny 2002). The urgency and course of the evaluation are based on
the likelihood of epidural spinal cord compression. Patients with stable back
pain without neurological symptoms are initially evaluated with plain X-
rays of the affected area that will detect approximately 70% of vertebral
tumors (Deyo and Diehl 1988). If pain persists and worsens or neurological
symptoms develop, more definitive imaging of the epidural space is warranted despite normal plain radiographs. Patients with mild myelopathy or
radiculopathy symptoms without evidence of spinal cord compression should
undergo an MRI (or another definitive imaging study) within 24 hours, with
consideration of treatment with steroids and hospitalization pending imaging

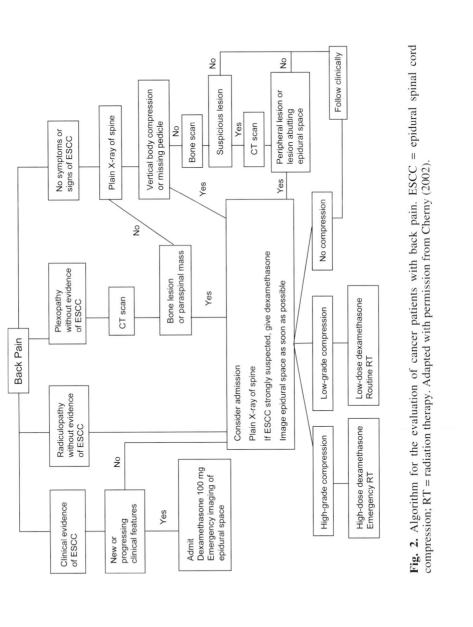

Fig. 2. Algorithm for the evaluation of cancer patients with back pain. ESCC = epidural spinal cord compression; RT = radiation therapy. Adapted with permission from Cherny (2002).

results. Strong suspicion or clinical evidence of epidural spinal cord compression requires emergent imaging of the epidural space, corticosteroids, and (typically) admission to the hospital. In patients with an absolute contraindication to MRI or when MRI is unavailable, CT scan or CT myelography should be substituted. If MRI is negative for an epidural mass despite neurological deficits or the presence of headache and meningismus, evaluation of the cerebrospinal fluid for leptomeningeal carcinomatosis is necessary.

If MRI confirms the presence of an epidural or spinal mass with neural compression, treatment with corticosteroids should be initiated or continued. Definitive evidence guiding corticosteroid dosing in spinal cord compression is limited, but many advocate high-dose steroids (dexamethasone 100 mg initially, followed by 96 mg/day in divided doses) for high-grade compression and lower doses (16 mg/day in divided doses) for low-grade compression (Greenberg et al. 1980; Posner 1995).

Patients with epidural spinal cord compression should be evaluated promptly for the possible need for radiation therapy or surgical intervention. Radiation therapy can inhibit tumor growth, restore and preserve neurological function, treat pain, and improve quality of life. Radiation therapy is effective in over 85% of cases of radiosensitive tumors (Perrin et al. 1996). Surgical intervention for epidural spinal cord compression is performed to decompress neural structures and stabilize the spine, to halt rapid clinical deterioration, or to determine a diagnosis in a new presentation of cancer (Galasko and Sylvester 1978; Byrne and Waxman 1990).

Prompt and attentive pain management is essential throughout the evaluation of the cancer patient with back pain. Nearly all patients with epidural spinal cord compression have severe pain requiring management with opioids with ongoing dose titration, adjuvant therapies for neuropathic pain, and consideration of nonpharmacological pain management modalities.

The ability to ambulate after treatment for epidural spinal cord compression predicts the patient's overall survival. Patients who remain unable to walk after treatment for spinal cord compression have only a 7% rate of survival at 1 year, probably due to more advanced disease and complications of their persistent paresis. Patients who remain ambulatory fare better, with a 1-year survival rate of over 30% (Perrin et al. 1996). Decisions regarding treatment for epidural spinal cord compression must take into account the patient's overall prognosis, quality of life, and goals.

PAIN MANAGEMENT AT THE END OF LIFE

Older adults living with chronic, life-threatening illnesses experience increasing symptoms including pain, dyspnea, nausea, and fatigue as death approaches. Studies confirm that between 40–60% of patients dying of a variety of illnesses in different settings suffer from pain and other distressing physical symptoms during the last days and months of life. A large study of hospitalized adults (median age 65 years) found that 50% of patients experienced moderate to severe pain during the last 3 days of life (SUPPORT Principal Investigators 1995). Another study of symptom prevalence in the hospital during the last 48 hours of life revealed high rates of multiple symptoms including severe pain, dyspnea, restlessness, agitation, fatigue, nausea, and anorexia across a variety of terminal diagnoses (Goodlin et al. 1998). A sample of 200 older adults dying at home found that pain increased over the last year of life, with 66% of patients experiencing pain frequently or all of the time during the last month of life (Moss et al. 1991). As many as 25% of cancer patients experience severe pain in the 3–6 months before death, and more than 40% are in severe pain during the last 3 days of life (McCarthy et al. 2000). Patients dying with congestive heart failure and chronic obstructive lung disease also suffer unrelieved symptoms in the last hours of life, with more than a quarter experiencing severe pain and 60% severe dyspnea in the 3 days before death (Levenson et al. 2000; Lynn et al. 2000). During the last 3 months of life, 61% of nursing home patients experience distressing physical symptoms including pain and dyspnea (Teno et al. 2004).

Untreated symptoms at the time of death are detrimental not only to a patient's quality of life, but also to family members and loved ones. Caregiver stress strongly correlates with increased patient distress and can also result in caregiver depression, distress, and even death (Redinbaugh et al. 2003; Tilden et al. 2004). Increased caregiver stress is associated with complicated bereavement (Kelly et al. 1999). Careful attention to pain and symptom management through a patient's final hours can ease the stress and burden of caregivers (Tilden et al. 2004).

Pain assessment in end-of-life care can be especially challenging for several reasons. Clinicians must distinguish pain mediated by typical physiological nociception from the global distress and suffering often experienced by individuals facing the end of life. The concept of suffering or "total pain" has been used to describe this complex experience of pain in patients approaching the end of life—encompassing not only the physiological symptoms but also emotional, social, economic, and spiritual distress. Studies of existential and spiritual distress in terminally ill patients are largely descriptive, consisting of personal reflections and patient interviews (Strang et al. 2004). Interviews of caregivers suggest that unaddressed existential and spiritual concerns are often expressed as physical pain (Strang et al. 2004). Conversely, some patients deny physical pain but present with significant distress manifested as fatigue, depression symptoms, and anxiety (Rao and Cohen 2004). A comprehensive pain assessment in patients approaching the end of life must target each of these domains to effectively alleviate pain and suffering. Health care providers must at minimum be able to screen for spiritual, existential, and family issues and involve appropriate members of a multidisciplinary team as needed to fully address identified issues. Table I lists helpful screening questions for identifying and exploring existential and spiritual issues (Quill and Byock 2000).

Palliative care and hospice teams have the expertise to thoroughly explore the full range of issues facing terminally ill patients and their loved ones. Their involvement should be sought early for patients exhibiting significant distress as death approaches. Hospice services can be provided at home, in skilled nursing facilities, and in hospitals or designated palliative care units. Hospice services include skilled nursing visits for physical assessment and expert symptom management, home health aide visits to assist with physical needs, medications for symptom control, social work and pastoral care assessments, and bereavement services for the patient's family. Bereaved family members of patients who receive hospice services at home or in a facility report higher satisfaction, fewer concerns with care, and fewer unmet needs (Baer and Hanson 2000; Teno et al. 2004). In the nursing home setting, hospice care has been shown to improve pain management and to reduce the likelihood of re-hospitalization (Miller et al. 2001; Miller and Mor 2002). Hospice care is underutilized and often initiated too late (in the last week of life), especially for nursing home residents (Happ et al. 2002). Early referral for hospice services allows the patient to benefit maximally from the available services and to form a comfortable relationship with the hospice team.

Dying patients typically experience a cognitive decline that further complicates efforts at pain assessment. Half of advanced cancer patients are unable to use a typical pain assessment tool (Shannon et al. 1995). Clinicians

Table I
Representative questions for exploring existential and spiritual concerns

"How have you tried to make sense of what is happening to you?"
"Given the severity of your illness, what is most important for you to achieve?"
"What are some of the things that give you a sense of hope?"
"As you look back on your life, what has given your life the most meaning?"
"If you were to die sooner rather than later, what would be left undone?"
"What do you want your loved ones to remember about you?"
"Is faith or spirituality important to you in this illness?"
"Are there any spiritual issues you are concerned about at this point"
"Would you like to explore religious or spiritual matters with someone?"

often rely on a patient's family members or caregivers to assist with pain assessment. However, caregivers tend to overestimate the symptom intensity of dying patients (McMillan and Moody 2003), and their reporting of the patient's pain is often influenced by their own experience (Redinbaugh et al. 2002). Multiple scales to assess discomfort in nonverbal patients have been used to assess patients with dementia (Stolee et al. 2005); however, their role in assessing pain in dying patients has not been established (Plonk and Arnold 2005).

As death approaches, pain management strategies must adapt to rapidly changing clinical conditions. Most studies suggest that pain tends to decrease during the dying process, although patients may experience new pain in the last hours of life (Mercadante et al. 2000). A careful history and physical examination may reveal reversible causes of pain (bladder distension, rectal impaction, or decubitus ulcers) for which simple interventions may provide significant relief. Analgesic requirements in the last 48 hours of life may actually decrease due to various factors including worsening organ dysfunction, ketosis, and build-up of exogenous opioid metabolites.

Close to the end of life, oral intake becomes unreliable, and medications must be delivered by alternative routes. Many medications can be administered by rectal, transdermal, sublingual, or parenteral routes in the final stages of life. Table II lists some of the different formulations available. Morphine and oxycodone are available in concentrated elixirs that can be administered sublingually (Coluzzi 1998). Morphine and hydromorphone are available as rectal suppositories. Fentanyl can be given transdermally for continuous opioid action or as a transmucosal lozenge for episodes of incident pain (Ellershaw et al. 2003). Intravenous and subcutaneous infusions can be used if other routes are impractical. Doses should be based on a patient's previous opioid use and current symptoms. Skilled use of equianalgesic conversion tables facilitates appropriate dosing as routes are changed.

Other features of the dying process must be distinguished from pain and treated accordingly. Terminal delirium occurs in many patients near the end of life and may be interpreted as pain by family and other caregivers (Casarett and Inouye 2001). Terminal delirium can be hyperactive (with restlessness, agitation, moaning) or hypoactive (with somnolence) (Plonk and Arnold 2005). Frequent symptoms of hyperactive delirium are distressing to the majority of families and can hamper effective end-of-life care (Morita et al. 2004). Two recent reviews of treatments for terminal delirium supported a role for haloperidol and chlorpromazine (Jackson and Lipman 2004; Kehl 2004). Benzodiazepines and other typical and atypical antipsychotics were also found to be effective.

Table II
Examples of useful drugs for pain management during the dying process

Drug	Formulation	Strength	Route	Typical Dose Range	Comments
Morphine	Liquid; suppository	20 mg/mL; 5, 10, 20, 30 mg	s.l., p.r.	2.5–20 mg q 1–4 h p.r.n.	Determine starting dose based on previous opioid use. Titrate dose and frequency until effective.
Oxycodone	Liquid	20 mg/mL	s.l.	5–20 mg q 1–4 h p.r.n.	
Hydro-morphone	Suppository	3 mg	p.r.	3–6 mg q 3 h p.r.n.	
Fentanyl	Transdermal patch	25, 50, 75, 100 µg/h	t.d.	25–300 µg q 72 h	Base initial dose on previous use of opioids. Slow onset of action; not effective for acute pain.

Abbreviations: p.r. = rectal; s.l. = sublingual; t.d. = transdermal.

In rare cases, distress in an actively dying patient remains refractory despite every effort to effectively control ongoing symptoms with conventional symptom management strategies. In such cases, sedation—usually with parenteral benzodiazepines, barbiturates, or other sedatives—may be employed to address the persistent suffering. The chosen medication is initiated and rapidly titrated until the patient is comfortably sedated. The optimal level of sedation is usually maintained until the patient's death. This practice, termed palliative or terminal sedation, represents a final effort to relieve extreme suffering. The purpose of the sedation is to render the patient unconscious in an effort to relieve refractory suffering, not to hasten death (Quill and Byock 2000). While clinical practice guidelines exist for palliative sedation (Quill and Byock 2000), decisions to use palliative sedation are complex and are often best made in consultation with a palliative care specialist.

CONCLUSIONS

Cancer pain management in older adults relies on many of the same principles of chronic nonmalignant pain management in this population. Careful pain assessment and design of an appropriate pain treatment plan employing pharmacological, interventional, and nonpharmacological modalities is essential. Clinicians must be able to recognize and promptly treat specific cancer pain syndromes to achieve optimal outcomes. Growing attention to how to optimally manage cancer and its consequences in older adults may provide more guidance to clinicians as our evidence base grows.

Older adults in the last year of life experience more pain as death approaches. Effective pain management near the end of life requires frequent reassessment, adjustment of pain regimens, and attention to other components of suffering, including existential and spiritual issues. Coordinated care provided by a multidisciplinary clinical team can best meet the diverse needs of a patient approaching death.

REFERENCES

Abrahm JL. Management of pain and spinal cord compression in patients with advanced cancer. *Ann Intern Med* 1999; 131:37–46.

American Geriatrics Society Panel on Persistent Pain in Older Persons. The management of persistent pain in older persons. *J Am Geriatr Soc* 2002; 50:S205–224.

Baer WM, Hanson LC. Families' perception of the added value of hospice in the nursing home. *J Am Geriatr Soc* 2000; 48(8):1017–1018.

Balducci L. Management of cancer pain in geriatric patients. *J Support Oncol* 2003; 1(3):175–191.

Benedetti C, Brock C, Cleeland C, et al. National Comprehensive Cancer Network. NCCN practice guidelines for cancer pain. *Oncology (Williston Park)* 2000; 14(11A):135–150.

Berenson JR, Lichtenstein A, Porter L, Dimopoulos MA, et al. Efficacy of pamidronate in reducing skeletal events in patients with advanced multiple myeloma. Myeloma Aredia Study Group. *N Engl J Med* 1996; 334(8):488–493.

Berger A, Koprowski C. Bone pain: assessment and management. In: *Principles and Practice of Palliative Care and Supportive Oncology,* 2nd ed. Philadelphia: Lippincott Williams & Wilkins, 2002, pp 53–67.

Bernabei R, Gambassi G, Lapane K, et al. Management of pain in elderly patients with cancer. *JAMA* 1998; 279(23).

Byrne TN, Waxman SG. *Spinal Cord Compression: Diagnosis and Principles of Management,* Contemporary Neurology Series, Vol. 45. Philadelphia: Davis, 1990, p 164.

Caraceni A, Zecca E, Bonezzi C, et al. Gabapentin for neuropathic cancer pain: a randomized controlled trial from the Gabapentin Cancer Pain Study Group. *J Clin Oncol* 2004; 22(14):2909–2917.

Casarett DJ, Inouye SK. American College of Physicians–American Society of Internal Medicine End-of-Life Consensus Panel. Diagnosis and management of delirium near the end of life. *Ann Intern Med* 2001; 135(1):32–40.

Cherny N. Cancer pain: principles of assessment and syndromes. In: *Principles and Practice of Palliative Care and Supportive Oncology,* 2nd ed. Philadelphia: Lippincott Williams & Wilkins, 2002, pp 3–52.

Clotfelter CE. The effect of an educational intervention on decreasing pain intensity in elderly people with cancer. *Oncol Nurs Forum* 1999; 26:27–33.

Coluzzi PH. Sublingual morphine: efficacy reviewed. *J Pain Symptom Manage* 1998; 16(3):184–192.

Deyo RA, Diehl AK. Cancer as a cause of back pain: frequency, clinical presentation, and diagnostic strategies. *J Gen Intern Med* 1988; 3:230–238.

Eisenberg E, Berkey CS, Carr DB, Mosteller F, Chalmers TC. Efficacy and safety of non-steroidal anti inflammatory drugs for cancer pain: a meta-analysis. *J Clin Oncol* 1994; 12:2756–2765.

Ellershaw JE, Kinder C, Aldridge J, Allison M, et al. Care of the dying: is pain control compromised or enhanced by the continuation of the fentanyl transdermal patch in the dying phase? *J Pain Symptom Manage* 2003; 26:589–590.

Ferrell BR, Grant M, Chan J, Ahn C, Ferrell BA. The impact of cancer pain education on family caregivers of elderly patients. *Oncol Nurs Forum* 1995; 22:1211–1218.

Foley KM. The treatment of cancer pain. *N Engl J Med* 1985; 313(2):84–95.

Galasko CS, Sylvester BS. Back pain in patients treated for malignant tumours. *Clin Oncol* 1978; 4(3):273–283.

Gloth FM III. Concerns with chronic analgesic therapy in elderly patients. *Am J Med* 1996; 101(Suppl 1):19S–24S.

Goodlin S, Winzelberg G, Teno J, et al. Death in the hospital. *Arch Intern Med* 1998; 158:1570–1572.

Grant R, Papadopoulos SM, Greenberg HS. Metastatic epidural spinal cord compression. *Neurol Clin* 1991; 9(4):825–841.

Greenberg HS, Kim JH, Posner JB. Epidural spinal cord compression from metastatic tumor: results with a new treatment protocol. *Ann Neurol* 1980; 8:361–366.

Grond S, Zech D, Schug SA, et al. Validation of World Health Organization guidelines for cancer pain relief during the last days and hours of life. *J Pain Symptom Manage* 1991; 6:411–422.

Hall S, Gallagher R, Gracely E, Knowlton C, Weschules D. The terminal cancer patient: effects of age, gender, and primary site on opioid dose. *Pain Med* 2003; 4(2):125–134.

Happ MB, Capezuti E, Strumpf NE, Wagner L, et al. Advance care planning and end-of-life care for hospitalized nursing home residents. *J Am Geriatr Soc* 2002; 50(5):829–835.

Helweg-Larsen S, Sorensen PS. Symptoms and signs in metastatic spinal cord compression: a study of progression from first symptom until diagnosis in 153 patients. *Eur J Cancer* 1994; 30A(3):396–398.

Hipp JA, Springfield DS, Hayes WC. Predicting pathologic fracture risk in the management of metastatic bone defects. *Clin Orthop* 1995; 312:120–135.

Hortobagyi GN, Theriault RL, Porter L, et al. Efficacy of pamidronate in reducing skeletal complications in patients with breast cancer and lytic bone metastases. Protocol 19 Aredia Breast Cancer Study Group. *N Engl J Med* 1996; 335(23):1785–1791.

Jackson KC, Lipman AG. Drug therapy for delirium in terminally ill patients. *Cochrane Database Syst Rev* 2004; 2:CD004770.

Jacox A, Carr DB, Payne R, et al. *Management of Cancer Pain,* Clinical Practice Guideline No. 9, AHCPR Publication No. 94-0592. Rockville, MD: U.S. Department of Health and Human Services, Public Health Service, Agency for Health Care Policy and Research, 1994.

Jadad AR, Browman GP. The WHO analgesic ladder for cancer pain management: stepping up the quality of its evaluation. *JAMA* 1995; 274(23):1870–1873

Kehl KA. Treatment of terminal restlessness: a review of the evidence. *J Pain Palliat Care Pharmacother* 2004; 18:5–30.

Kelly B, Edwards P, Synott R, et al. Predictors of bereavement outcomes for family carers of cancer patients. *Psycho-oncology* 1999; 8:237–249.

Leggon RE, Lindsey RW, Panjabi NM. Strength reduction and the effects of treatment of lung bones with diaphyseal defects involving 50% of the cortex. *J Orthop Res* 1988; 6(4):540–546.

Levenson J, McCarthy E, Davis R, Phillips R. The last six months of life for patients with congestive heart failure. *J Am Geriatr Soc* 2000; 48:S101–S109.

Lynn J, Ely EW, Zhong Z, et al. Living and dying with chronic obstructive pulmonary disease. *J Am Geriatr Soc* 2000; 48(Suppl 5):S91–S100.

Mantyh PW. A mechanism-based understanding of bone cancer pain. *Novartis Found Symp* 2004; 261:194–214; discussion 214–219, 256–261.

Marinangeli, F, Ciccozzi A, Leonardis M, et al. Use of strong opioids in advanced cancer pain: a randomized trial. *J Pain Symptom Manage* 2004; 27:409–416.

McCarthy E, Phillips R, Zhong Z, Drews R, Lynn J. Dying with cancer: patients' function, symptoms, and care preferences as death approaches. *J Am Geriatr Soc* 2000; 48: S110–S121.

McMillan SC, Moody LE. Hospice patient and caregiver congruence in reporting patients' symptom intensity. *Cancer Nurs* 2003; 26(2):113–118.

McNicol E, Strassels SA, Goudas L, Lau J, Carr DB. NSAIDS or paracetamol, alone or combined with opioids, for cancer pain. *Cochrane Database Syst Rev* 2005: 2: CD005180.

McQuay HJ, Collins SL, Carroll D, Moore RA. Radiotherapy for the palliation of bone metastases. *Cochrane Database Syst Rev* 2000; 2:CD001793.

Mercadante S. Malignant bone pain: pathophysiology and treatment. *Pain* 1997; 69:1–18.

Mercadante S, Casuccio A, Fulfaro F. The course of symptom frequency and intensity in advanced cancer patients followed at home. *J Pain Symptom Manage* 2000; 20:104–112.

Miaskowski C, Cleary J, Burney R, et al. *Guidelines for the Management of Cancer Pain in Adults and Children.* American Pain Society, 2005.

Miller SC, Mor VN. The role of hospice care in the nursing home setting. *J Palliat Med* 2002; 5(2):271–277.

Miller SC, Gozalo P, Mor V. Hospice enrollment and hospitalization of dying nursing home patients. *Am J Med* 2001; 111(1):38–44.

Morita T, Hirai K, Sakaguchi, Tsuneto S, et al. Family perceived distress from delirium-related symptoms of terminally ill cancer patients. *Psychosomatics* 2004; 45:107–113.

Moss MS, Lawton MP, Glicksma A. The role of pain in the last year of life of older adults. *J Gerontol* 1991; 46(2):51–57.

Patrick DL, Ferketich SL, Frame PS, et al. National Institutes of Health State-of-the-Science Conference Statement: symptom management in cancer: pain, depression, and fatigue, July 15–17, 2002. *J Natl Cancer Inst Monogr* 2004; (32):9–16.

Perrin RG, Janjan NA, Langford LA. Spinal axis metastases. In: Levin VA (Ed). *Cancer in the Nervous System.* New York: Churchill Livingstone, 1996, p 259.

Plonk WM, Arnold RM. Terminal care: the last weeks of life. *J Palliat Med* 2005; in press.

Posner JB. Back pain and epidural spinal cord compression. *Med Clin North Am* 1987; 71(2):185–205.

Posner JB. *Neurologic Complications of Cancer,* Contemporary Neurology Series, Vol. 45. Philadelphia: Davis, 1995, p 112.

Quill TE, Byock IR. Responding to intractable terminal suffering: the role of terminal sedation and voluntary refusal of food and fluids. *Ann Intern Med* 2000; 132:408–414.

Rao A, Cohen HJ. Symptom management in the elderly cancer patient: fatigue, pain and depression. *J Natl Cancer Inst Monogr* 2004; 32:150–157.

Redinbaugh EM, Baum A, DeMoss C, Fello M, Arnold R. Factors associated with the accuracy of family caregiver estimates of patient pain. *J Pain Symptom Manage* 2002; 23:31–8.

Redinbaugh EM, Baum A, Torbell S, Arnold R. End-of-life caregiving: what helps caregivers cope? *J Palliat Med* 2003; 6:901–909.

Repetto L, Venturino A, Fratino L, et al. Geriatric oncology: a clinical approach to the older patient with cancer. *Eur J Cancer* 2003; 39:870–880.

Roodman GD. Mechanisms of bone metastasis. *N Engl J Med* 2004; 350(16):1655–1664.

Roque M, Martinez MJ, Alonso P, et al. Radioisotopes for metastatic bone pain. *Cochrane Database Syst Rev* 2003; 4:CD003347.

Ruff RL, Lanska DJ. Epidural metastases in prospectively evaluated veterans with cancer and back pain. *Cancer* 1989; 63(11):2234–2241.

Shannon MM, Ryan MA, D'Agostino N, Brescia FJ. Assessment of pain in advanced cancer patients. *J Pain Symptom Manage* 1995; 10:274–278.

Smith TJ, Staats PS, Deer T, et al. Randomized clinical trial of an implantable drug delivery system compared with comprehensive medical management for refractory cancer pain: impact on pain, drug-related toxicity, and survival. *J Clin Oncol* 2002; 20(19):4040–4049.

Stark RJ, Henson RA, Evans SJW. Spinal metastases: a retrospective survey from a general hospital. *Brain* 1982; 105:189–213.

Stewart BW, Kleihues P. *World Cancer Report*. Geneva: WHO Press, 2003.

Stolee P, Hillier LM, Esbaugh J, et al. Instruments for the assessment of pain in older persons with cognitive impairment. *J Am Geriatr Soc* 2005; 53(2):319–326.

Strang P, Strang S, Hultborn R, Arner S. Existential pain—an entity, a provocation, or a challenge? *J Pain Symptom Manage* 2004; 27:241–250.

SUPPORT Principal Investigators. A controlled trial to improve care for seriously ill hospitalized patients: the study to understand prognoses and preferences for outcomes and risks of treatments (SUPPORT). *JAMA* 1995; 274:1591–1598.

Teno J, Clarridge B, Casey V, et al. Family perspectives on end-of-life care at the last place of care. *JAMA* 2004; 291:88–93.

Tilden V, Tolle S, Drach L, Perrin S. Out-of-hospital death: advance care planning, decedent symptoms, and caregiver burden. *J Am Geriatr Soc* 2004; 52:532–539.

Urch C. The pathophysiology of cancer-induced bone pain: current understanding. *Palliat Med* 2004; 18:267–274.

Ventafridda V, Tamburini M, Caraceni A, et al. A validation study of the WHO method for cancer pain relief. *Cancer* 1987; 59:850–856.

Vigano A, Bruera E, Suarez-Almazor ME. Age, pain intensity, and opioid dose in patients with advanced cancer. *Cancer* 1998; 83:1244–1250.

Wagner G. Frequency of pain in patients with cancer. *Recent Results Cancer Res* 1984; 89:64–71.

Wai MS, Mike S, Ines H, Malcolm M. Palliation of metastatic bone pain: single fraction versus multifraction radiotherapy—a systematic review of the randomised trials. *Cochrane Database Syst Rev* 2004; 2:CD004721.

Wiffen P, Collins S, McQuay H, et al. Anticonvulsant drugs for acute and chronic pain. *Cochrane Database Syst Rev* 2000; 3:CD001133.

Wong R, Wiffen PJ. Bisphosphonates for the relief of pain secondary to bone metastases. *Cochrane Database Syst Rev* 2002; 2:CD002068.

Correspondence to: Linda A. King, MD, 5230 Centre Avenue, Pittsburgh, PA 15232, USA. Tel: 412-623-1702; email: kingl@msx.upmc.edu.

Index